Yoga *and* Multiple Sclerosis

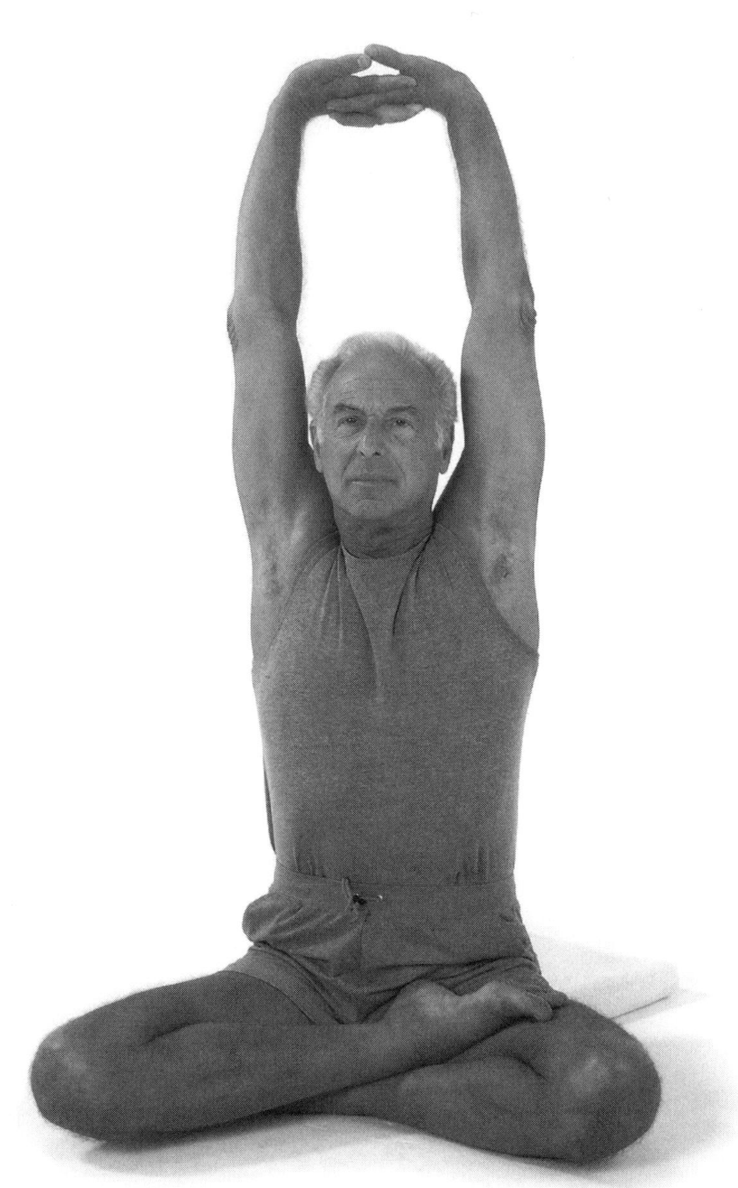

Yoga *and*

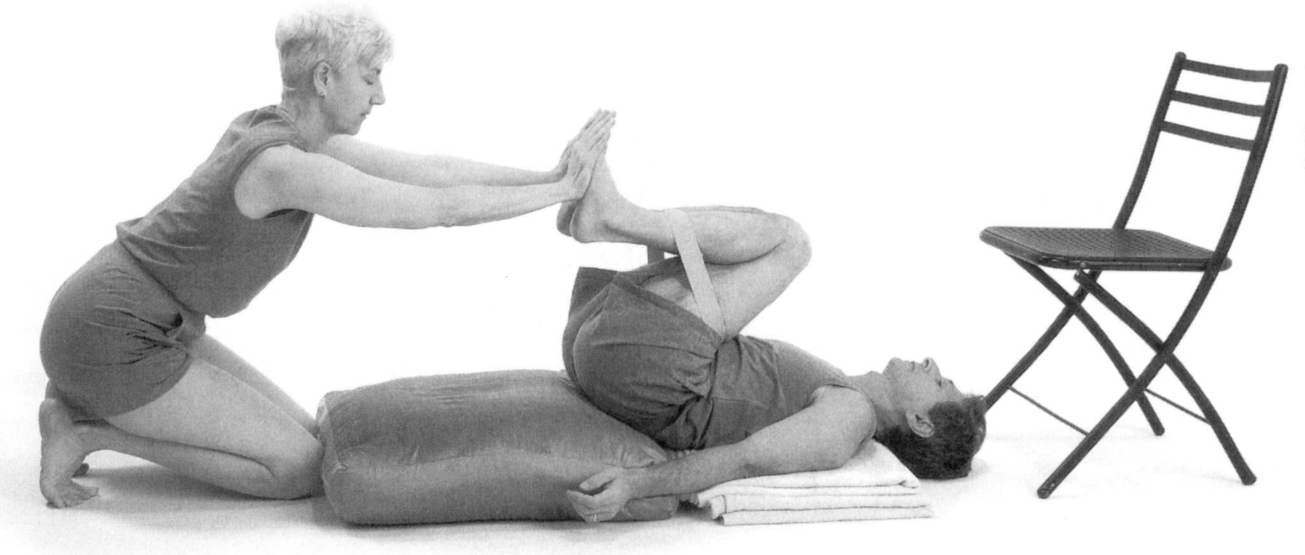

Multiple Sclerosis

A Journey to Health and Healing

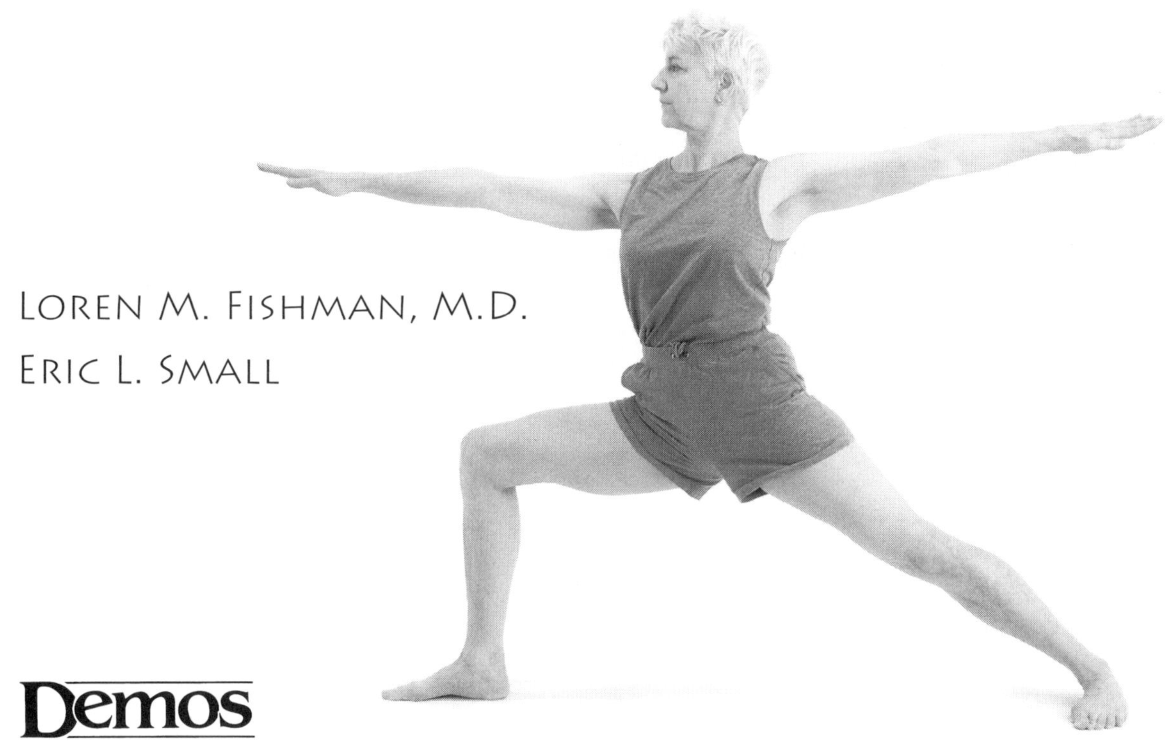

LOREN M. FISHMAN, M.D.
ERIC L. SMALL

Demos

Special discounts on bulk quantities of Demos Medical Publishing books are available to corporations, professional associations, pharmaceutical companies, health care organizations, and other qualifying groups. For details, please contact:

Special Sales Department
DEMOS MEDICAL PUBLISHING
386 Park Avenue South, Suite 301
New York, NY 10016

Phone: 800-532-8663, 212-683-0072
Fax: 212-683-0118
Email: orderdept@demosmedpub.com

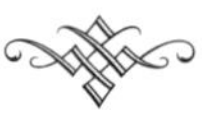

Visit our website at www.demosmedpub.com

LIBRARY OF CONGRESS CATALOGING-IN-PUBLICATION DATA
Fishman, Loren M.
Yoga and multiple sclerosis : a journey to health and healing / Loren M. Fishman, Eric L. Small.
p. ; cm.
Includes bibliographical references and index.
ISBN-13: 978-1-932603-17-0 (pbk. : alk. paper)
ISBN-10: 1-932603-17-4 (pbk. : alk. paper)
1. Multiple sclerosis—Patients—Rehabilitation. 2. Yoga—Therapeutic use. I. Small, Eric L. II. Title.
[DNLM: 1. Multiple Sclerosis—rehabilitation. 2. Yoga. WL 360 F537y 2007]
RC377.F57 2007
616.8'34062—dc22
2006030464

Designed by Steven Pisano

MANUFACTURED IN CANADA

08 09 10 11 5 4 3

Dedication

Mr. Iyengar has led the quest for the authentic yoga of antiquity no less than for its refinement and adaptation to current times and the needs of living people. As a teacher and researcher, a creative and disciplined leader, a conceptual inventor and a physical presence in classes and out, he is our master. To express our intellectual debt and heartfelt gratitude to Mr. Iyengar, language fails. But it is easy to state that the authors are fully responsible for everything in this book.

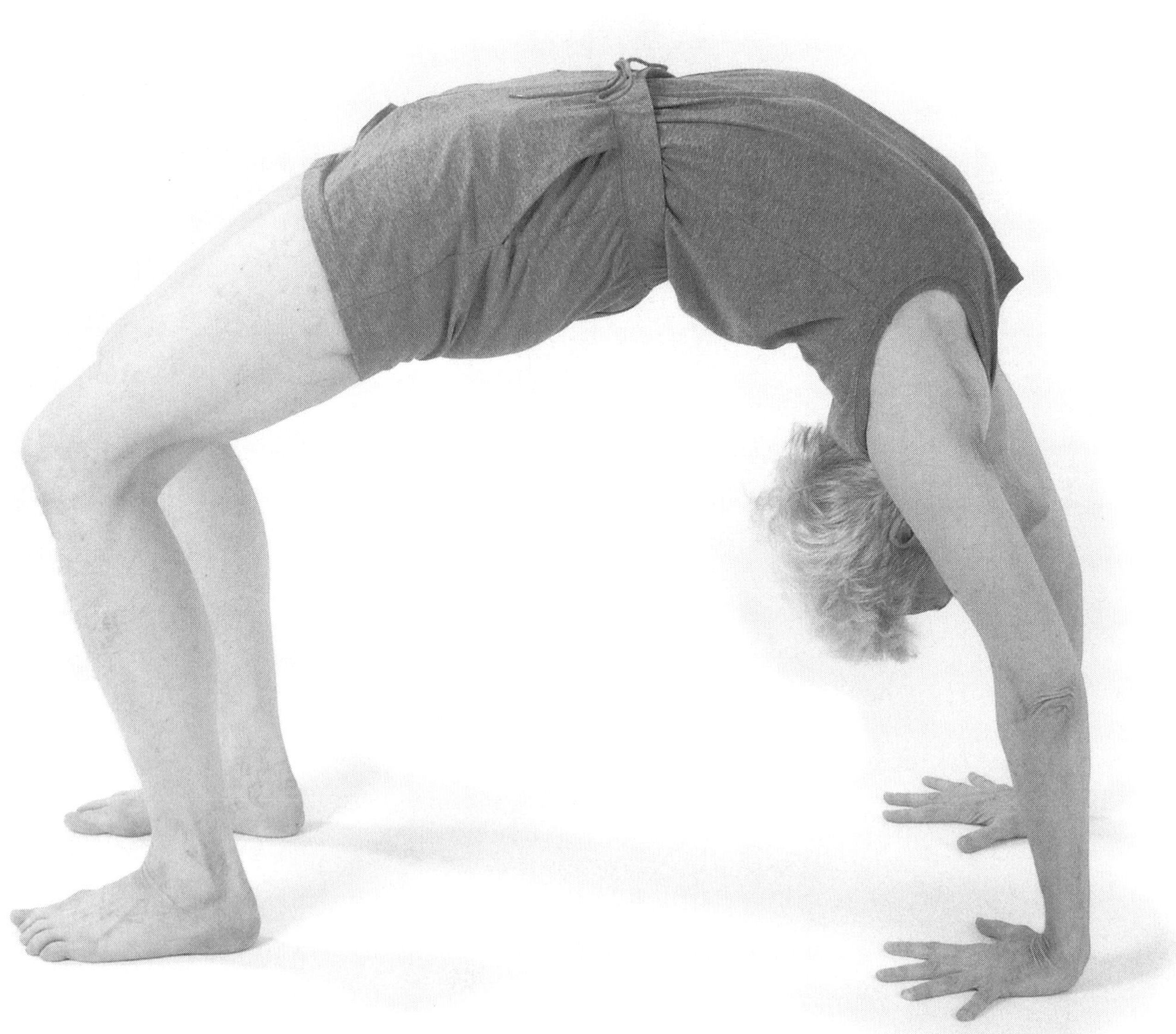

Contents

CHAPTER 2. WHEELCHAIR SERIES

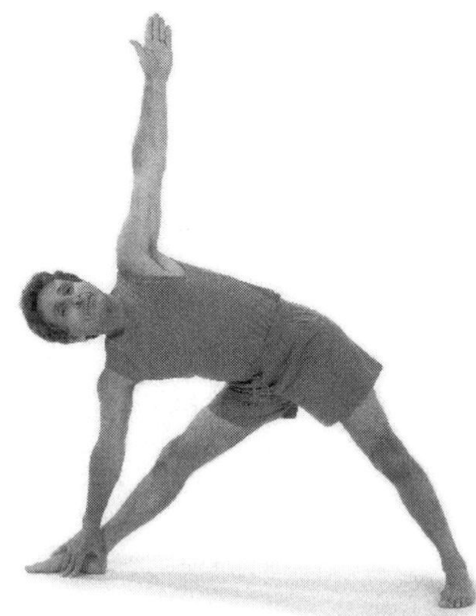

CHAPTER 3. CHAIR SERIES

CHAPTER 4. SEATED POSES

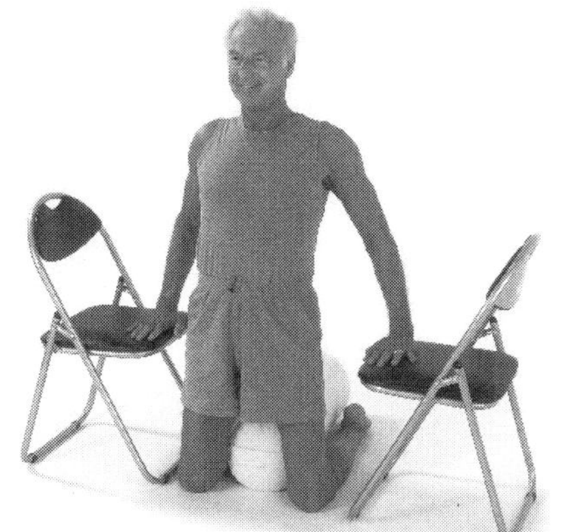

CHAPTER 5. SEATED/FLOOR SERIES

CHAPTER 6. PRANAYAMA AND RELAXATION

PART II

FUNCTION-DIRECTED YOGA FOR FUNCTIONALLY IMPAIRED INDIVIDUALS

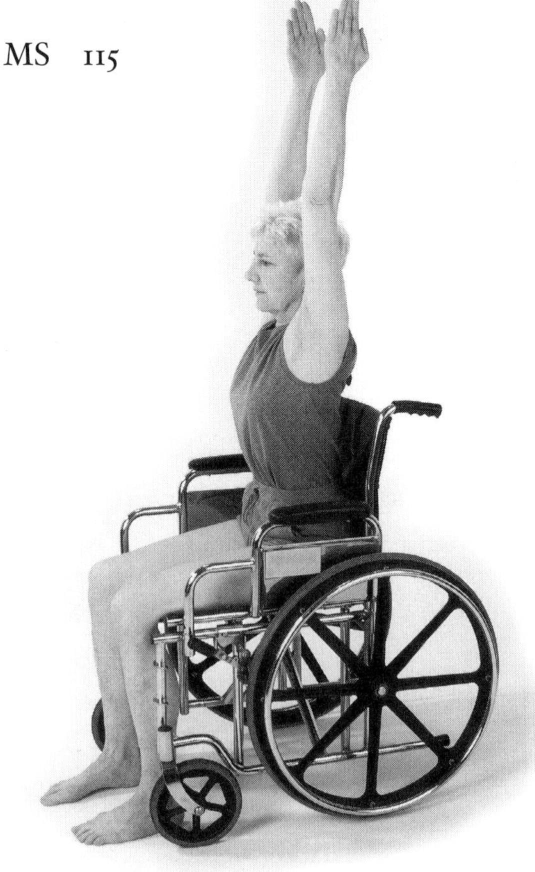

CHAPTER 8. IMPROVE RANGE OF MOTION

CHAPTER 9. SPASTICITY

CHAPTER 10. STRENGTH

CHAPTER 11. COORDINATION AND BALANCE

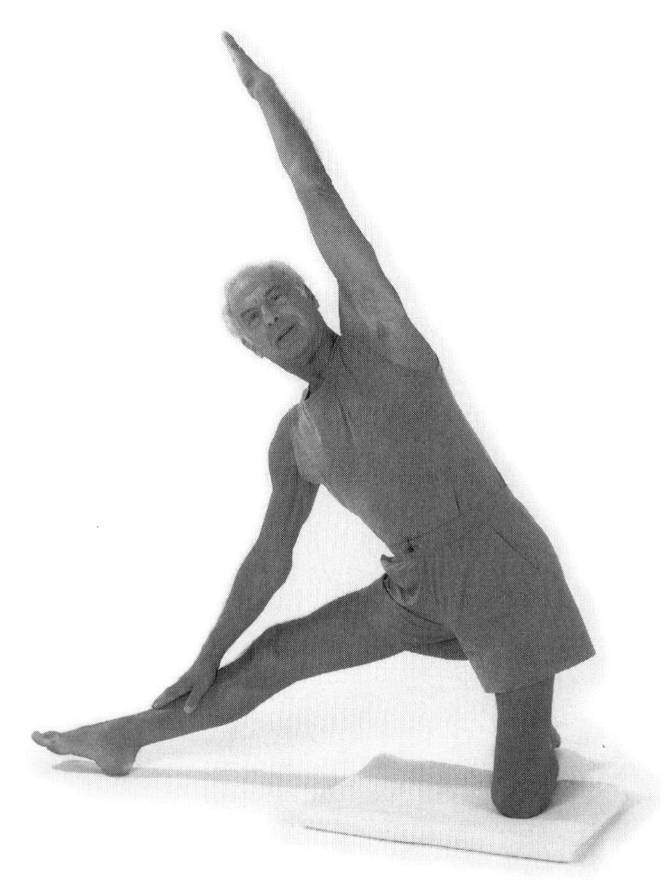

Preface

It is paradoxical that yoga, thousands of years old and originating in India, a warm country where multiple sclerosis is almost nonexistent, is both utterly contemporary and of great benefit in the treatment of multiple sclerosis (MS). Fatigued by modern medicine's sharp compartmentalization, contemporary medicine has rebelled and claims interest in the whole person. Yoga and its goals have always addressed the whole person; there is no such thing as "yoga of the thigh."

But there are also distinct differences between medicine and yoga. With the exception of public health, medicine is only brought in when things go wrong, and only until the status quo has been reached again. Yoga, always concerned with the individual, takes up for no reason at any stage along the continuum of health and disease, and does not relinquish its hold when illness does. On the contrary, it continues to take practitioners beyond mere absence of disease toward a goal of wisdom and peace.

Yoga is not science. The constellation of physics, chemistry, and biology, from which medicine is an offspring, gathers data empirically and uses logical methods of proof. Empirical and deductive means combine to determine the diagnoses and progress of individuals. If yoga is to be rationally valued, it must be evaluated in terms of the sciences: it will not do anyone any good to conclude that yoga is beneficial in MS because more people learn to do the shoulder stand. They must be shown to ambulate more safely, have better visual evoked potentials, or score better on the Kurtzke Scale. Science's services are then needed again to explain how yoga works.

Yoga is changing along with the global culture of which it forms a part. While yoga has been passed on from teacher or guru to individual student for all of its many generations, today's mobile societies require a certification program to distinguish the serious practitioner from other types. There are a large number of written texts, movies, tapes, videos, and web sites, but it is part of the credo of yoga that it actually be taught.

The precious gift that Mr. B. K. S. Iyengar has given us, in the form of his work and the distinguished striving his life represents, has enabled large numbers of people to avail themselves of a very refined and detailed teaching that would not have been possible using the old-time methods. Many quotes, techniques, and almost all the poses in this book derive from his books and teaching.

In this context, this book is offered as a guide and helpmate to those who would use yoga, be they physicians, physical therapists, nurses, parents, children, students or, perchance, teachers.

The book is divided into two sections: the first is a straightforward but gentle introduction to yoga for people with significant MS involvement. It is a therapeutic approach to the practice itself. Without this, the rest of the book might be just an academic exercise.

The second part is functionally oriented: different yoga poses are assembled that work toward a common goal, such as combating fatigue, reducing spasticity, and increasing range of motion. It is intended for people with MS and other neurological conditions, people who undertake yoga on their own, and for members of the medical and yoga communities. It begins with a more detailed analysis of how yoga appears to work: describing basic physiological means by which it helps people with MS and similarly affected patients. It then sorts out which poses are helpful for which conditions, and it guides teachers, students, and patients on how to use the physiological considerations to adapt the poses to individual patients' needs. It is intended for people that have or readily could have completed Part I.

Yoga was begun thousands of years ago as the science of quieting the mind. Patanjali, the man attributed authorship of the first text on yoga, was also the first grammarian and a physician. His *Yoga Sutras* (*Threads of Yoga*) begins, "Yoga chitta-vritti-nirodhah," "Yoga is inhibition of different states of mind." The goal of a completely unmodified consciousness pervades every aspect of yoga. It is held up as the best arbiter for individual decision-making and the ultimate aim of life. The idea is that an unprejudiced and unemotional examination of a situation is the most successful. Yet the principle of unattached evaluation is itself recommended not on empirical or rational but rather on intuitive grounds. The science of yoga has never endeavored to prove the value of nonattachment. Those who value yoga simply believe it.

While yoga is therefore something people believe in, it is nonsectarian. There is no faith that opposes it, and yoga has gathered devoted practitioners from many faiths, and from every land. Yoga is also by and large theistic—with reverence for a supreme being—but it is without a hierarchical clergy. It has no established church; there are no religious personnel. Rather, yoga has been passed down for thousands of years in a personal way, from teacher to pupil, without institutional support of any kind. It is perhaps a tribute to Patanjali's brilliance and clarity that, while there are many branches and approaches to yoga, it has remained an eminently recognizable discipline, with principles and practices that present an integral whole. In classical Indian philosophy, yoga is divided into eight limbs.

The first limb of yoga is Yama, or universal moral commandments having to do with our relations with other people:

- Ahimsa, or nonviolence
- Satya, truth, deemed by some to be the highest commandment
- Asteya, honesty
- Brahmacharya, continence
- Aparigraha, noncovetousness

The second limb, Niyama is not universal but rather contains individual moral directives:

- Saucha, or purity
- Santosa, contentment
- Tapas, austerity
- Svadhyaya, introspection
- Isvara pranidhana, dedication to a higher being

The third limb of yoga is Asana, or postures, and is what we in the West typically identify as yoga. They are meant to bring steadiness, health, and lightness of limb. "The young, the old, the extremely aged, even the sick and infirm obtain perfection in Yoga by constant practice. Constant practice alone is the secret of success."

Many asanas have been practiced and refined for hundreds of generations; all are still in evolution. Many poses have biological names based on the gestalt of the position, such as "the tree," or "the scorpion," or "the lotus." Others are named for their "attitude," after heroes or gods in Hindu mythology, such as Hanumanasana or Virabhadrasana. Still others are named for anatomical parts that figure prominently in their execution, such as "headstand" or "arm balance."

Asana is considered a prerequisite for the fourth limb, Pranayama. This concerns the apparatus and technique of breathing, extending from the nostrils through the diaphragm, and involving inhalation, exhalation, and the periods before and after each. While useful in a variety of respiratory and psychiatric conditions, pranayama is intended to carry the student beyond mere health, closer to a state of liberation. "When the prana (breath) and the manas (mind) have been absorbed, an indefinable joy ensues."

Pratyahara, control of the senses, is the fifth limb, wherein the yogic aspirant becomes absorbed in self-examination or introspection. It is by this means that the yogi confronts envy, deceit, greed, lust, and hatred, the roots of which lie inside the individual.

Dharana begins after the body has been tempered through asanas, the mind is invigorated through pranayama, and the seductive powers of the senses are controlled through pratyahara. In a nutshell, this is concentrating and focusing on "the bullseye," the still point of the turning wheel, the very heart of the matter. This single-pointedness, or ekagrata, is essential for the final two stages.

Dhyana, "total dedication to the goodness of the world," is meant to convey a blissful state in which one selflessly devotes all of one's time and boundless energy to seeing the spiritual essence in each aspect of reality. While the concentrated exclusivity of dharana has the possibility of producing an egotistical reaction, the humble, total absorption in seeing the best essence of things is its antidote.

Samadhi is the famous destination of the yogi's journey: in the manner of a Mother Theresa, people that have reached samadhi are a great blessing and benefit to the world. In the words of Sankaracharya, "ever serenely balanced, I am neither free nor bound."

The object of yoga is the attainment of liberation or enlightenment. Once this state is attained, things are experienced as they truly are, without any particular point of view or preconception. There is no reason to leave this state, and it is permanent. This gives yoga a different orientation than most of the healing sciences. It not only aims to bring people from below normal, from illness or injury, back to normal. Yoga keeps on going, striving toward inner and outer perfection, well beyond the levels of normal or average or merely healthy.

Viewed broadly, the more advanced stages of yoga can be seen as extending the domain of consciousness, of conscious control, into regions generally left to the autonomic nervous system. It may start with pranayama, the study, manipulation, and mastery of breathing, which is a process that is clearly autonomic in the sense that it goes on unbidden during sleep and when we are not paying attention to it. Yoga makes increasingly profound forays of control and command into the process of breathing. It is all, ultimately, part of an effort to limit the "modifications of the mind."

In other words, yoga entails mastery of our very human attention span through steadfast resistance of both sensory temptations and our inherent distractibility. For example, it is difficult to restrain our attention from darting to moving objects at the edges of our visual fields. This and other neurophysiological facts of life can be mastered when we resolve consciously and with great determination to concentrate on the goals of yoga and, with the help that yoga offers, to eventually achieve ekagrata, one-pointedness.

The dedication and liberation that complete the yogi's journey are overwhelming draughts of the same wine: conscious mental effort toward increasing consciousness until there are no surprises.

Possibly because yoga's basic program brings its practitioners from any condition at all back through "normal" to elevated physical, mental, and spiritual states, it has long been known for the extraordinary feats of its advocates. Voluntarily stopping and then restarting their hearts, holding their breath for extended periods, remaining motionless for months or even years, and prolonging life itself are well-known examples. But with or without these astonishing abilities, all yoga involves self-discipline. All yoga promotes a peaceful, purely conscious individual.

Many poses that appear originally in ancient texts have been adapted by nineteenth- and twentieth-century physical therapeutics. Physicians and physical therapists may recognize many of the postures and techniques described here. It is then their individual choice to react by saying, "I already know all this, it's nothing new," or "We already do this, we know it is effective, let's see if there are additional maneuvers, combinations, applications, or refinements here that can benefit our patients." It is along the lines of the second attitude that this book is offered.

Acknowledgments: We are grateful to Sally Hess, Lindsey Clennell, Mary Dunn, Joan White, Victor Oppenheimer, Tova Ovadia, Rama Patela, yoga models and consultants; to Donal Holloway and Luis Ramirez, photographers; and to Robert Troy, photographer, commissioned by Eric Small; Max Tzinman, artist; Desmond Gomes, office manager; Carol Ardman and Flora Thornton, indulgent wives; and the many patients and students who have, wittingly or not, but always willingly, allowed us to attempt to help them, and in this way permitted us to learn what we offer here.

Loren M. Fishman, MD
Eric L. Small

Part I

Yoga for People with Multiple Sclerosis

This yoga program was introduced by and derives from the teachings of B. K. S. Iyengar of Poona, India, who has been practicing therapeutic yoga for the past fifty years. Mr. Iyengar has always focused on therapeutics and directed his countless refinements of classical yoga to people who have special problems.

It was the authors' honor and privilege to be able to synthesize the classic hatha yoga each of us learned from Mr. Iyengar in various trips to India and during Mr. Iyengar's visits to the United States. Eric Small has done a great deal in the past twenty-five years on the West Coast to apply and further develop Mr. Iyengar's work to create and teach a yoga program that is appropriate for every MS patient, no matter what the individual's level of mobility or ability to perform. Dr. Loren Fishman has used yoga in his medical practice for more than twenty-five years, adapting it to all sorts of needs of patients and analyzing the physiological means by which it is so helpful.

There are many benefits to be gained from practicing hatha yoga, especially the asanas, or poses, described in this book. Some of those gains could be increased motility for digestion, increased circulation, and in many cases significant relief from the depression that often accompanies the symptoms of MS. Yoga is not a cure for MS. Eric is not cured. But he certainly is handling his MS in a much more effective manner than before. In our joint experience, over eighty years altogether, yoga has been a singular godsend to young and old alike. In Eric's case, in the past fifty-four years since he was diagnosed with MS, yoga has enabled him to maintain a life that sometimes surprises even him. Part I includes five sequences or series, each with a different goal. These are the restorative series, wheelchair series, chair series, floor series, and pranayama and relaxation series. Choose the options that best suit your needs.

Each yoga session should include some poses from most of the sequences. A family member, friend, or a certified Iyengar Yoga instructor may be required to help you in certain poses. We recommend consulting with a certified yoga instructor or connecting with a yoga program or physical therapist if you can. If you have the accompanying DVD from the National Multiple Sclerosis Society, use the remote control to pause the DVD as needed.

No matter what your range of motion or your present abilities, each of these yoga postures can be approached with the use of props. These props may be necessary to modify the poses to meet your personal needs. Recommended props, along with their household equivalents, are:

- Straps: bathrobe ties or neckties
- Blocks: phone books or hardcover books
- Taps for stability
- Sticky mat or yoga mat
- Sleeping bag or sticky bath mat
- Blankets: firm cotton or wool blankets
- Bolsters: couch or chair pillows
- Sandbags: five-pound bags of flour, brown rice, or dry beans
- Eye bag: folded hand towel
- Armless folding chair: any stable chair without arms

These props are going to be used throughout this book. We want to stress that they do not need to be purchased. Many of them are in your home—chairs, tables, walls, and even the kitchen counter. Old telephone books bound together with scotch tape make a very good substitute for blocks and lifts. If you find that the props described or shown are something you want to purchase, they are easily available in stores or over the Internet.

Why use props? The props enable you to receive full benefit of the postures without causing any strain or stress or overheating of the body. Unlike most other physical disciplines, hatha yoga encompasses the whole body. If you are doing a posture that involves twisting or moving forward, for instance, not only the front of the body is involved. With the use of props, all of the body is brought into the activity. This is important because it brings back to you the full power of your body, and it is a very challenging and interesting part of this discipline.

It is important to remember that, due to the risk of injury, you should never force or strain in a pose. Consult your physician before you work on this or any other exercise regimen. Instructions and advice presented in this program are in no way intended as a substitute for medical counseling. Women who are menstruating should not practice inverted poses, backbends, or vigorous standing poses. Read the entire pose at least once before doing it. Never practice after eating. Allow two hours after snack and four to five hours after a large meal. Practice on a nonskid surface.

Now let us begin.

Restorative Series

Restorative poses refresh body and brain, calm the nervous system, and open the chest to oxygenate the lungs, heart and liver.

PROPS

As we stated in the introduction, props are important. Here we use a regular folding chair, blankets, blocks, a strap, a sticky mat, a bolster, and an eye bag. Lots of props are specially designed for use in therapeutic yoga, but many of them can be substituted by using chairs, tables, telephone books, blankets, towels, bathrobe ties, or old neckties.

In the restorative series, we are using props to help your body to assume the postures in a manner that is restful. The goal for all the body's systems, particularly the nervous system, is to restore themselves. This goal of restoration is where you start in your yoga practice. It teaches you to relax and to reduce the stress and strain of the day. It also allows you to restore activity to your nervous system by using your breath to ease your body into the postures.

SAVASANA

Reclined Pose

The first restorative pose is the supine posture. You will need 2 or 3 blankets, a strap, and eye bag, and possibly a bolster. Start by

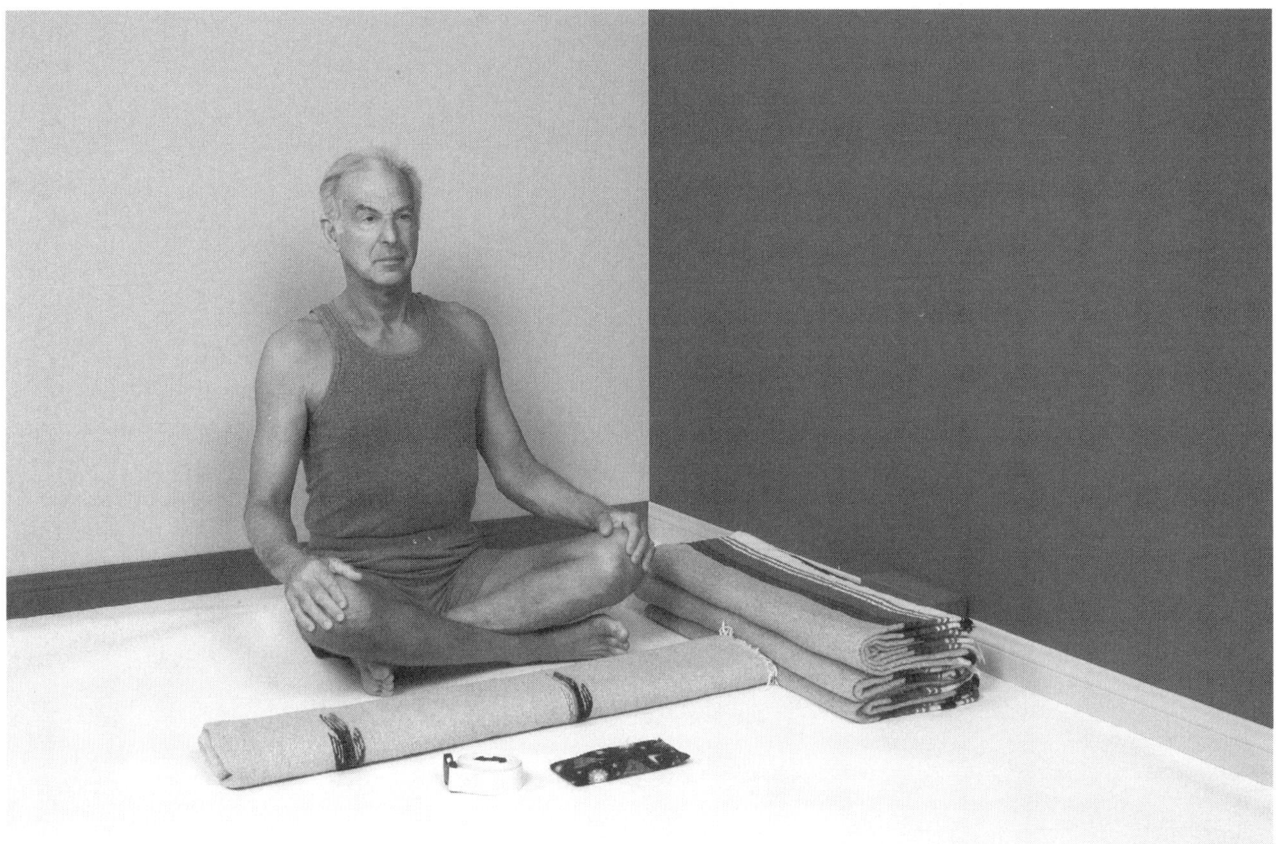

Blanket folded into quarters

folding 2 or 3 blankets into quarters, remembering that each person has a different body. (Your teacher, trainer, or therapist, if you have one, can help you adjust this pose for your particular body.)

1. Sit. Place the strap across your thighs and place your hands on the floor, slightly behind the hips, fingers pointing forward.

2. Raise your chest, keeping your chin tucked toward the collarbone. Begin to bend the elbows toward the floor, as you slowly lower the torso onto the blankets.

3. As your hands slip toward your hips, slide them under the buttocks, pressing the flesh toward the knees. This is important in order to place the sacrum, the spinal column, and the head into proper alignment. This will enable you to fully relax the body and brain.

When women lie supine on the floor, it is important that the blanket does not lie beneath the lower back. (For men it is perfectly all right for it to do so.) Women's organs are arranged a little differently than men's, and they need to avoid any pressure against the kidneys, colon, or reproductive organs. Women should position the bottom edge of the blankets just at the bottom of the ribs, so the lower back is free from any pressure.

The head, from the shoulders (not from the ears) upward, is supported by the blankets. If it

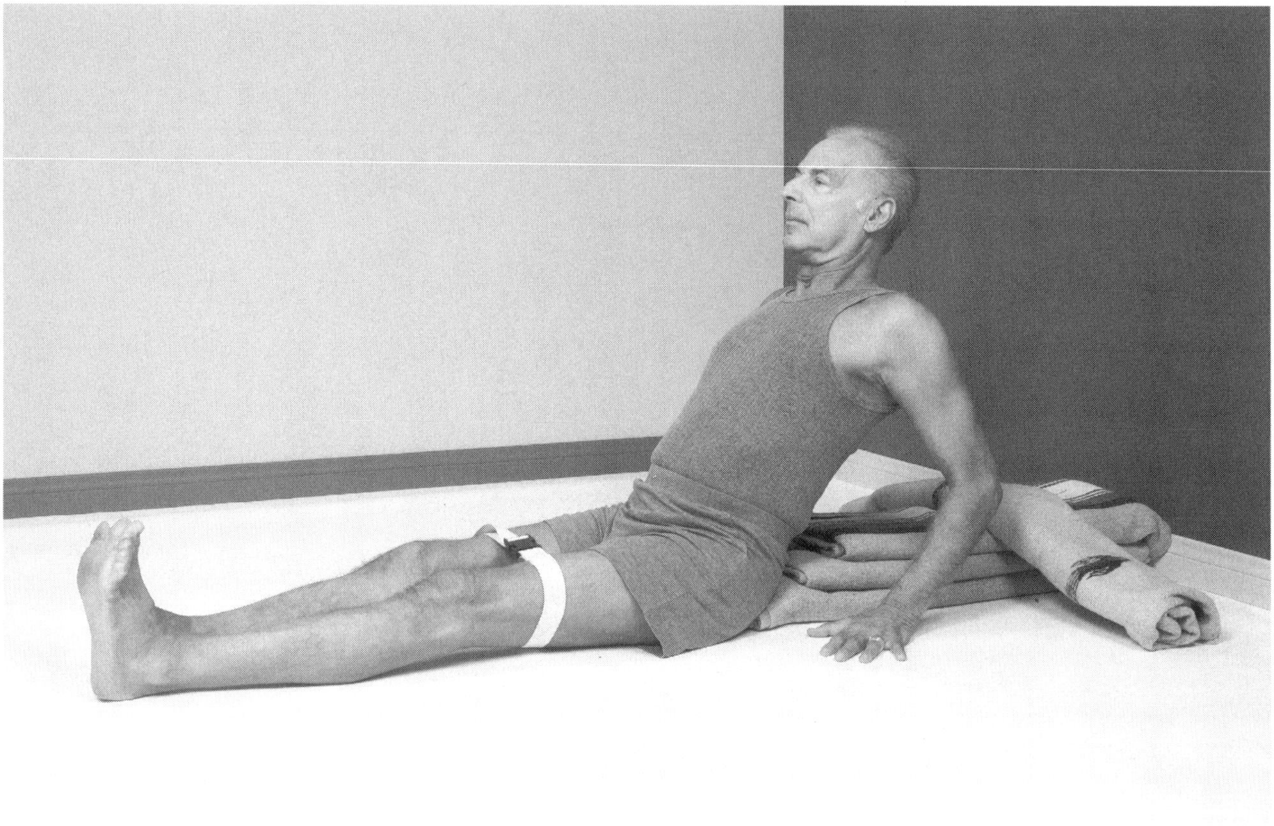

Blanket reaching only to upper iliac crest

is difficult to relax your legs, fasten the strap at the middle of the thigh, to hold the legs firmly into their joints within the pelvis, allowing the weight of the leg and pelvis to descend.

You can enhance the pose even more by putting a bolster under the knees. You can use either bolster or a folded blanket, depending on your size.

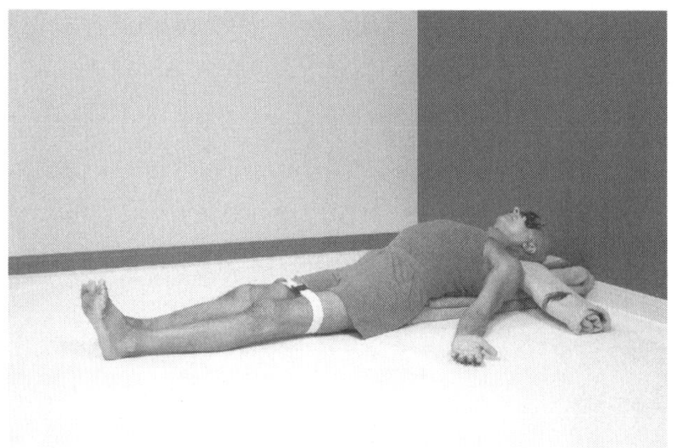

At this point your legs and pelvis should be very relaxed. The sacrum, the bottom of the spinal column, is well supported. Your shoulders are moving back and away from the front of the chest. With just with this very small adjustment this whole area of the thorax, the place where we breathe, has been opened.

4. Now place your arms 30 degrees away from your sides, with the palms up. Allow the weight of the thumbs to move toward the floor, externally rotating your arms and rotating your shoulders even farther away

from the ribs at the front of the torso. Do not force the thumbs to go to the floor. Allow them to do so at their own pace.

5. As the thumbs and palms open, the upper parts of the lungs are less constrained, and breathing capacity increases accordingly.

The breath in this posture begins from behind the navel as it moves toward the spine, allowing the diaphragm to pull downward in the lumbar region, opening the chest, and helping the ribs to catch the breath and bring it toward the sternum.

The breath in the restorative postures should always come in through the nose in a particular way:

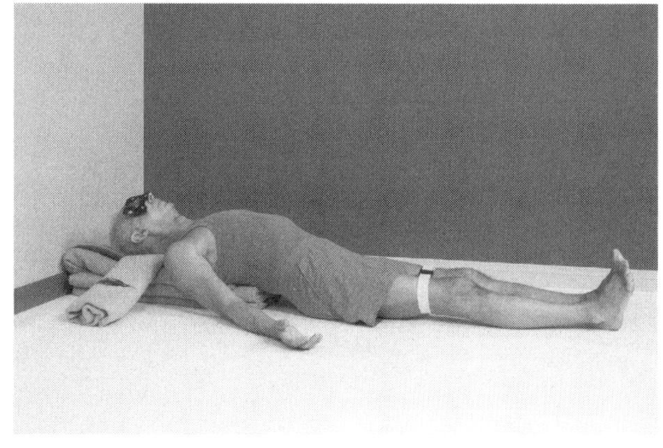

With strap

1. As you inhale, air enters through the bottom of the nose near the upper lip.

2. As you exhale, the breath comes out at the tip of the nose. Within just a few

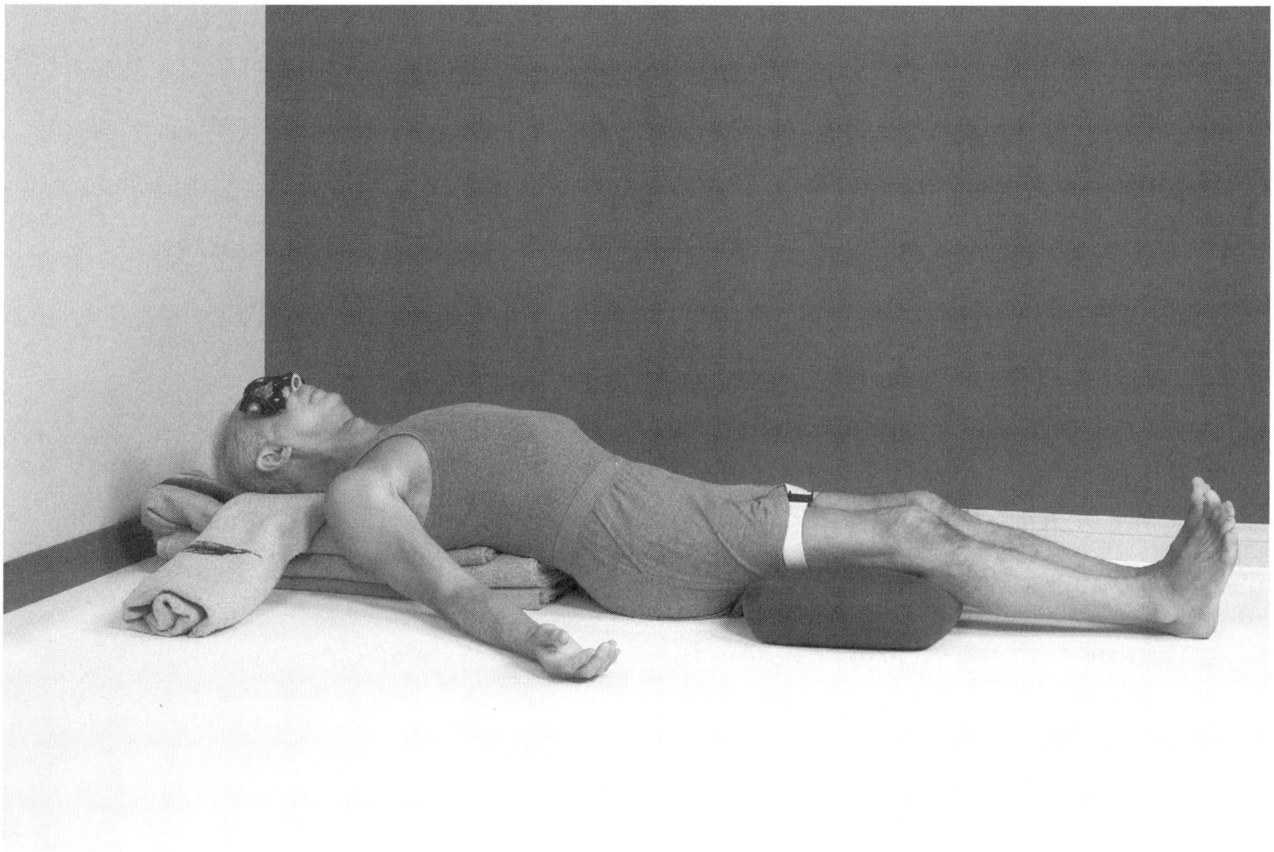

With bolster

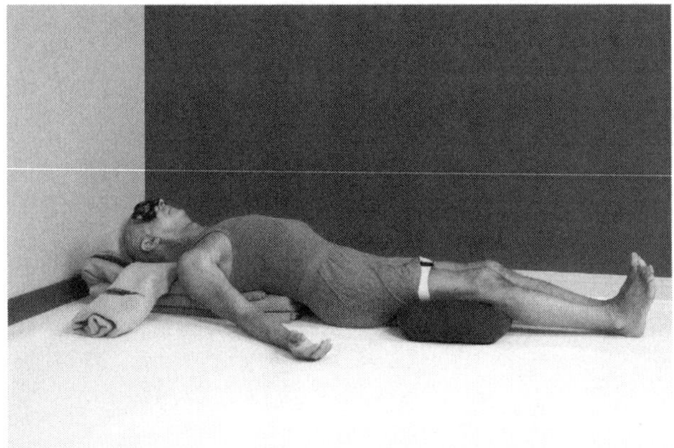

With eye bag

moments you will notice that the breath changes its rhythm from a short inhalation-exhalation to a fuller inhalation and a long, slow exhalation.

Mr. Iyengar has explained that inhalation energizes the body, and exhalation is a matter of surrender. This permits the physical body to reconstitute and relax, especially the central nervous system. In this posture, the body is well-supported by the blankets, and we are gently opening the breathing apparatus, which is the lungs, the bronchial tubes, and the diaphragm. The pose is also kind to the liver; the breathing itself gently increases blood flow to the brain.

In addition, an eye bag can be applied at any point during this pose. It is applied from the eyebrow. Gently draw the skin of the forehead down toward the nose and just allow the weight of the eye bag to go toward the temples and ears. The eyes do not look into the bag or into the lid. The eyes look down toward the heart, in order to release tension from the frontal lobes of the brain.

By eliminating stimulation that comes through the eyes and by activating your ears to listen to the breath, you have reduced the outside stress that comes to the body and are starting to explore the power of the mind.

DANDASANA

Supported Bridge Pose

This restorative pose opens the chest and releases pressure in the cervical, thoracic, and lumbar spine. The most important effect of the pose is to completely enhance the breathing process. It is aimed at the heart, lungs, and liver. You will need one or more blankets and a block.

1. Sit on a blanket with the spine completely elongated out of the base of the pelvis. In most cases sitting on to the floor causes the spine to round and the chest and heart to draw back and together. Instead, sit up on the blanket so that you have enough of a lift that the spine and central nervous system are ver-

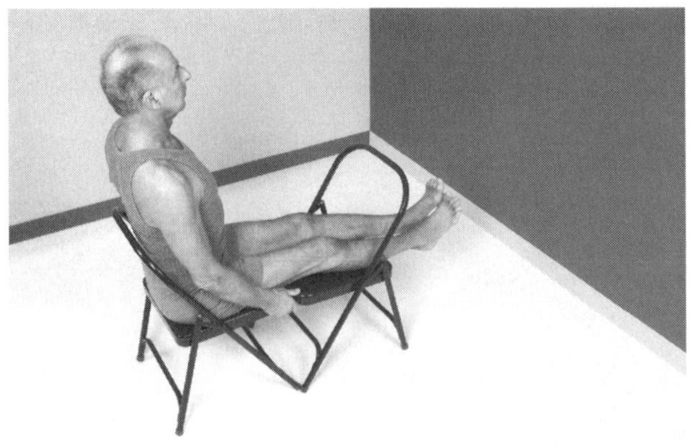

With rounded back (incorrect)

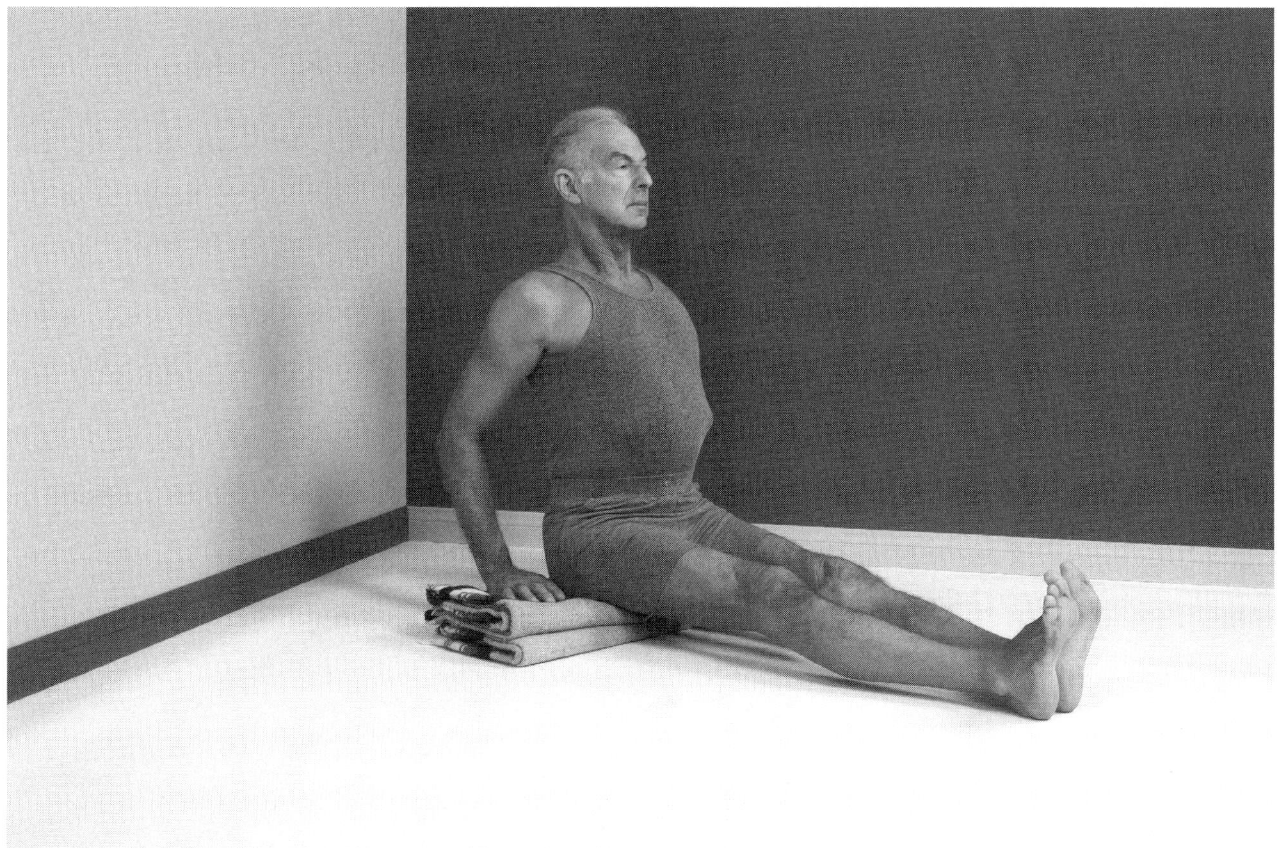

Dandasana (correct)

tical and completely at ease. To correct, place a blanket, rolled sticky mat, or block between the thorax and the back of the chair.

2. Place your hands on the floor, and release your head as you lie down on the floor, making sure that your hips are well supported on the blanket. Roll to the right on the way down.

Now the hips are elevated. In order to keep the thighs and the pelvis relaxed, fasten a strap around the middle of the thighs. Pull the strap so it is comfortably firm but not tight. To completely release the leg you can place a block underneath your feet, so that there is a nice relationship between the releasing of the legs and the opening of the chest.

This is considered a backbend. The benefit of backbending is that it encourages the rib cage and chest to open. If the shoulders are slightly high, as is frequently the case, just draw the shoulders down and, most importantly, draw the armpit and the shoulder blades back.

3. Move the shoulder blades toward the spine and down toward the waist to bring the outer shoulder down to the floor.

4. Very gently adjust your head so the skull is resting evenly on the floor. Breathe as in Reclined Pose. Maintain the pose for 3–5 minutes.

In this pose, the abdomen drops gently toward the spine. The diaphragm, which arises in the lumbar spine and rises in a curve to the sternum, is relaxed and calm. The intercostals, the muscles between the ribs, are encouraged to relax and open rhythmically as the breath is cycled. By this gentle opening of the ribs upwards toward the sternum, the space in the chest is increased more quickly than the pressures of the diaphragm rise. That reduces any tension around the heart, and blood flows more copiously yet gently toward the brain. Because we do not always know where our plaques are and they can be anywhere—sometimes only in the cerebral hemispheres, sometimes in the stem of the brain—we want the whole brain to become flushed and irrigated with oxygenated blood.

Also, by slightly opening the body, the weight of the brain within the skull drops toward the floor, and that dropping allows the nervous system to give up any tension or tightness it may have acquired.

5. To come out, release the strap, bend your knees, and roll gently to your right side.

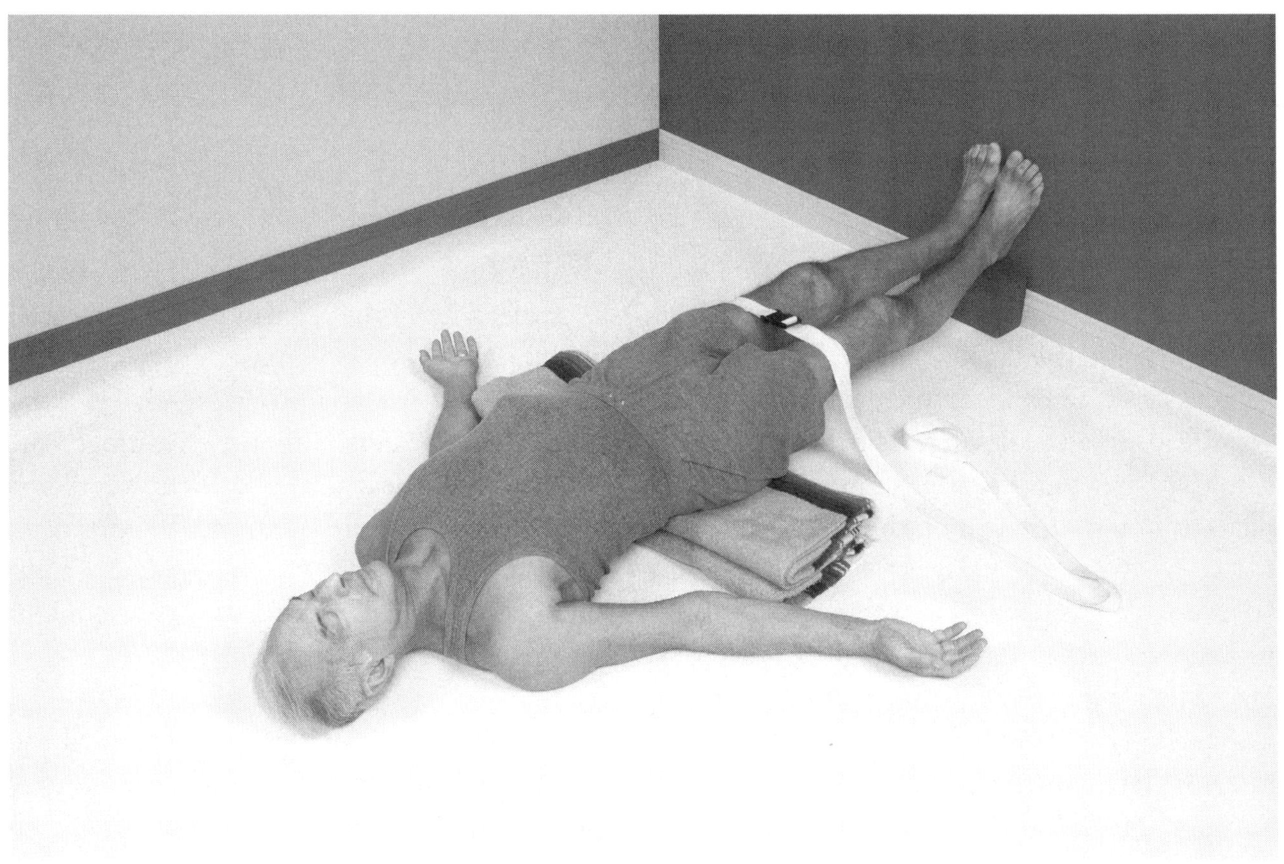

With strap and heel block

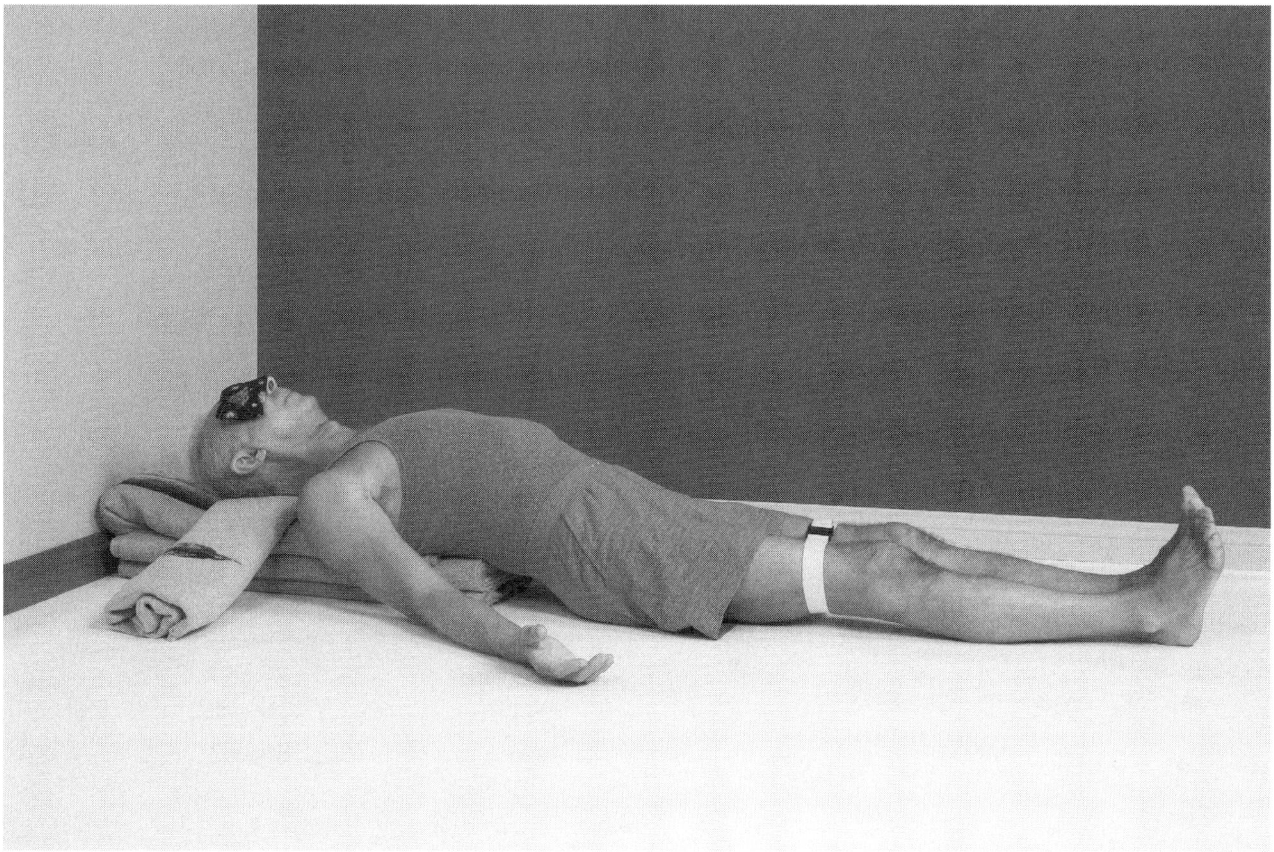

Final pose

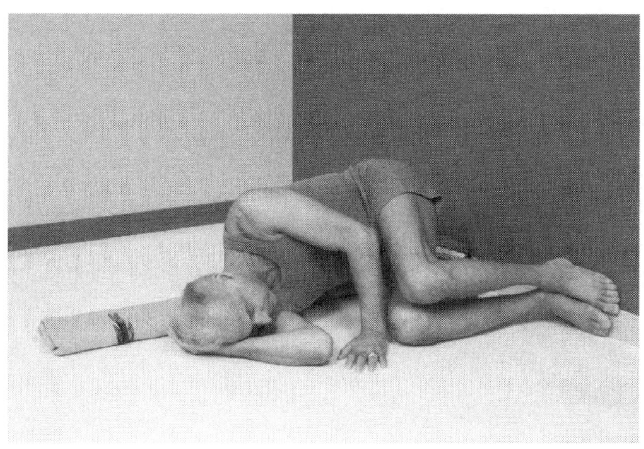

Cradling your head into your right arm helps the left hand to lie gently on the floor.

Spend an equal amount of time in this posture as you spent in the backbend. This permits the blood to reregulate itself between the liver, the heart, the lungs, and the brain. After 3 minutes, using your left hand, press yourself up off the floor and come to a comfortable sitting position on your mat. Using the wall for support, cross your legs comfortably and sit quietly.

Supta Baddha Konasana

Supine Bound Angle Pose

This asana is perhaps one of the most important of the restorative poses. It is preparation for the supported inverted pose Viparita Karani. The pose relaxes the central nervous system. All the major organs receive additional circulation and are relieved of compression. The strap passing over the groins increases flexibility and reduces tightness in the hips and pelvis. The interior adductor muscles are strengthened and lengthened, reducing spasticity and tightness in the legs. Additional circulation of blood in the pelvis invigorates both the male and female reproductive organs and enhances the digestive and elimination processes.

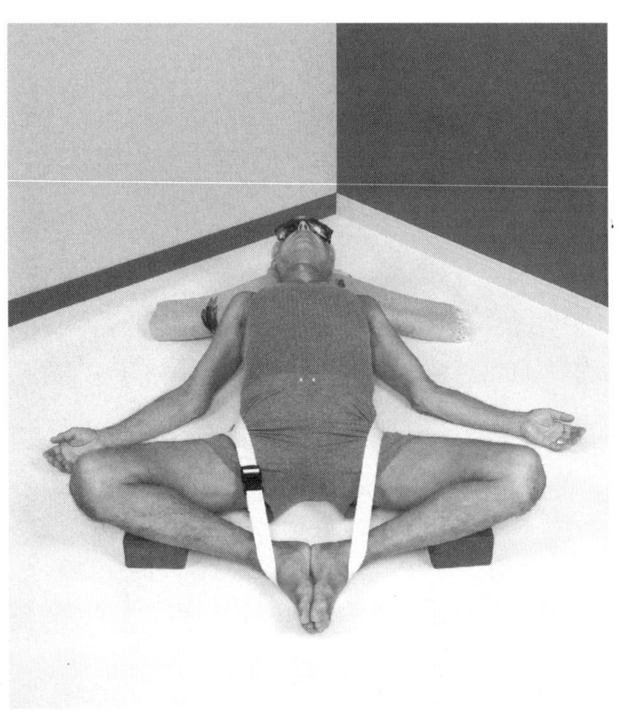

1. To begin, sit on the floor with the bolster behind you. For men, the bolster should touch the back of the hips. For women, the bolster is placed at the bottom of the rib

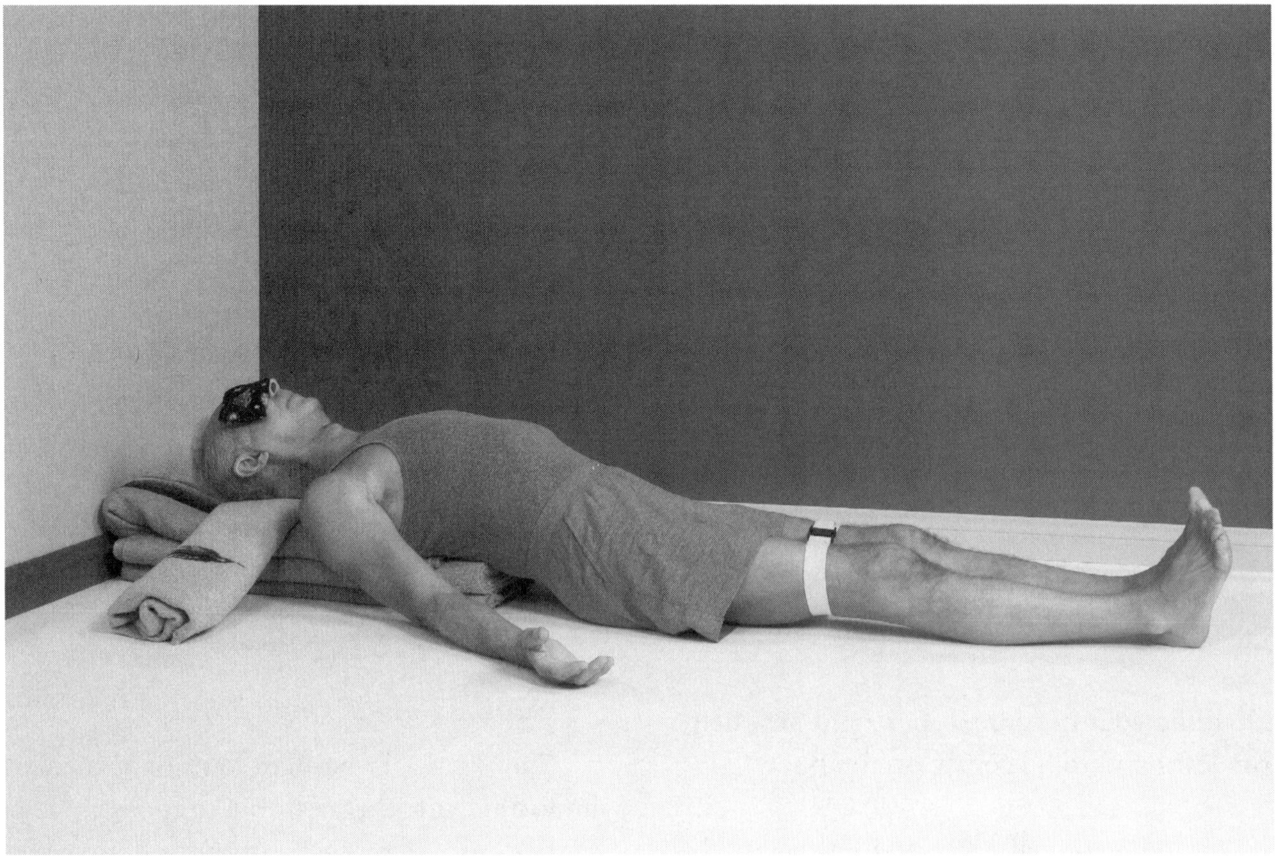

Position of the torso on the bolster only

cage. This avoids any undue pressure against the female reproductive organs.

2. Place the strap around the hips below the upper rim of the pelvis. Draw the heels back toward the pubis, with the soles and heels of the feet together.

3. Place the blocks under the outside of the knees.

4. Put a folded blanket at the top of the bolster, approximately where your head will come to rest.

5. Pass the strap around your feet, and fasten the strap so the buckle does not touch the flesh of the legs and the tail of the strap faces your upper body. That way, adjustments can be made easily while you are in the pose. Do not draw the strap too tight in the beginning. Place your hands by your hips.

6. Lean back, open the chest, and bring the shoulder blades close to the spine. Keep the chest open as you lower the torso onto the bolster and place your head on the folded blanket. The blanket should touch the tops of the shoulders and fully support the neck and head.

7. Place an eye bag onto the eyes. It is important that the eye bag be placed on the eyebrows and then softly lowered over the eyes. The weight of the bag should be adjusted so that the rim of the eyes carries the weight of the bag. This can be achieved by placing the thumb and forefinger on the bag over the bridge of the nose and then spreading the thumb and finger outward to distribute the weight of the bag to the outer eye.

8. Place the arms 30 degrees away from the hips, palms up. Rotate the biceps toward the ceiling, to bring the shoulder blades under and behind the lungs to support the upper chest.

9. Breathe evenly, bringing the breath from beneath the navel into the side ribs. Try to maintain the distance of the sternum from the pubis. Encourage the inhalation to enter the bottom edge of the nostril and the exhalation to exit the tip of the nose. Remain in this asana for at least two to five minutes.

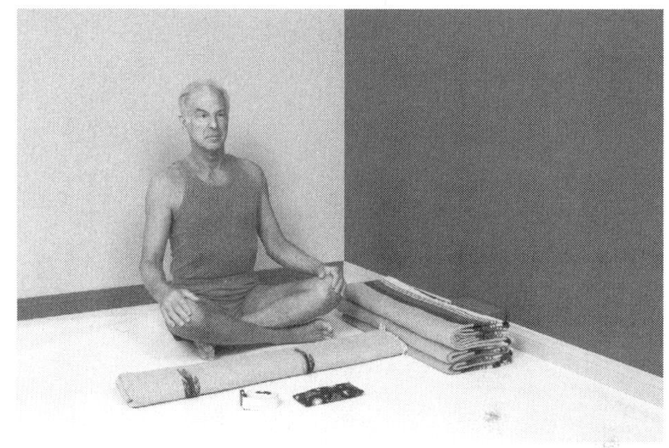

Set-up

VIPARITA KARANI

Supported Inversion Pose

The last of the restorative poses is perhaps the most important—a supported inversion. Over the past few years we have noticed that inverting the body with students who have MS seems to allow them to completely and totally refresh and restore the function of their internal organs and their nervous system.

You will need a bolster, a blanket folded into thirds, so that it only supports the spine, and a wall or headboard or any vertical surface, an eye bag, and a sandbag to weigh the shoulders down to the floor. In place of a

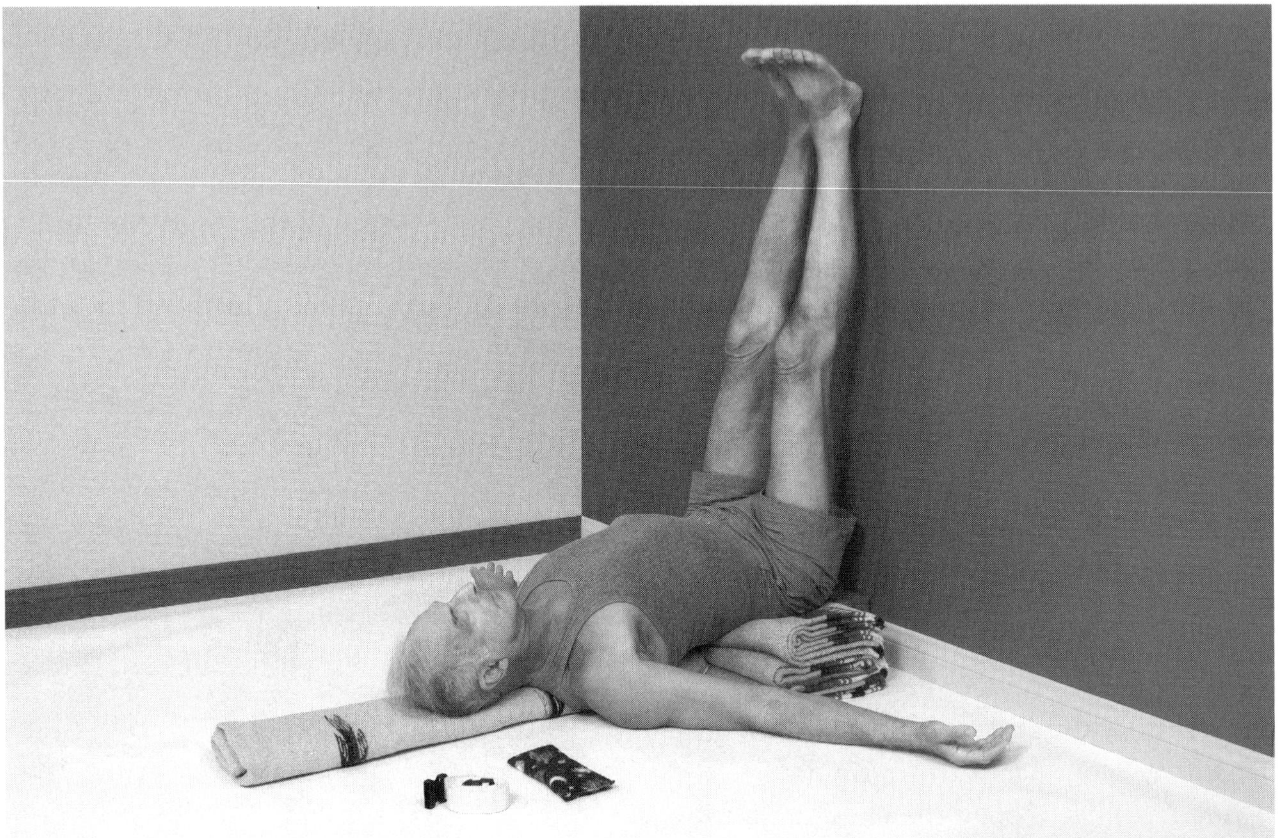

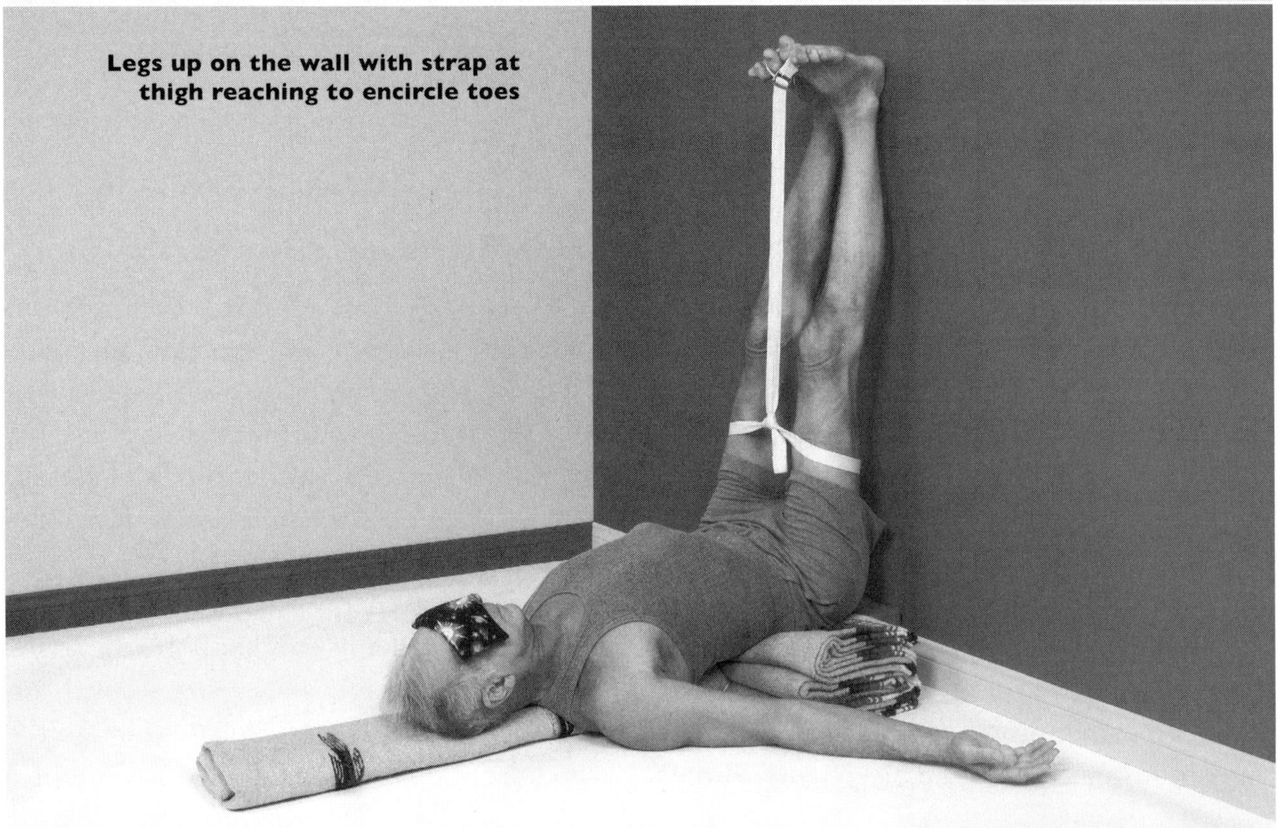

Legs up on the wall with strap at thigh reaching to encircle toes

sandbag, a five-pound bag of flour or rice can be used.

1. Sit on the blanket against the wall. Place your right elbow on the floor. Press both buttocks to the wall. Roll over to the left onto your back, supporting the spine from hip to head on the long folded blanket.

2. Keep your head on the blanket under the spine. Shift your hips into a spine position on the blanket and then gently bring your legs up onto the wall. The chest is supported on the blanket. There is arching across the chest, which opens the upper torso. This releases tension in the front part of the chest and allows it to relax.

If you have a condition in which the shoulders are pitched far forward, it is important to press the shoulders down with a sandbag.

Put an eye bag over the eyes, as described above, by placing it above the eyebrows, pulling the skin gently down toward the nose, and then distributing the bag across the eyebrow lines so that the weight is not directly on the eyeball but is on the bone surrounding the eye.

3. Place your hands (palms up) on the floor, about 30 degrees away from the hips, again with the thumb dropping toward the floor to open the chest and calm the tension in your shoulders.

If there is a problem maintaining the legs in this posture and they seem to turn out, you may want to fasten the strap around the midthigh region and loop one end around the big toes. You or an instructor or assistant can pull the strap gently in order to raise the legs up away from the pelvis and settle the back of the heels onto the wall. (This is essentially the same process we used in the backbend when we put the heels on top of the block.)

4. Breathe as in the other restorative poses. Inhalation is through the base of the nostril; exhalation is through the tip of the nose. Remain in the pose for three to five minutes.

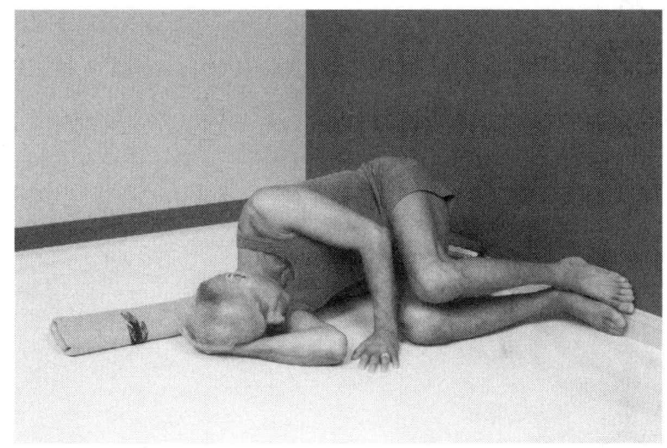

5. Remove the eye bag and strap. Roll over onto your right thigh. Bring your hips completely off your blanket or pad, cushion your head in your right arm, and allow your left arm to drop gently onto the floor. (When you lie on your right side, the liver, which is heavy, is supported by the floor, so the return flow of blood is even and gentle.)

6. Remain in this position for at least the same amount of time that you were inverted. Then sit up, cross your right leg in front your left, put your hands gently onto your thighs, and allow the total effect of the pose to come to you.

BENEFITS

In this posture, gravity gently enhances venous blood return. The blood flows "northward," back through the pelvis, with some possible additional cleansing because the liver is open to all the blood vessels coming up from the lower body. Blood flow through the hepatic portal system and venous blood flow are promoted through inversion.

Breathing in this position, which changes the pressures in the thoracic cavity with every inhalation and exhalation, massages the heart and brain gently through "waves" in the blood flowing through these organs. The practitioner becomes completely relaxed. If you look at the series of pictures, you may notice that he becomes quieter as the series advances. You can see that his face is very relaxed and gentle.

Five minutes of this pose once a day or if possible twice a day will offer you the utmost benefit. Remember, you are introducing a very effective modality to your system, and it must be taken in small doses. It is better at the introductory level to stay only three to five minutes in the pose. This posture should never be done after eating; it can be done before going to bed provided that the stomach is empty. But to do it early in morning after the bowels and bladder are empty is perhaps the most beneficial time. It will help move the bowels if they are constipated.

2 Wheelchair Series

This chapter deals with increasing the availability of our own energies to do things. That is important to many of us who have MS, because often at some time during the day our energy runs out. On some days we wake up in the morning without much vim. The poses in this chapter help with the very simple, gentle process of bringing oxygen into the body, making more oxygen available to the cells, thus promoting metabolism and enabling us to be more active. The poses are intended to enhance the circulation of blood, stimulate the nervous system, and increase range of motion in shoulders, spine, and hips.

If at any time during these movements your body starts to tremble or shake, then please stop, take a breath, and wait until the tremor stops. Then start again.

Wheelchair Urdhva Hastasana

Upward Hand Pose

1. Sit in a wheelchair with the back of the torso away from the back of the chair, if possible, or place a rolled sticky mat or blanket between the shoulder blades and the back of the chair to maintain a lifted spine and chest.
2. Place a strap around the arms, slightly above the elbows, with the buckle away from the flesh of the arm.

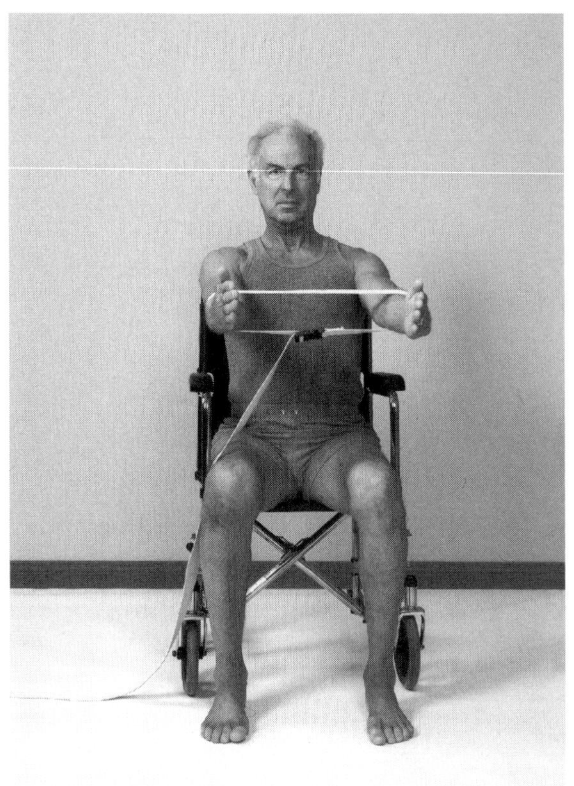

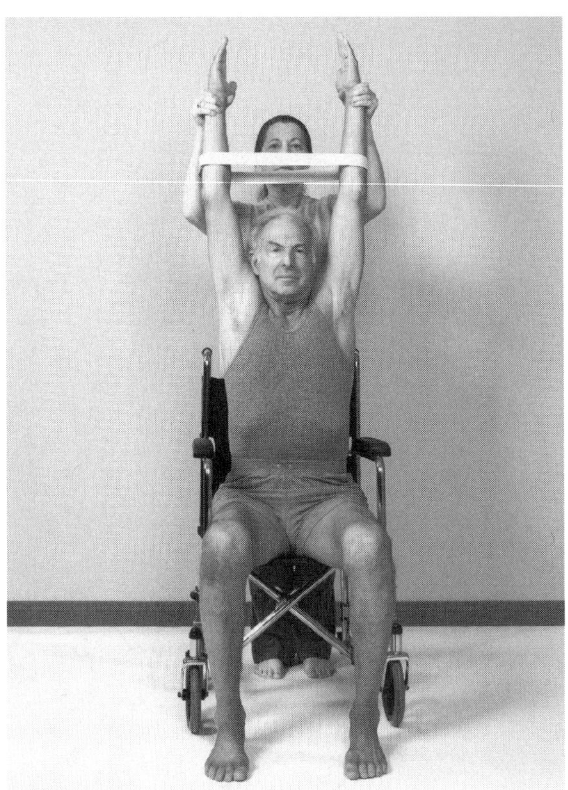

3. Extend the arms forward at shoulder height, with the palms facing each other.

4. On inhalation, raise the arms up. Bring them even with the ears, and rotate the biceps to the outside. This will enable the shoulder blades to support the back of the ribs.

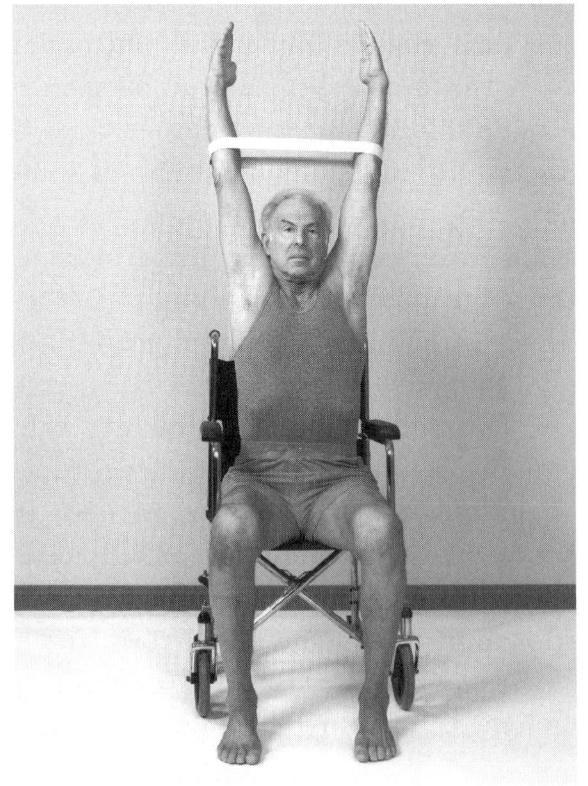

If you are using an assistant, he must first rotate the biceps away from the ears, then gently encourage the shoulders to descend away from the ears. Then he may place his hands just above the strap at the elbows, and with a lifting motion encourage the elbow joint to open from the inside to the outside, in order to fully extend the arm.

5. Hold for three to four breaths, and then return the arms to the starting position.

VIRABHADRASANA II

Warrior Pose II

1. Sit safely forward in a wheelchair.

2. Separate the thighs, with feet flat on the floor. Bend the right knee 90 degrees. Fully straighten the left knee.

3. Make a small loop at one end of a strap. Insert the right hand or thumb, keeping the buckle free.

4. With your left hand, grasp the strap behind the left side of your neck.

5. Stretch the arms apart. Simply slip the strap through your left hand until it is taut.

6. Lift the chest and back waist. Hold this position for a few breaths. Then slowly lower your arms. Sit quietly. Then repeat on the left.

BENEFITS

Strengthens and stretches legs, torso, and arms. Relieves thigh and calf cramps, and revitalizes abdominal organs.

PARIVRTTA VIRABHADRASANA

Wheelchair Lateral Twist

This is a variation on Warrior Pose. The instructor can stabilize the arms by supporting the wrist bones, as the practitioner turns first the abdomen, then the sternum, and finally the shoulders.

1. Take the strap and again lace it around the hand or thumb. Start at the

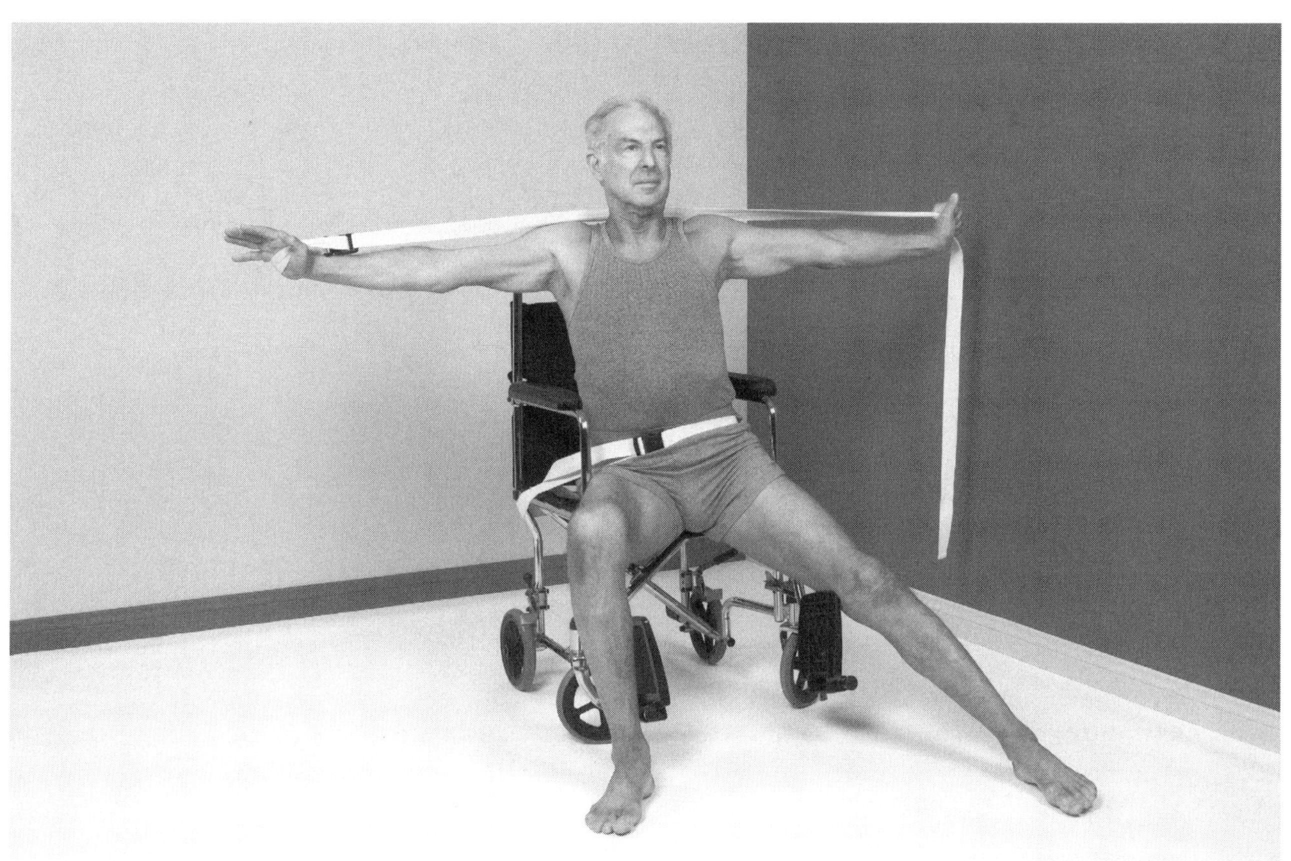

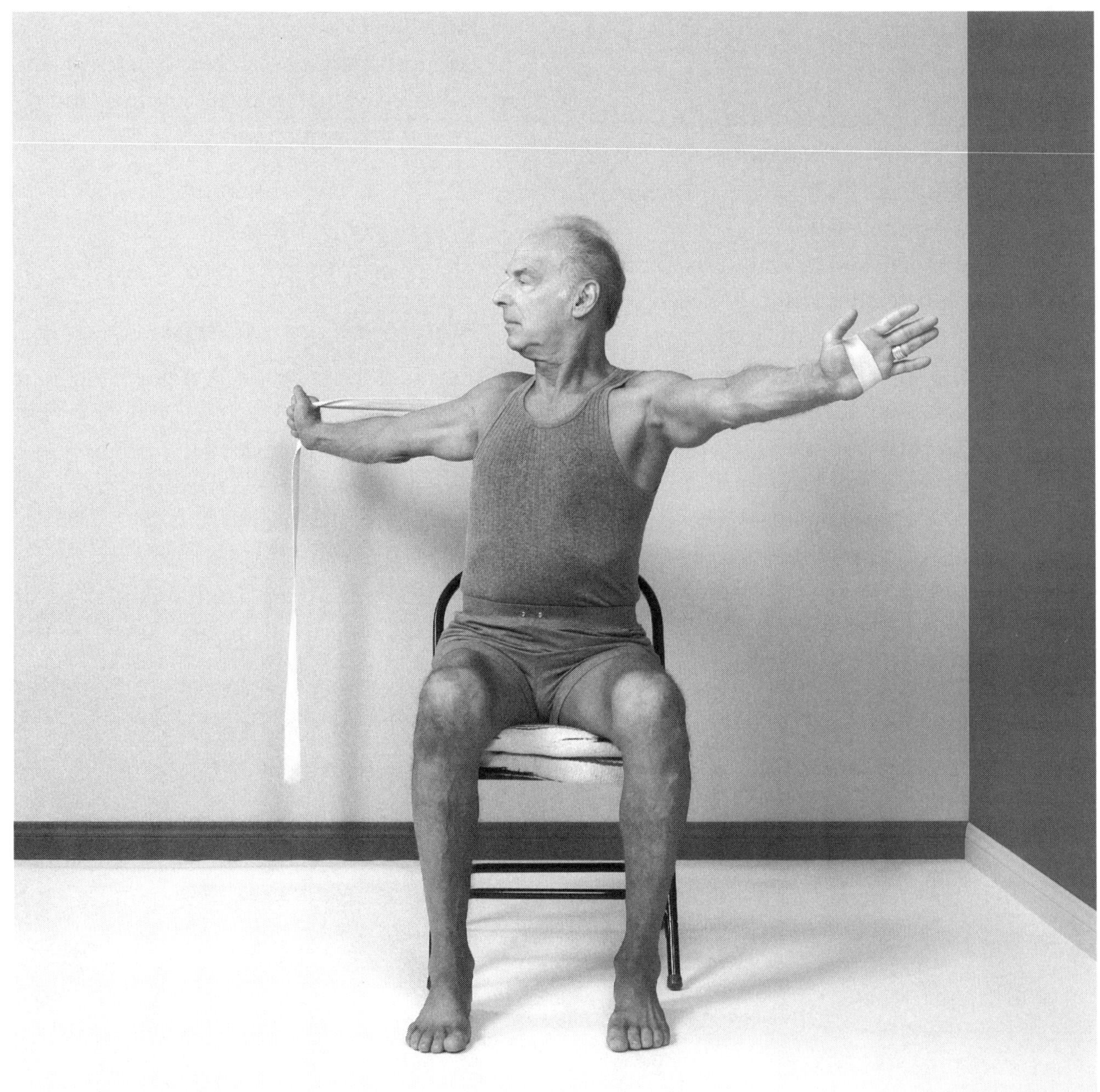

navel or the center of the abdomen, keep the legs firm, and turn the chest with the shoulder. Hold the arms horizontally, and breathe comfortably for 3 to 5 breaths. Keep your nose and sternum in line, without tightening the clavicles (collarbones), shoulder blades, ears, face, or eyes.

2. Inhale as you untwist back to the center. Then turn and repeat on the left.

Once again, the breath comes in from the base of the nostril and out of the tip of the nose, reaching into your center with the force of each inhalation. The inhalation should charge the chest, and the exhalation should descend into the legs.

BENEFITS

Improves hip and lumbar range of motion; counters abdominal cramps and constipation; plus benefits of untwisted Virabhadrasana II.

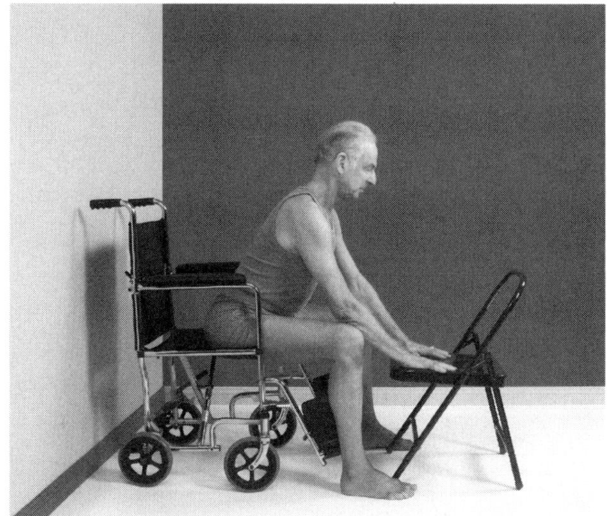

Wheelchair Adho Mukha Svanasana

Downward-Facing Dog Pose

1. Align the wheelchair securely against a wall. If needed, secure the safety belt.
2. Put your feet directly under the knees.
3. Place your palms on the seat of the chair.
4. On the inhalation, raise the top of your head, keeping the chin parallel to the floor.
5. Release the shoulders away from the ears. Exhaling, push the chair forward, and press the hips back.
6. On the next exhalation, push the chair forward to bring your arms in line with your ears.
7. Continue to press the hips back, press the heels down, lift the inner elbows, and press the palms and fingers firmly into the chair seat.
8. Try to move the breath from the low back around the ribs into the front of the sternum, allowing the abdomen to remain soft and free of pressure. After completing 3 to 5 inhalations and exhalations, return to an upright position, place the hands on the top of the legs, and breathe slowly and evenly.

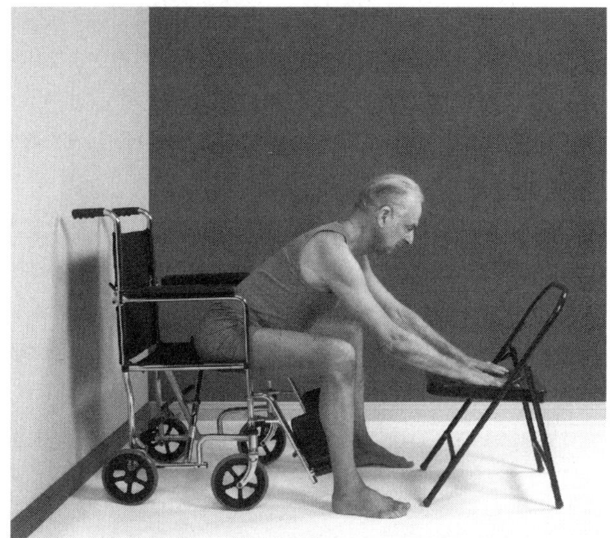

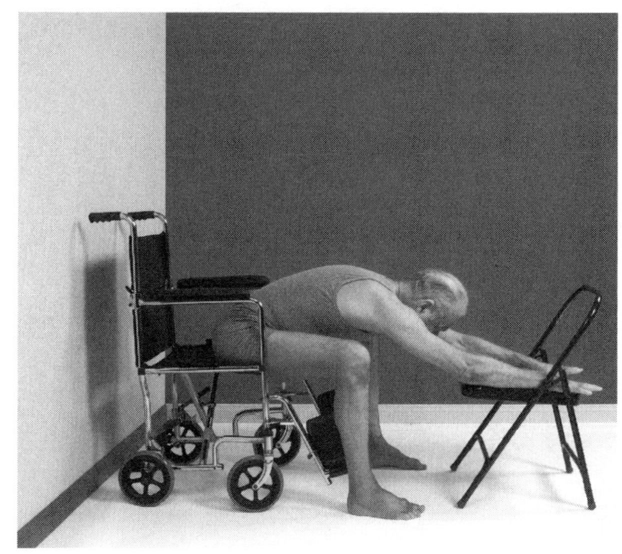

BENEFITS

This pose aids digestion, reduces gas, engages lower back muscles, relieves discomfort from long periods of sitting, realigns the thoracic spine, and reduces tension in the shoulders and neck. It can be used to reduce stress and anxiety by calming the frontal brain.

Wheelchair Parsva Adho Mukha Svanasana

Sideward Downward-Facing Dog

1. Align your wheelchair securely with its back against a wall. Be sure the safety belt is in place if one is needed. Move the yoga chair to the right outside the knee.

2. Place your palms on the seat of the chair, keeping the knees in alignment with the hips. Stretching the left arm slightly more than the right, keep the left hip pressed into the chair seat.

3. Push the chair diagonally to the right on an exhalation. Hold the position and breathe smoothly and evenly for 3 to 5 breaths.

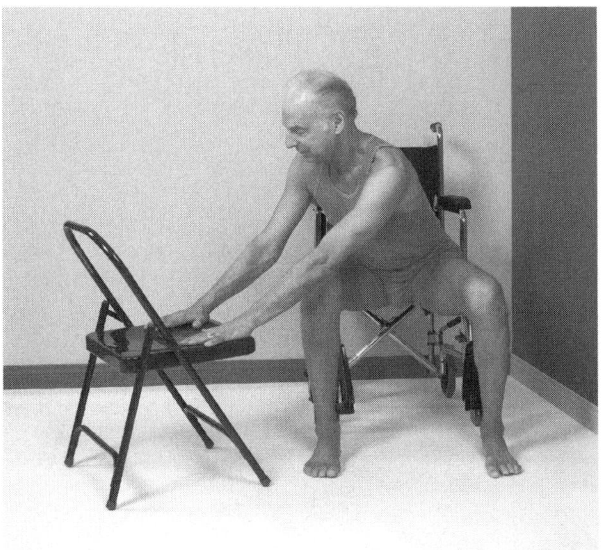

4. Return to the sitting position with the next inhalation. Lift the crown of the head, sit quietly, and then repeat on the other side.

BENEFITS

This pose is an aid to digestion, it engages the lower back muscles, and realigns thoracic spine, neck, and shoulders. It enhances the circulation of blood to the liver, kidneys, spleen, pancreas, intestines, heart, and lungs, allowing more oxygen to flow toward the brain and prompting the bowel to empty.

Wheelchair Adho Mukha Svanasana at Wall

Downward-Facing Dog Pose at Wall

1. Place your chair facing the wall, so that the knees are near the wall, with the feet slightly behind the knees, to gently stretch the Achilles tendon and the thigh muscles.

2. Then place the hands as high up on the wall as possible. Keep the arms in line with the ear canals, opening the outer edge of the armpits as much as possible.

3. Then rest the forehead on the wall, and allow the eyes to drop in to the cheekbones.

4. Press the hips back into the chair seat, and lift the bottom edge of the sternum, allowing the diaphragm to drape softly out to the sides of the rib cage.

5. Extend the fingers away from the palm of the hand; breathe normally for 3 to 5 breaths. Then lift the head and move the arms out to the sides of the torso.

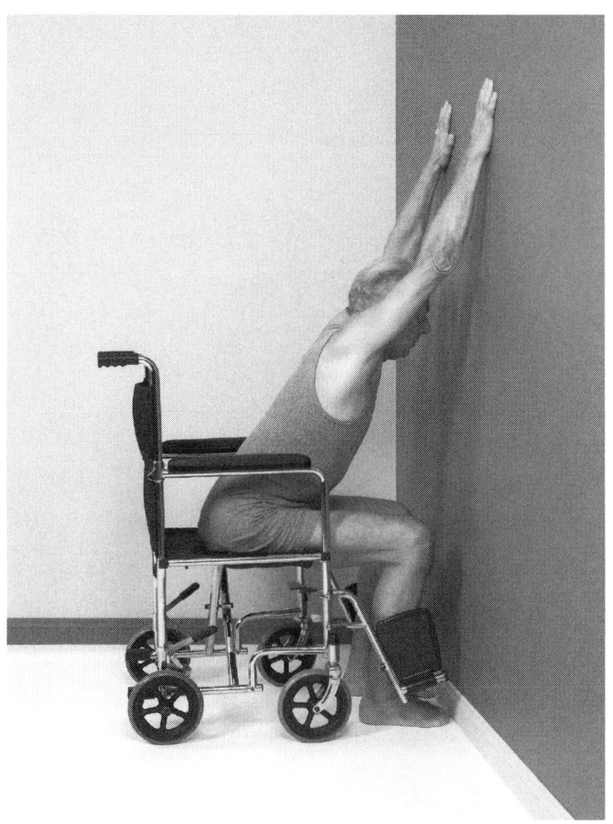

Wheelchair Surya Namaskar

Sun Salutation

This adaptation of the classic Sun Salutation effectively works most areas of the body. This develops the ability to coordinate the breath with measured movement of the limbs and torso. This series of asanas is usually used as a warmup to a practice session. Caution: Resist the temptation to press the tongue against either the roof of the mouth or the lower palate. Keep the breath even and without effort. Try to move smoothly from one position to the next without hesitation. Remember, practice is the key to success.

1. Begin by bringing the hands up to rest in front of the heart, with the elbows raised

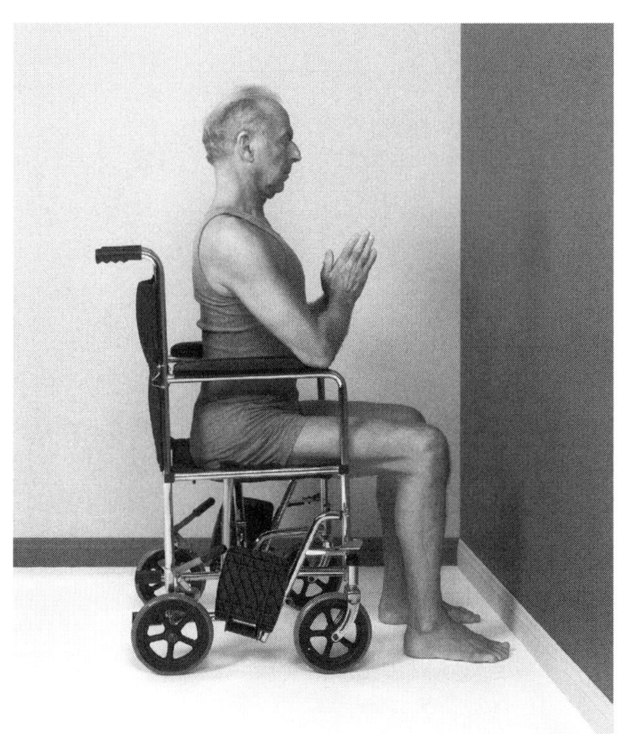

6. Turn the palms up to rotate the shoulder blades inward to support the back and lungs. Then lower the arms to rest the palms on the thighs and breathe evenly.

BENEFITS

This pose reduces tension in the low back, opens the chest and lungs to obtain more oxygen, engages the upper back and shoulders and neck, relieves tightness in the skull, and coordinates the digestive process. It increases hip joint range of motion, helps bowel elimination, and relieves pressure on the prostate gland. The pose also relieves pressure around and in the female reproductive organs. This is one of the essential asanas for those using wheelchair or walkers.

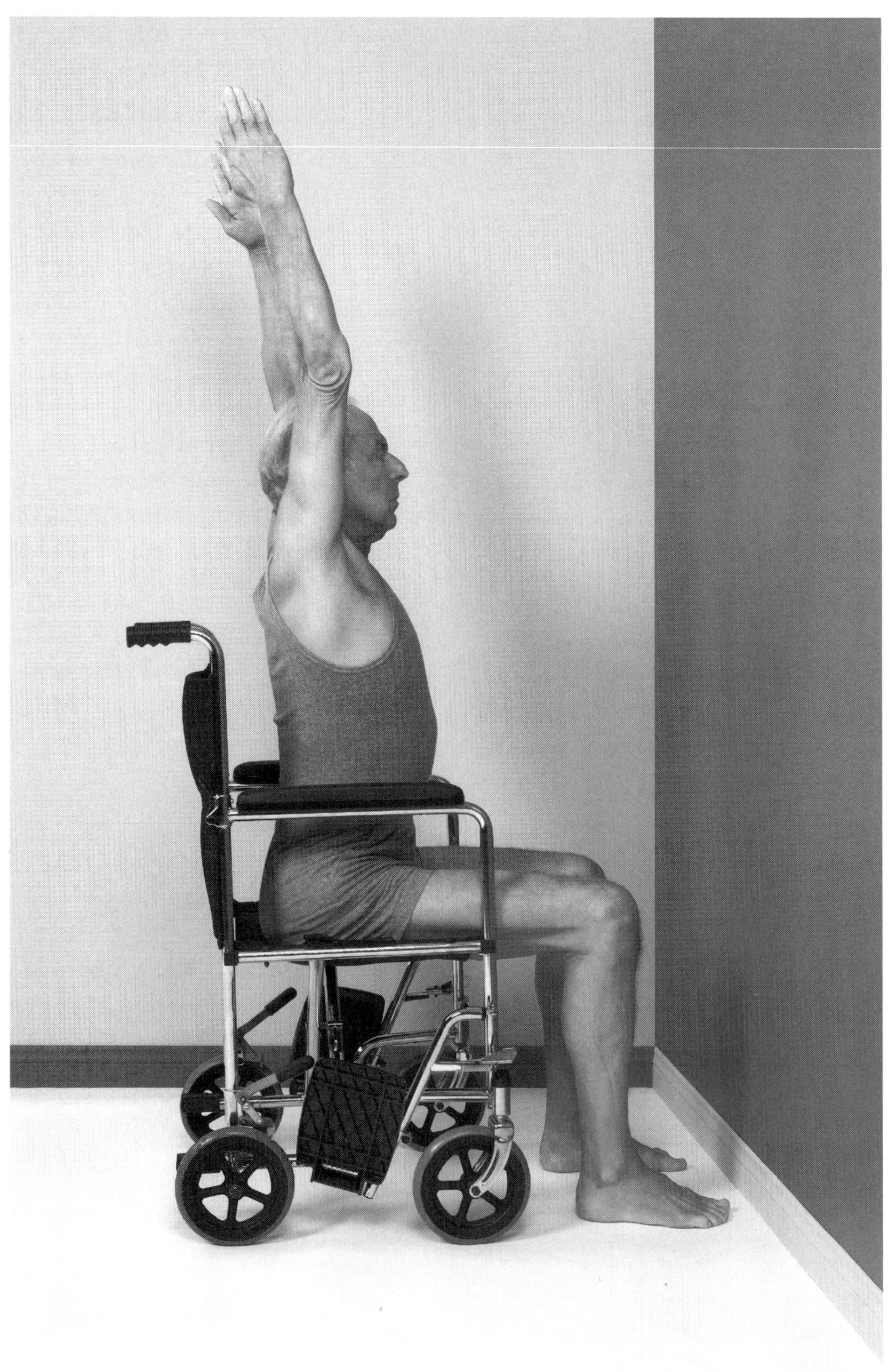

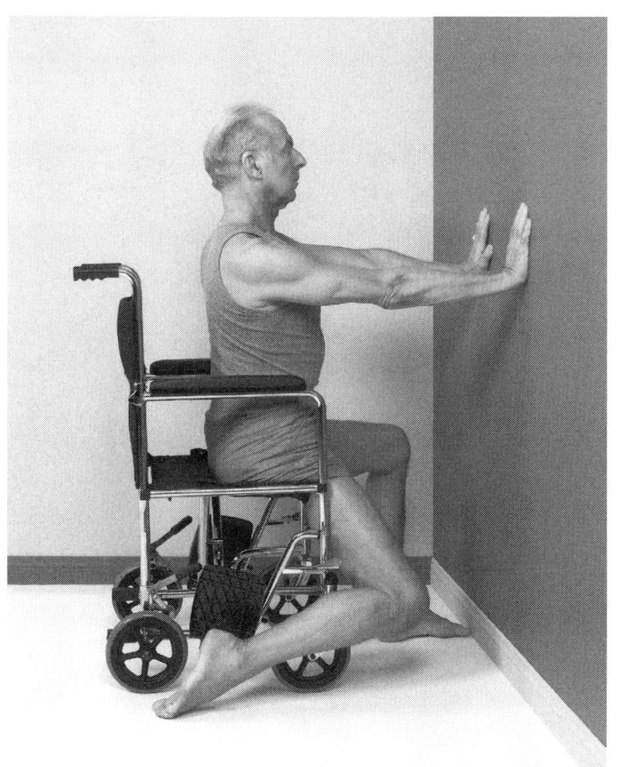

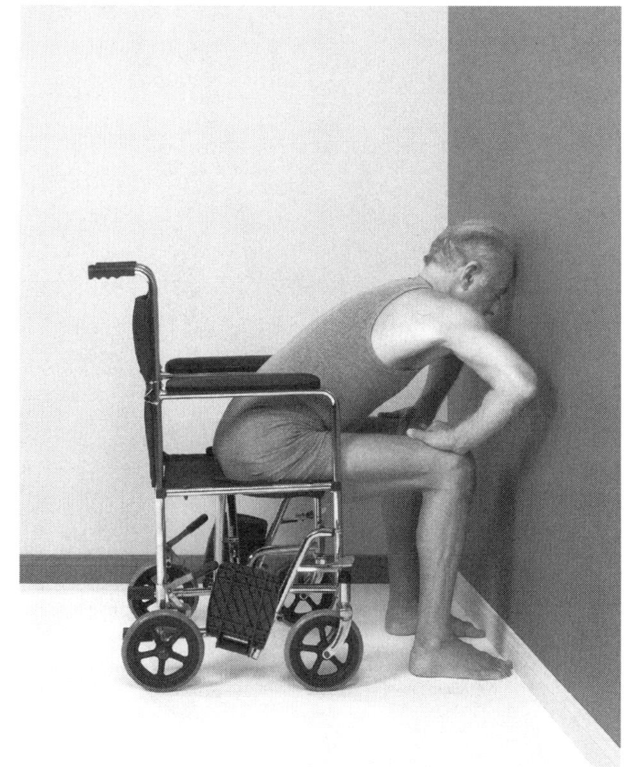

until they are parallel to the floor. Press the fingers together firmly, pointing slightly away from the chest.

2. Bring your feet to rest under the knees, distributing the weight from the balls of the big toes across the sole of the foot. Draw the outer edge of the foot back to the middle of the heel. Keep the knees in line with the hip joint.

3. Extend the arms forward, with the palms facing each other. If you have a shoulder joint problem, extend the arms out to the side with the palms facing up.

4. On the inhalation, bring your arms up alongside your ears.

5. On an inhalation, place your hands on the wall at shoulder height, drawing the wrists up and the shoulders down. At the same time, draw the right leg back outside the wheel of the chair and drop the right knee toward the floor.

6. As you raise the lower right leg forward, grip both hands under the knee, and with an exhalation, lift the leg up sharply toward your chest.

7. Then with the next inhalation, place the right foot on the floor beside the left. Breathe smoothly, lift the back waist, and try to bring the inhalation into the sides of the chest.

8. On an exhalation, place your hands on the top of the knees, and press the elbows forward, as you rest the forehead against the wall.

9. Next, inhale and raise your arms out to the side with the palms facing up, continuing until you place your arms over your head, which still rests on the wall.

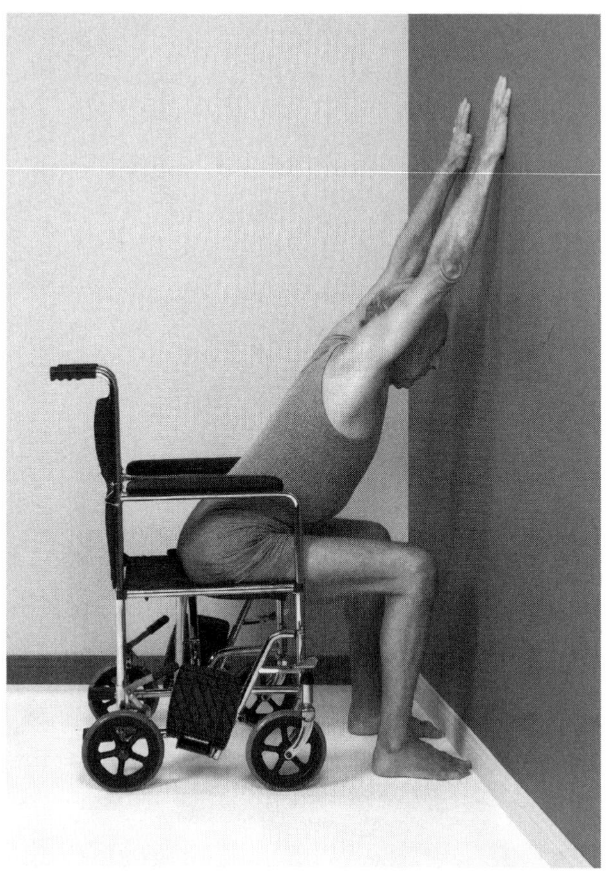

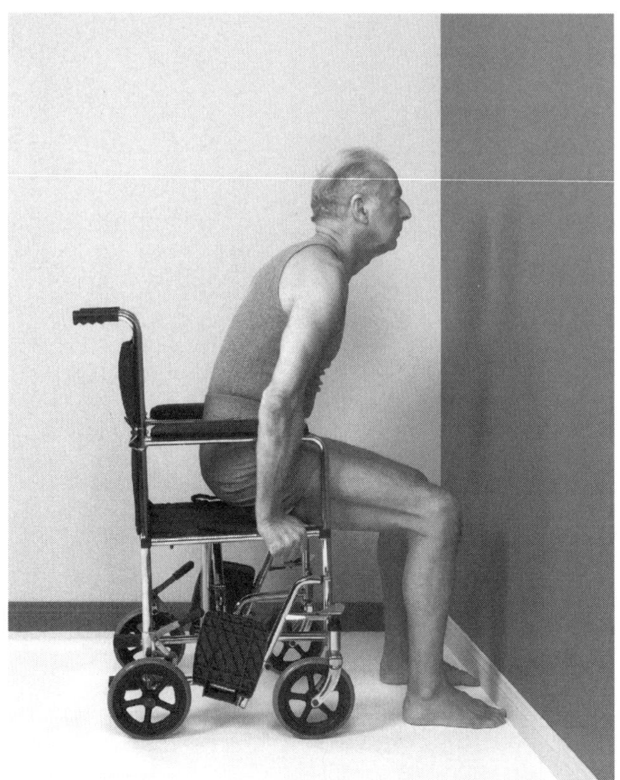

10. Press the palms firmly against the wall. Take several smooth breaths, extending the arms as much as possible and opening the sides of the chest and rib cage.

11. Swing the arms out to the sides of the chair, grip the seat firmly. Then push the hips back as you exhale. Following this, lift the buttocks as best as you can off the seat, and hold the position for 3 breaths.

12. On the 4th exhalation, return to a sitting position. On the next inhalation, press the hands to the wall, draw the left leg back, and drop the left knee toward the floor.

13. Raise the left leg, gripping both hands under the knee. As you exhale, lift the left leg up sharply toward your chest. Then with an inhalation, place the left leg on the floor beside the right.

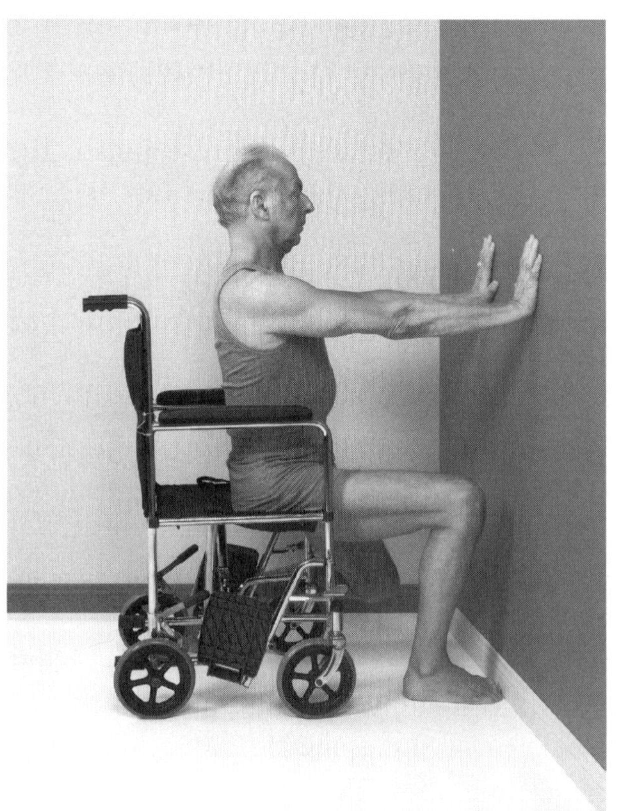

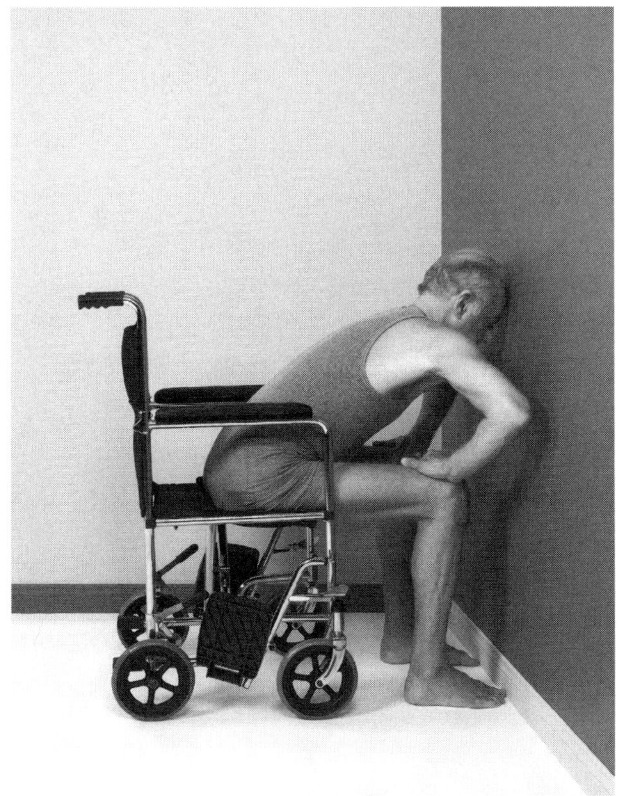

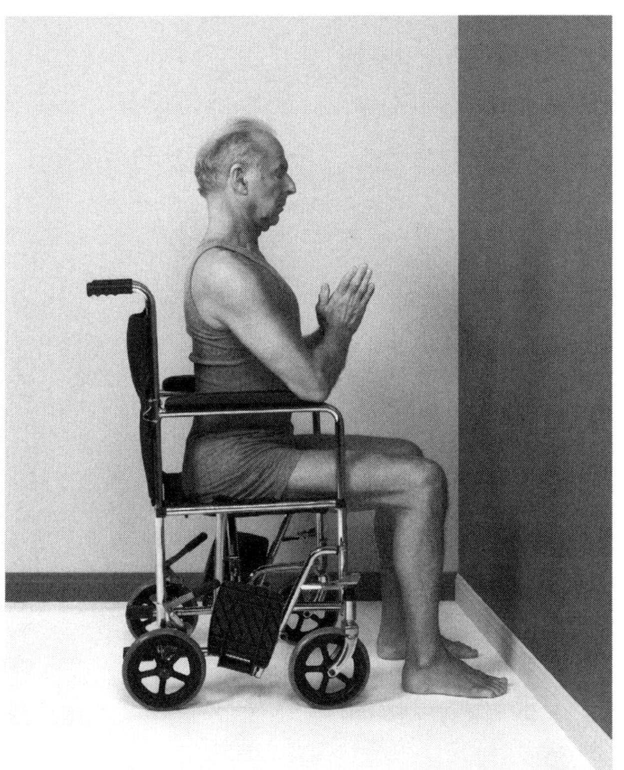

14. Breathe smoothly, lift the back waist, and try to inhale into the sides of your chest. On the exhalation, place your hands on top of the knees, and press the elbows forward, still resting your forehead against the wall.

15. Bring the arms down, lean forward, and rest your head on the wall.

16. Drop the arms down, place your hands on the floor, either outside the feet or between the feet, depending on your flexibility. On an inhalation, sit up and return to the first position, with hands resting in front of the heart, palms together.

17. Sit quietly, observe your breath and the balance of the body, and observe any changes in the spinal column, chest position, and softness of the shoulder girdle. Allow the eyes to gaze forward, releasing any tension in the forehead or temples. This asana can be repeated, starting by moving the left leg back first.

BENEFITS

This asana energizes and also calms the nervous system, depending on the intent of the practice. It increases flexibility, range of motion, and circulation of the limbs, particularly the legs. When you sit for a long time with little or no movement, blood tends to pool in the lower limbs, causing edema and hemostasis. This series helps reduce the swelling of the lower limbs, improves digestion, helps elimination become regular, and improves the volume, timing, and placement of the breath. It engenders a general feeling of contentment and accomplishment.

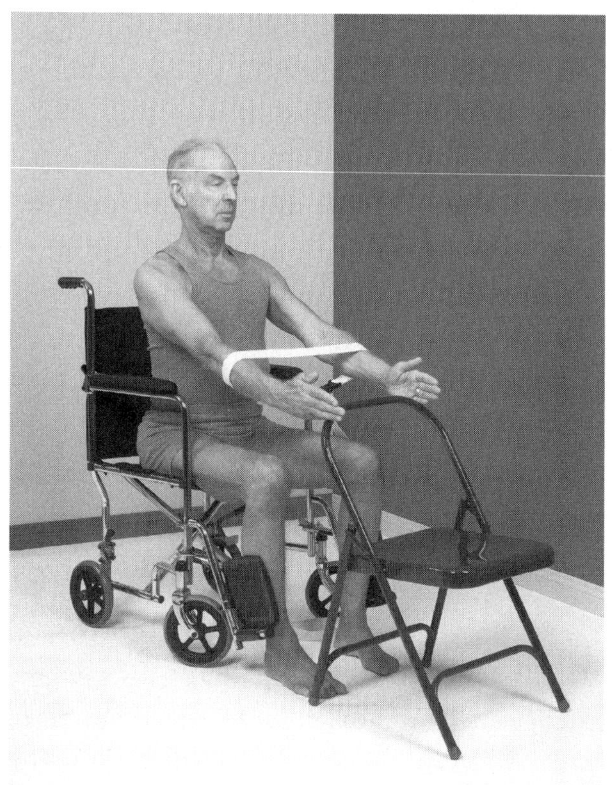

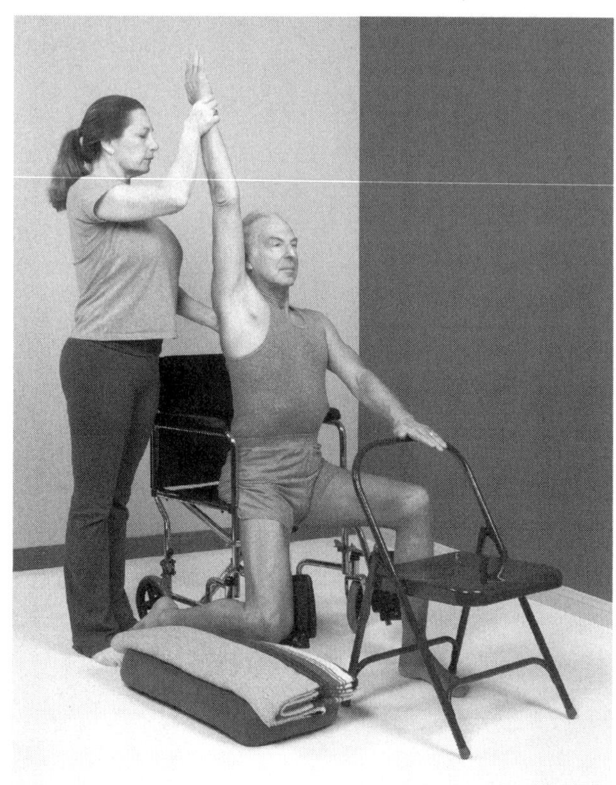

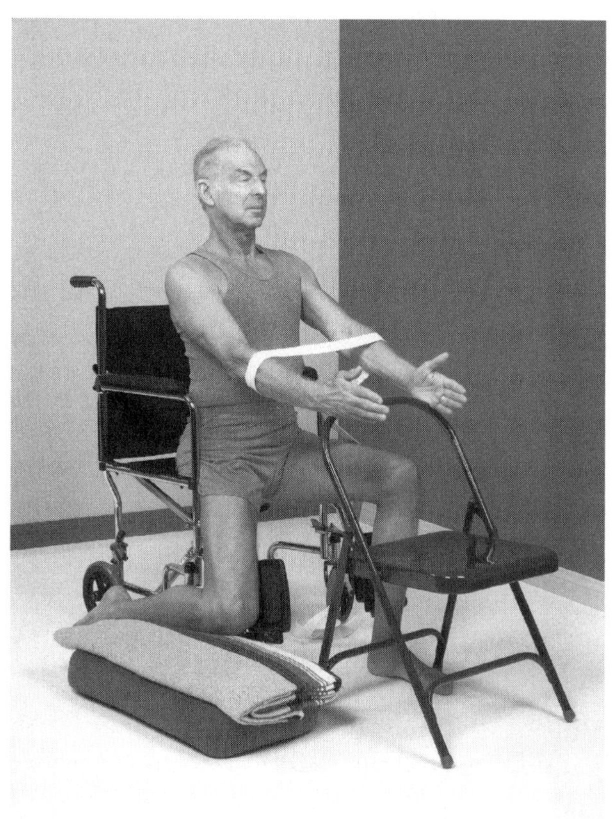

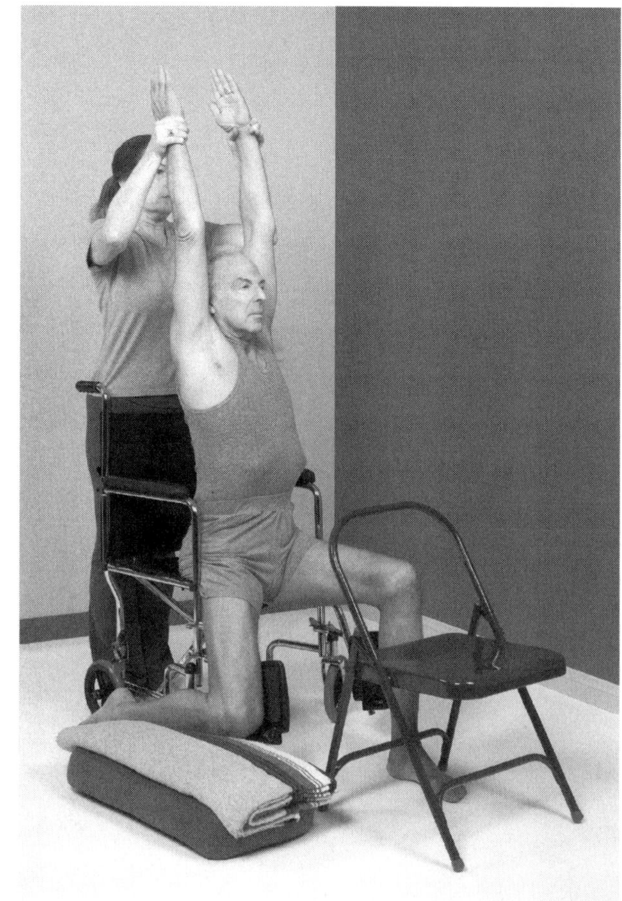

WHEELCHAIR VIRABHADRASANA I

Warrior Pose I

1. Sit upright in your chair, with the back of your torso away from the support of the chair. Place both feet directly under your knees, feet facing straight ahead.
2. Place a chair in front of your knees, with the seat facing forward.
3. Place a strap around the arms, just above the elbows, with the buckle away from your arms.
4. Move the hips to the right, raising the right buttock slightly off the seat of the chair.
5. Then draw the right leg back, using your hands if necessary, and drop the right knee toward the floor, as much in line with the hip as possible.
6. If the knee does not touch the floor, then place a folded blanket under the knee to stabilize the posture.
7. Rest the outside of the palms on the top of the chair. On an inhalation, lift the back waist together with the sternum.
8. Raise the arms up until they are even with the ears, if possible. Hold the position for 3 inhalations and exhalations, and then lower your arms. If using an assistant, raise one arm at a time.

Note that the assistant is encircling the wrist with a thumb and forefinger, thus enabling the student to extend the rib cage. Press the sit bones deeper into the chair, stretching the middle back muscles to counteract the effects of sitting for long periods of time with a soft, rounded back support. Flexing the knee on a folded blanket encourages additional blood flow into the pelvic cavity.

9. Return to the original sitting position with an exhalation, sit quietly for a few moments, and then repeat to the other side.
10. After completing the asana to both sides, remain sitting as much as possible away from the back of the chair.

BENEFITS

The pose helps to develop deeper breathing by expanding the chest. It relieves stiffness in shoulders, neck, back. hips, and knees, and strengthens ankles and knees. In most instances, it improves the sense of

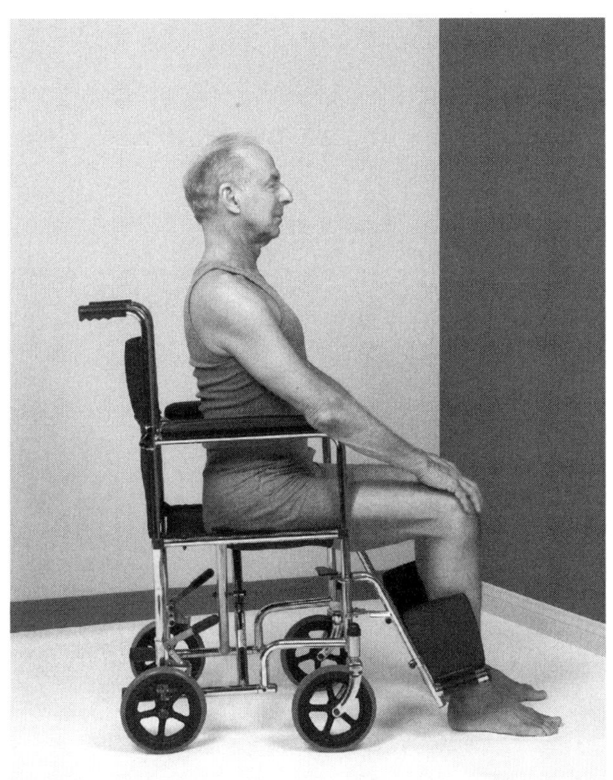

balance and builds stamina in the legs and arms.

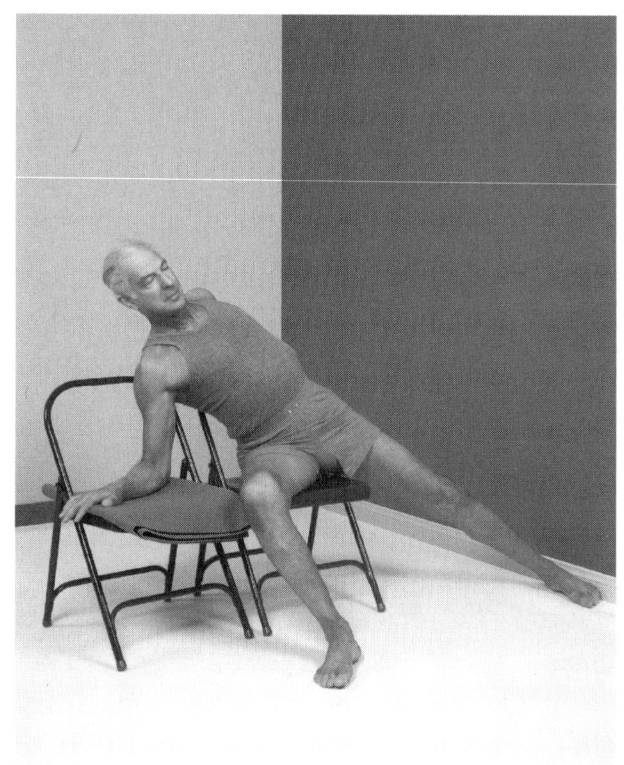

Wheelchair Utthita Trikonasana I

Extended Triangle Pose I

1. Place a folding chair to the right side of your wheelchair, and fasten a safety belt around your waist. Position a folded sticky mat with the folded edge even with the edge of the folding chair seat.

2. Bring your right leg to the right side of the wheelchair, with your foot as flat to the floor as possible. Move your left leg to the left as much as the chair allows.

3. Move your hips to the left as much as possible, and lean over and place the right elbow on the sticky mat.

4. Place your left hand on your hip, and drop the elbow backward, to open the chest cavity. Breathe into the upper ribs and chest area.

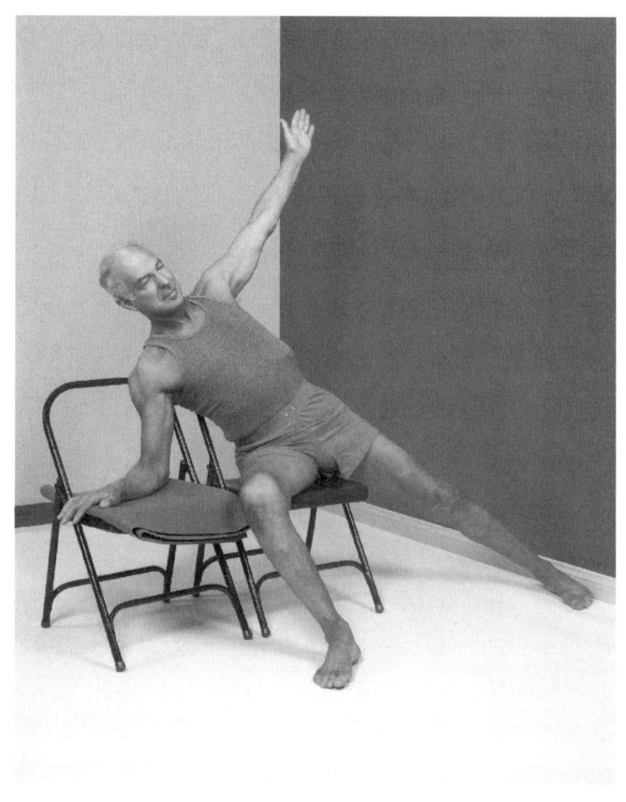

Do not distort the ribs in order to place the right elbow, instead use blankets under the elbow to maintain the alignment of the spine and rib cage. Take a few breaths. With an inhalation, raise the left arm parallel to the right arm.

5. Hold the position for 3 to 5 breaths. Then, retaining the left hand and arm firmly aloft and to the left, press up into a sitting position. Remain seated quietly before repeating to the left.

Wheelchair Utthita Trikonasana II

Extended Triangle Pose II

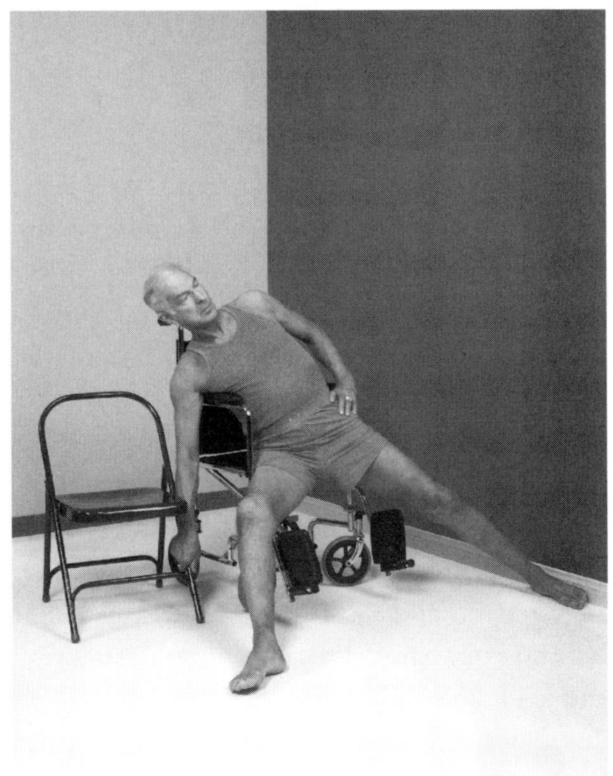

1. Sitting upright in the wheelchair with a safety belt around the waist, bring a second folding chair to your right side.

2. Bring the right leg to the right side of the wheelchair, as far as is comfortable, with the foot flat on the floor.

3. Move the left leg to the left as much as is allowed by the chair. Move the hips to the left as much as possible. Lean over and place the right hand on the bar of the front legs of the folding chair. Do not distort the ribs in order to place the right hand.

4. Place your left hand on the left hip, and drop the elbow backward, to open the chest cavity. Breathe into the upper ribs and chest area. Take a few breaths.

5. With an inhalation, raise the left arm parallel to the right arm. Hold the position for 3 to 5 breaths. Then maintaining the left hand and arm firmly to the left, press up into a sitting position. Remain seated quietly before repeating on the left.

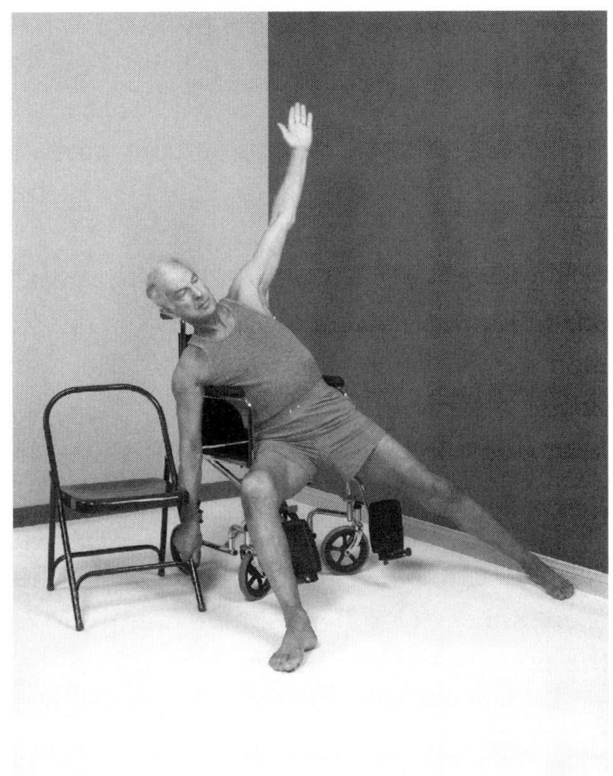

BENEFITS

Both versions of Extended Triangle Pose create a dynamic change in circulation in both the pelvis and the torso. The kidney functions are stimulated, together with the digestive system and the elimination process. Tension in the spinal column and surrounding muscles is reduced. The lower back and pelvis are realigned, thereby counteracting the effects of long periods of sitting. The pose revitalizes the ligaments and tendons and tones the leg muscles.

VIPARITA DANDASANA

Wheelchair Backbend

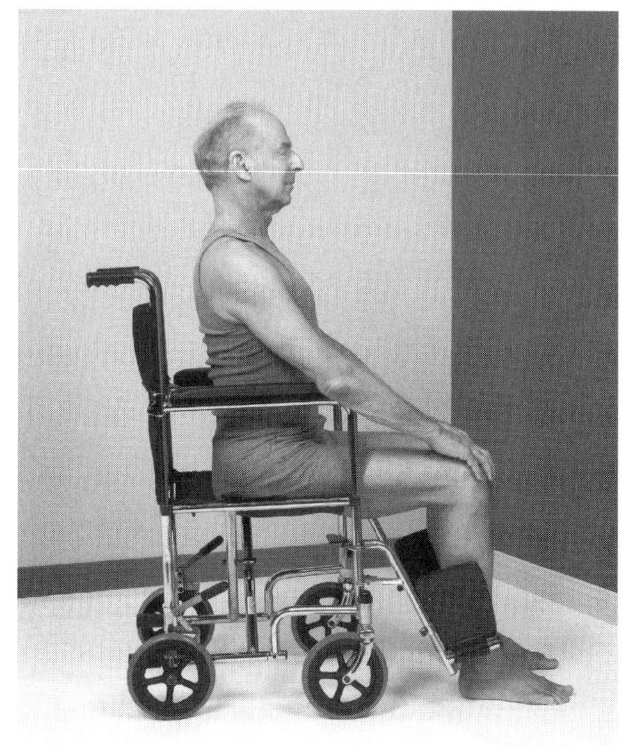

1. To start, roll a sticky mat into a tight roll. This can be achieved by opening the sticky mat, folding over one end about a foot, then rolling the mat very tightly.

2. Sit up as much as possible away from the back of the wheelchair. The buttocks should be in the middle of the seat.

3. Lean back to make sure that the bottom edges of the shoulder blades can be supported against the back of the chair. Then sit up again and insert the rolled sticky mat behind you. parallel to the spine, supporting the neck and the back of the head.

4. Press your feet into the wall, with the heels 3 inches away from the wall and the toes up on the wall, with slightly bent knees.

5. Interlock your fingers firmly in front of you, and if possible place the hands behind your neck, with the little finger on the occipital bone and the thumbs coming around to the sides of the throat and resting on the collarbones.

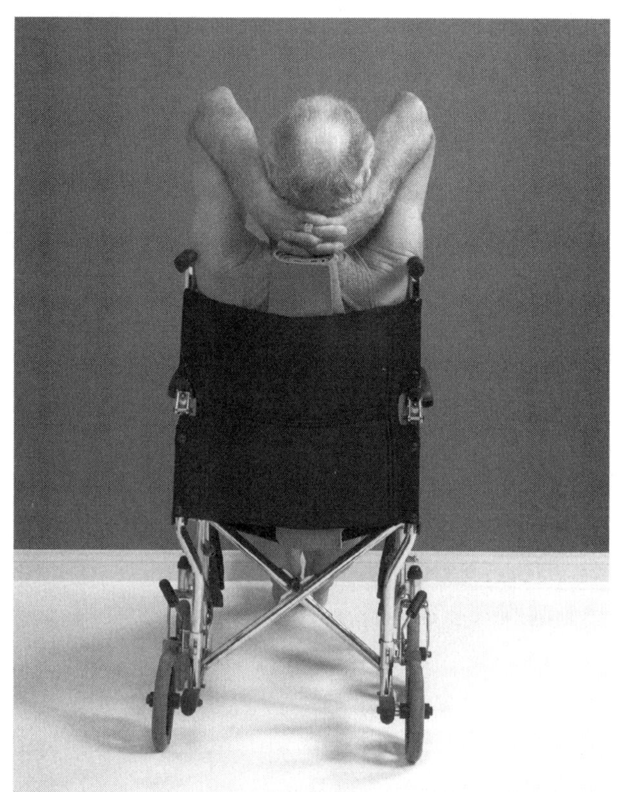

6. Bring your elbows close to your ears and point them up to the ceiling.

7. Allow the head to rest in the palms, as you press the feet into the wall.

8. Gently release the head into the hands, with the sticky mat supporting the neck and back of the skull.

9. Let your eyes settle gently into the cheekbones; the tongue should not press on the upper palate or the lower jaw. Breathe gently, allowing the breath to move up into the chest cavity. After 3 to 5 breaths, bring the head up first on the inhalation.

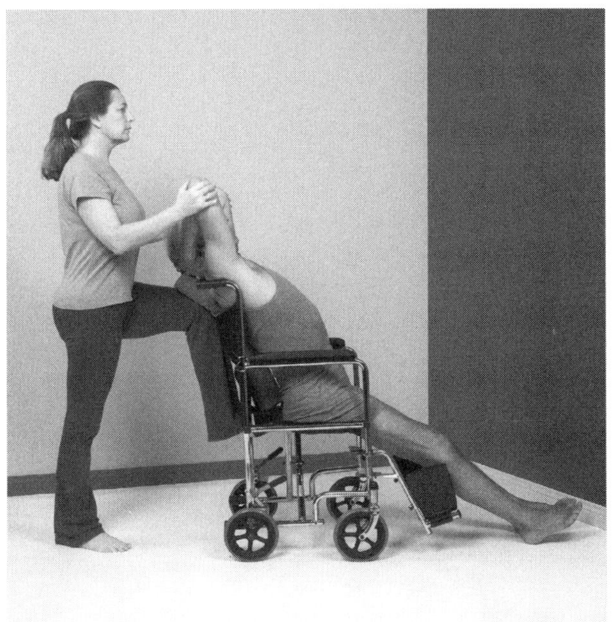

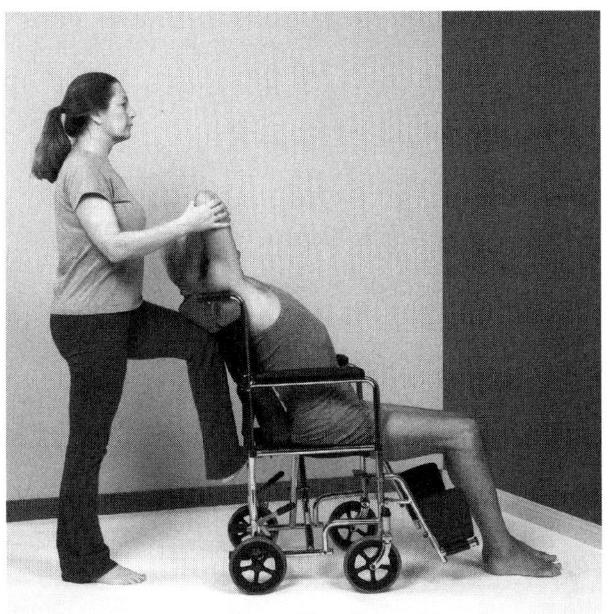

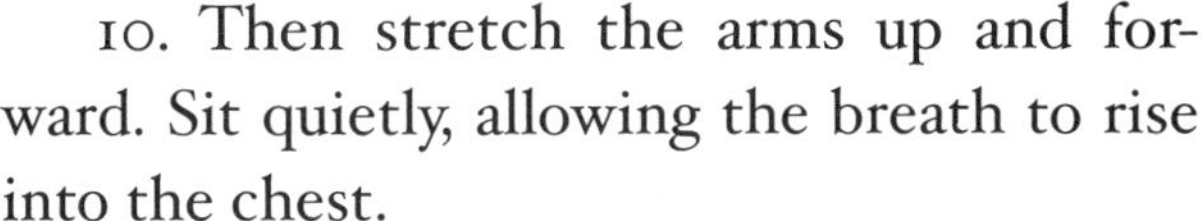

10. Then stretch the arms up and forward. Sit quietly, allowing the breath to rise into the chest.

Notice that the assistant has braced one leg on the bottom edge of the seat of the chair, placing the knee gently into the mid-back. Her hands are on the elbows, with thumbs rotating the bicep outward, and lightly lifting the arms up parallel to the ears.

Caution: Do not grip or tighten the throat.

Here the knees are bent. If extending the legs is a challenge, keep the feet under the knees as much as possible.

BENEFITS

This pose greatly relieves lower back issues. The diaphragm is freed from the constant pressure of resting against the abdominal organs. Digestion is improved by realigning and gently stretching the intestinal tract. And as digestion improves, so does elimination. The pose benefits the chest area by correcting the forward slump of the shoulders. Neck and shoulder discomfort is reduced. It is recommended that seated twists follow the backbends.

Wheelchair Marichyasana III

Wheelchair Seated Twists

1. Begin by placing a folding chair in front of your wheelchair, with the seat facing right. Then rest the right leg on the chair. If this causes any discomfort at the knee, place a rolled sticky mat or towel under the knee to release the hamstrings. If the leg is long, two chairs will be necessary, so the foot does not hang.
2. Then lift the left leg, resting the left foot on the seat of the chair.
3. Turn the navel toward the back of the folding chair, allowing the right hand

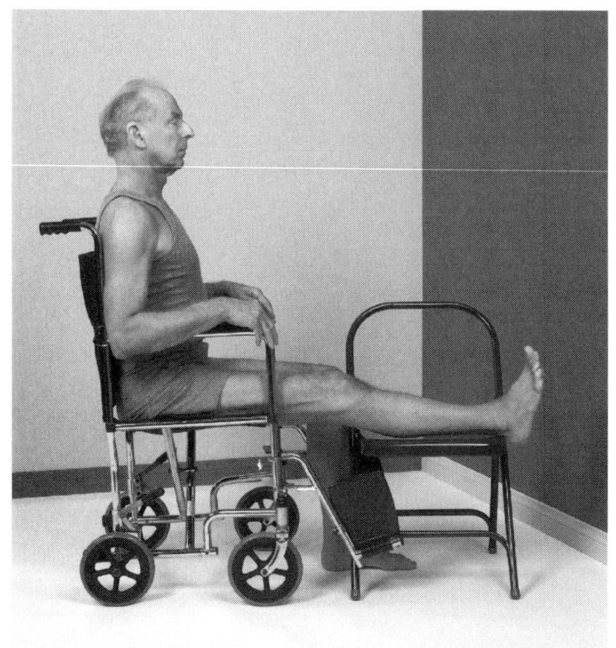

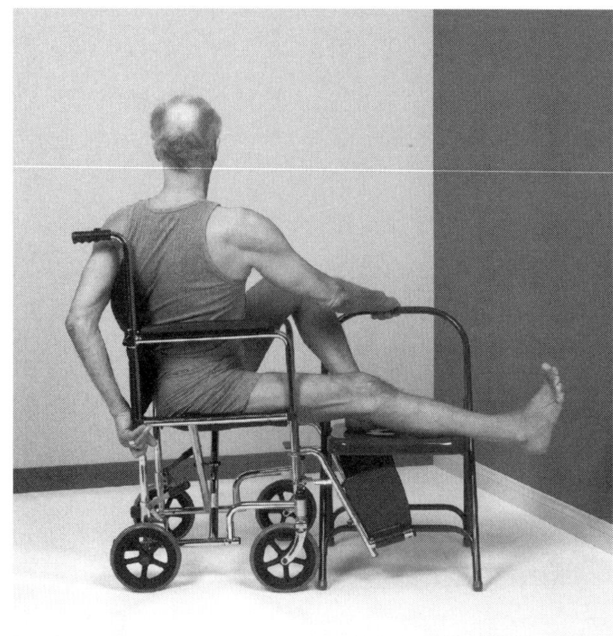

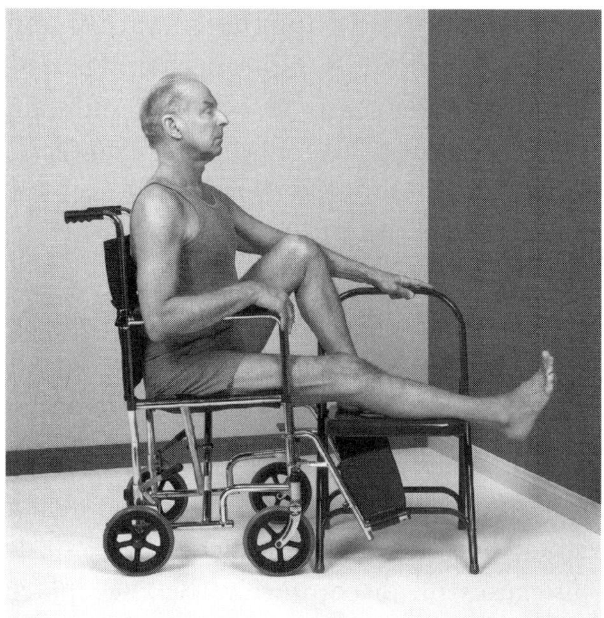

to follow and clasp the back of the chair. Press the left leg into the back of the folding chair.

4. With another exhalation, take the left hand around to the back of the wheelchair, so the top of the wheelchair is under the armpit, supporting the ribs.

5. Release and lower the shoulders away from the ears, and keep the nose in line with the heart.

6. Press down into the left foot, extend the right foot away from the right hip, and breathe in a smooth and easy manner, keeping the chest lifted and the shoulders back.

7. Release the right arm first, then the left arm.

8. Take each leg to the floor, and sit quietly. Then turn the folding chair in the opposite direction, and repeat to the other side

BENEFITS

This pose stimulates all the organs in the torso to improve their function. Sitting posture is improved, flexibility in the hips and legs is enhanced, and leg cramps are reduced. Tension in shoulders and neck is lessened, resulting in fewer headaches.

Wheelchair Pasasana

Wheelchair Twist with Bolster

1. Begin by securing the safety belt. Bring the feet under the knees. If the leg is long, place a folded blanket under the buttocks. If the leg is short, place a folded blanket under the feet.

2. Place a bolster or folded blankets on top of the thighs. This is important if the student is full-figured or has a limited range of motion, so as to not cramp or pinch the organs in the torso or pelvis.

3. Sit up, turn toward the bolster, and grasp the side of the wheelchair with the right hand in order to maintain balance.

4. Raise the left arm up level with the ear, and press the sit bones down into the chair seat.

5. Lift the rib cage, turn the navel toward the bolster, and bring the left elbow to the top of the bolster, as close to the right side as possible.

6. Keep your head in line with the spine, and try not to tighten the throat.

7. Extend the fingers of your left hand as if pressing against a wall, and breathe smoothly and evenly for 3 to 5 breaths.

8. Return the arm to the level of the left ear on the inhalation, bring the arm down on the exhalation, and sit quietly for 10 to 20 seconds. Then repeat on the other side.

Note that the left ear is more in line with the left leg, rather than leaning to the right or looking down or back. This ensures that the muscles of the mid and lower back are not strained.

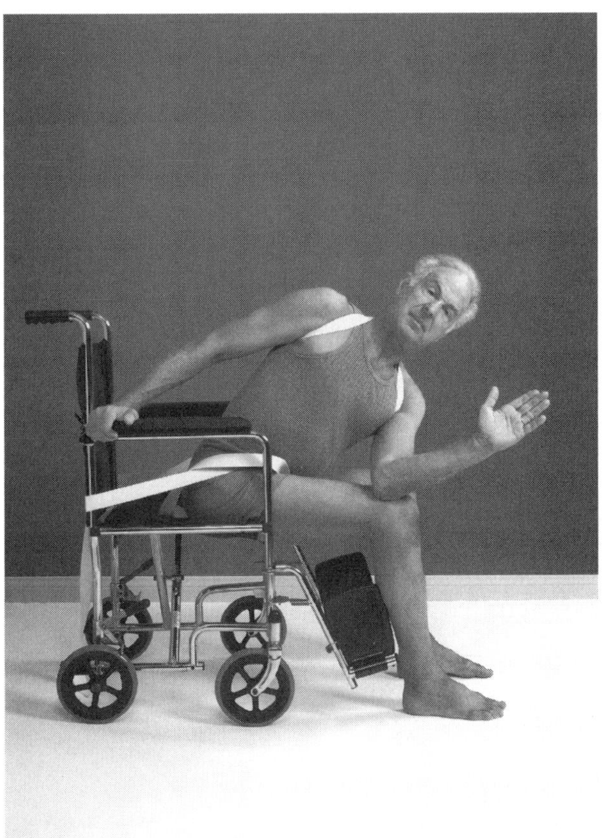

BENEFITS

This pose is excellent for the digestion. It relieves lower back discomfort from sitting for extended periods of time, aids elimination, and reduces constipation. It increases flexibility in the hip joints and increases circulation in the torso, pelvis, and limbs.

Wheelchair Baddha Konasana

Cobbler's Pose

1. Secure the safety belt and lock the wheels of the wheelchair. Place a folding chair with the seat facing the wheelchair.

If your range of movement is limited, turn the chair around so the back of the chair can act as a support, and place a folded sticky mat on the seat.

2. Raise the legs by holding behind the knee and relaxing the adductor muscles.
3. Place the feet together, with the toes and heels touching if possible.

If there is undue pressure in the groins, support the outer knee with the back of a chair placed under the leg.

4. Sit up away from the back of the wheelchair. If that presents a problem, place a rolled sticky mat, a folded blanket, or a block between the chair back and the mid back, behind the heart area.
5. Lift the rib cage and side chest with an inhalation, and exhale behind the navel.

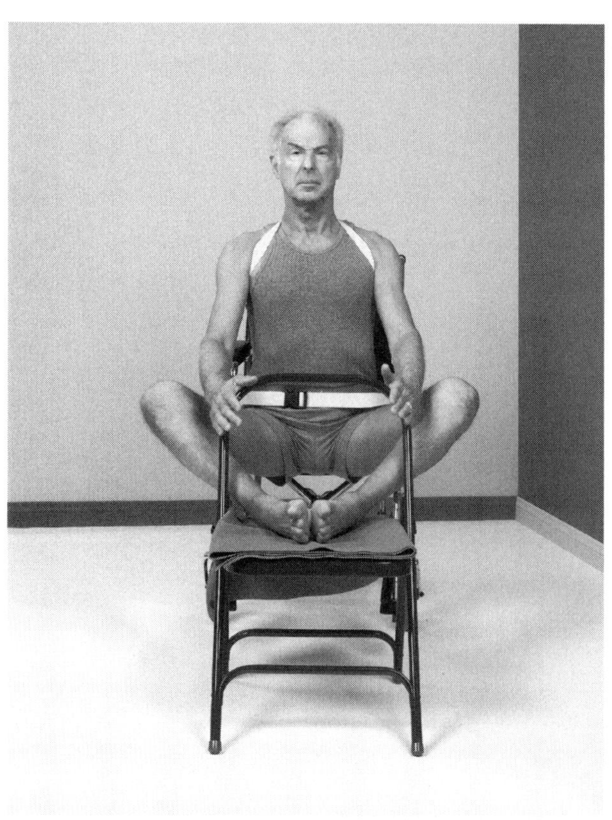

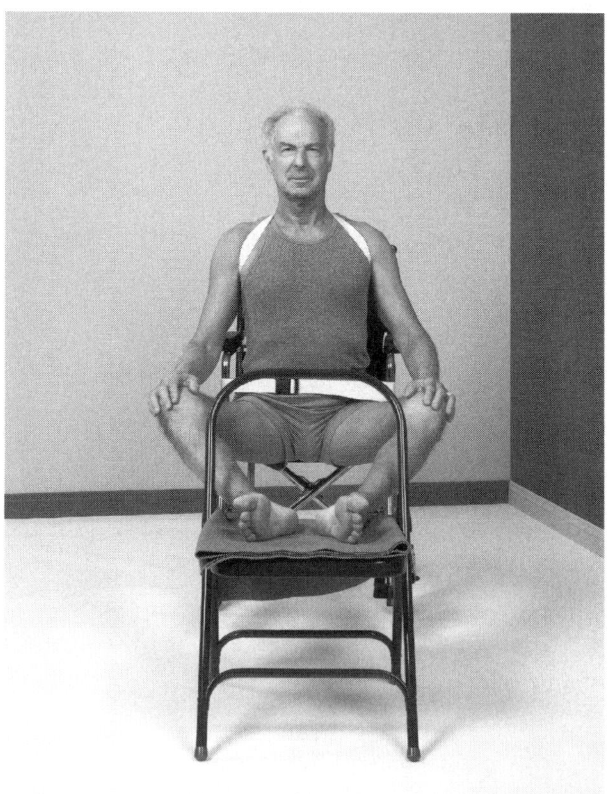

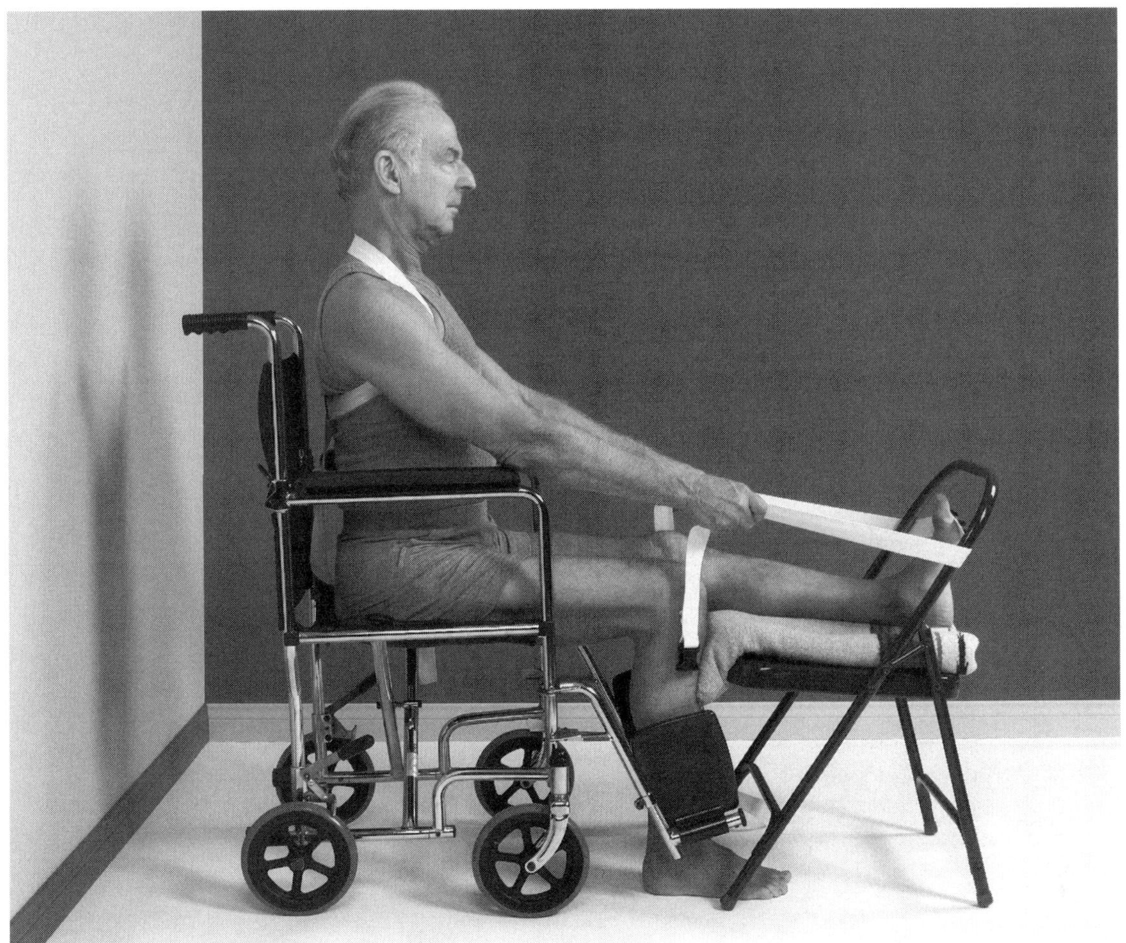

A strap can be looped around the back of the folding chair to facilitate lifting the torso. Hold the position for 10 breaths or whatever is comfortable.

6. Use your hands on the outer side of the knees to lift the legs up and together, slowly and carefully.

8. Then place your hands behind your knees, and draw the flesh of the knee back toward the hips as the legs stretch forward to rest on the seat of the chair.

9. Bring legs down. Sit quietly with both feet on the floor.

Wheelchair Preparation for Janu Sirsasana

Preparation for Head-to-the-Knee Pose

1. Sit up away from the back of the wheelchair, using a prop if necessary to support the torso.

2. Place the folding chair in front, with the seat facing toward the wheelchair. Please note that a strap has been placed around the shoulders and over the back of the neck, like a harness.

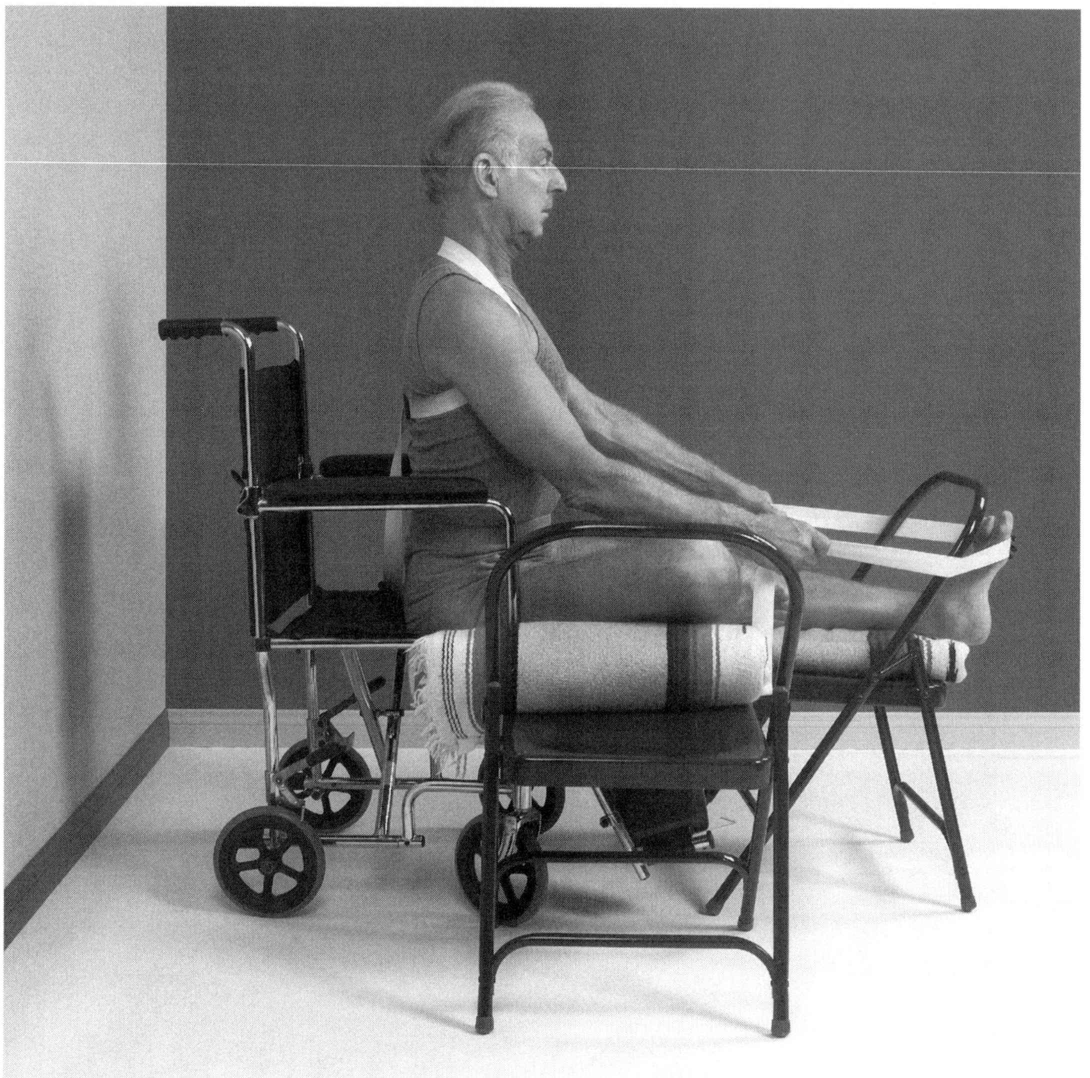

The buckle is in the middle of the back, and the tail of the strap can be used to tighten the strap in order to hold the shoulders back to improve the posture and strengthen the torso. This device can be used in many asanas throughout the book to enhance the posture and develop an awareness of alignment.

3. Loop a strap around the back of the folding chair, and with a moderate pull, sit up as tall as possible.

4. Encourage the inhalation to lift the ribs and side chest, lowering the shoulders away from the ears. If there is increased pressure behind the knee, use a rolled towel or sticky mat to reduce any tension.

WHEELCHAIR JANU SIRSASANA

Head-to-the-Knee Pose

1. Begin by locking the wheels of the chair. Place a folding chair in front, with the seat facing toward you.

2. Place a folded blanket on the seat of the chair. Bring a second folding chair to the right side.

3. Bending the right leg and placing the right foot against the left thigh, support the right leg with additional folded blankets.

4. Loop a strap around the left foot or the back of the first chair. Holding the strap in each hand, raise the torso away from the back of the wheelchair.

5. Raise the rib cage, lift the bottom edge of the sternum, and press the buttocks back and down into the seat.

6. Gently turn the navel toward the left leg without distorting the neck or head. Hold the position for at least 5 even breaths and then release.

7. Use the right hand outside the right knee to bring the right knee up.

8. Place both hands behind the right knee and stretch the right leg forward, placing it on the seat of the chair next to the left leg.

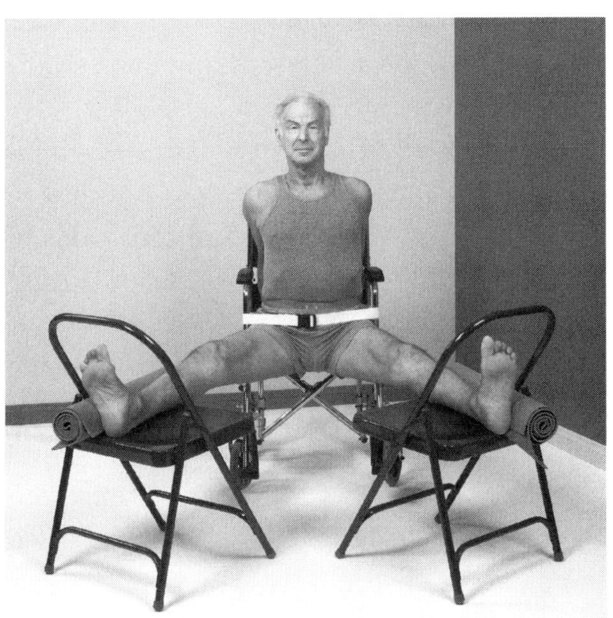

9. Bring the second chair with the folded blankets to the other side, and repeat the asana on the other side.

BENEFITS

This asana is a combination of Baddha Konasana, Paschimottanasana, and the seated twists. It greatly enhances digestion, elimination, flexibility of legs and arms, and it releases tension in the shoulders, neck, and spine. It tones the legs and arms and lengthens the hamstrings.

Wheelchair Upavistha Konasana

Seated Wide Angle Pose

1. Begin by securing the safety belt and locking the wheels.

2. Bring two folding chairs in front and to the side of the wheelchair, with the seats facing toward you.

3. Place the legs on the chair, with the back supports of the chair bracing the legs.

4. Place a rolled sticky mat between the chair and the legs, which helps to keep the legs and feet in alignment. Notice that the feet are pointing up as much as possible, and the inner knees are turning toward the seat of the chair.

5. Bring the back of the torso away from the back of the chair, using props if necessary. Sit on the tips of the sit bones, bracing your hands behind you.

6. Bring the breath into the side chest, press down on the hands, and lift the side chest as much as possible.

7. Remain in the posture for 5 to 10 breaths.

8. Return to center by bringing the chairs together slowly and carefully with your hands, and remain seated with the legs stretched forward supported on the chairs. Sit quietly and breathe.

BENEFITS

This pose will open the groins, increase circulation in the lower pelvis, and increase flexibility in the hips, adductors, and hamstrings. It reduces tension in the mid and lower spine and generally tones the legs and arms. Additional blood circulation in the hip joints strengthens the joints and reduces the brittleness and dryness of the bone, which can lead to spontaneous fracture.

WHEELCHAIR UTTANASANA

Forward Bend Pose

1. Begin by securing the seat belt, with enough slack to be able to bend forward. Lock the wheels. If necessary, use the shoulder harness, as illustrated.

2. Place a bolster between the feet, toes forward, ankles braced by the sides of the bolster.

3. Sit up and with a few breaths align your head with the center of the pelvis.

4. Place the hands palm down on top of the knees and lean forward 30 degrees.

5. Slip the hands down the inside of the legs to the mid calf, and lean forward 60 degrees.

6. Keep the head in line with the spine, and with an exhalation, place the palms down onto the bolster between the legs, if possible.

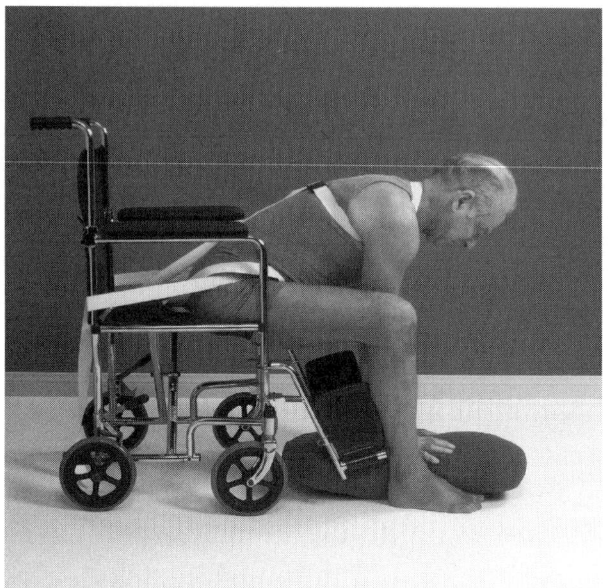

7. Then gently press the knees against the outer upper arm and the arms against the inside of the knees. This action releases tension in the lower spine and hips.

8. If there is any difficulty maintaining the head in line with the spine, a second chair can be placed under the head, with folded blankets or bolsters on the seat to support the head. Only the forehead rests on the support, so that the nose is free from pressure. Allow the eyes to rest against the cheekbones.

9. Hold for at least 30 seconds to 1 minute to start, and then build up to 2 minutes.

10. Return to a sitting position by keeping the head down and placing the hands on top of the knees, hold for several breaths, then use the hands to press up slowly on the count of 10 to a sitting position.

11. Sit quietly for 10 to 20 breaths.

BENEFITS

This pose irrigates the kidneys, liver and may reduce discomfort in the stomach . The heartbeat slows, and the spinal nerves are

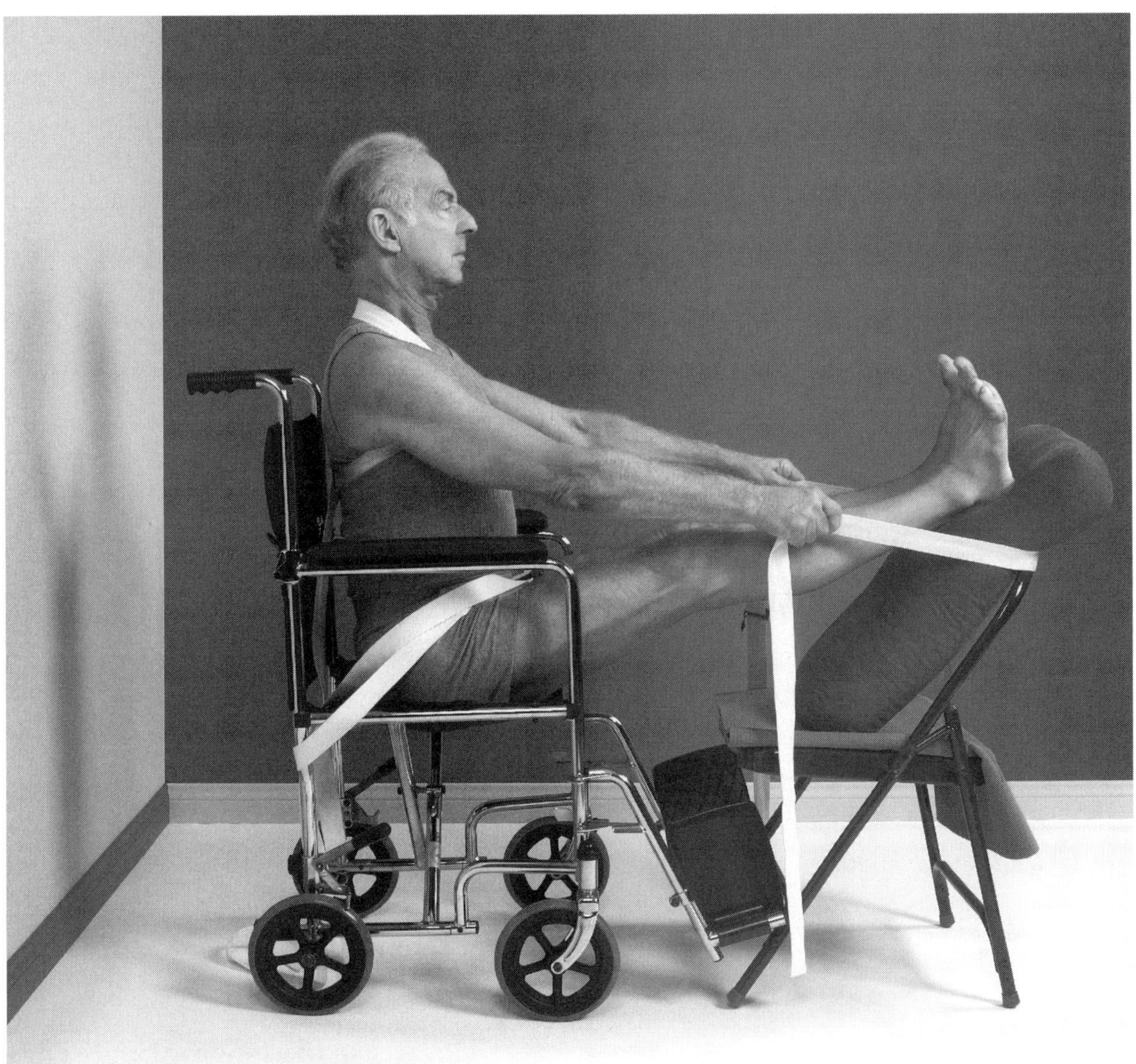

rejuvenated. The pose counters depression, and students that are easily excited often become calm and cool, with a sense of well-being. Vision often improves.

WHEELCHAIR ARDHA NAVASANA

Supported Boat Pose

Note: This asana is not to be done without at least three months of prior practice. Then it is usually performed toward the end of a practice or class session.

1. Begin with the safety belt secured. Lock the wheels. Bring a folding chair in front, with the seat facing you.
2. Place a folded sticky mat on the seat of the second chair. A blanket can be folded over the back of the wheelchair for comfort.
3. Lift both feet onto the edge of the folding chair, and place the bolster at the angle illustrated.

4. Extend the legs up toward the back of the folding chair, clasping a strap in each hand that has been placed midway on the back of the chair around the bolster. The bolster can be placed flat on the seat to accommodate those who are tight in the hamstrings or have a balance problem.

5. Raise the chest and side ribs. Keep the head parallel to the spine, and breathe easily.

6. Try not to hold the breath. If there is undue stiffness in the neck and shoulders, the wheel chair can be moved next to a wall and the back of the head will be supported.

7. Hold the posture for at least 10 breaths.

8. Release the strap, bend the knees, and rest the feet on the edge of the chair seat.

9. Lower the legs to the floor with manual support behind the knees to keep the groins soft.

10. Walk your hands bent to your sides. Return to a sitting position.

BENEFITS

This pose is very beneficial to the liver, gall bladder, and spleen. It strengthens the back muscles, which become flaccid due to the shape of the wheelchair and prolonged sitting. It opposes lumbar osteoporosis.

WHEELCHAIR SAVASANA

Relaxation Pose

1. Place a folding chair in front of the wheelchair and facing it. Put a folded sticky mat on the seat.

2. Rest one end of a bolster against the back of the folding chair, and place the other end in your lap or on your thighs.

3. Lean forward to rest the head face down, with a towel or blanket supporting the forehead, allowing the nose to be free from any pressure.

4. If possible, cross your arms over your head while it rests on the bolster. If it is difficult to rest your head on the bolster, then use folded blankets or another bolster to allow greater comfort. The arms can also rest on the seat of the chair if it is difficult to raise them over your head.

5. Allow the eyes to rest into the cheekbones, and release the tongue away from the upper and the lower palate.

6. Allow the breath to be smooth and even. Try to stay focused on the breath. It is natural to let the thoughts wander into the past, into the future, or to take in the events of the day. Part of Savasana is to learn to be in the moment.

This is also the time when the effects of yoga practice can be absorbed into the conscious mind. When it becomes difficult to remain in the rhythm of the breath, then it is time to begin slowly rising up from the support of the bolster.

7. Lift the head from the chest. Open the eyes on an inhalation.

3

Chair Series

This chapter enables students to perform many of the asanas that are important to maintaining their health. Not all possible asanas are included. It is feasible, with correct instruction, to adapt many of the asanas. This can be done by attending classes conducted by certified Iyengar instructors, many of whom are familiar with adaptive yoga. It is the intent of this book to illustrate the possibilities and to give a well-rounded series of asanas addressing many of the symptoms that we experience. The chair series requires chairs that have been altered to be safe props.

Chair Urdhva Hastasana

Arms-Above-the-Head Pose

1. Start by putting a strap around your hands. The strap stabilizes the arms to connect the movement of the arms with the breath.

2. Start the movement by bringing your shoulder blades back against the backs of the ribs, stabilizing the shoulder blades. The instructor can put his hands against the shoulder blades, supporting the chest from behind.

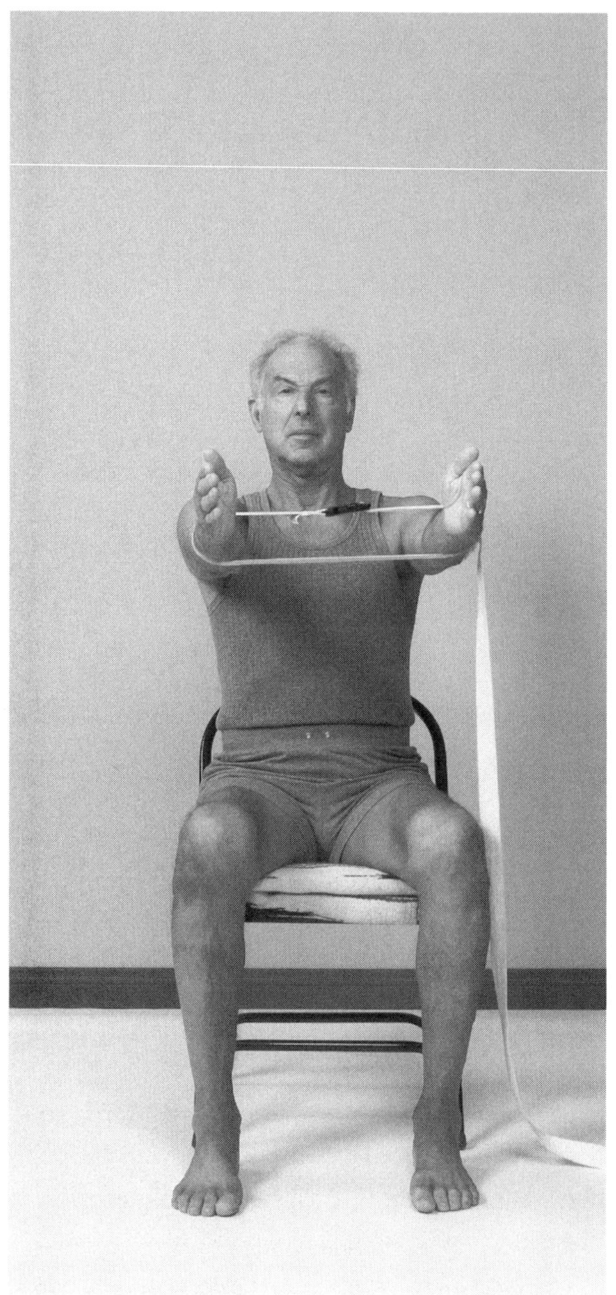

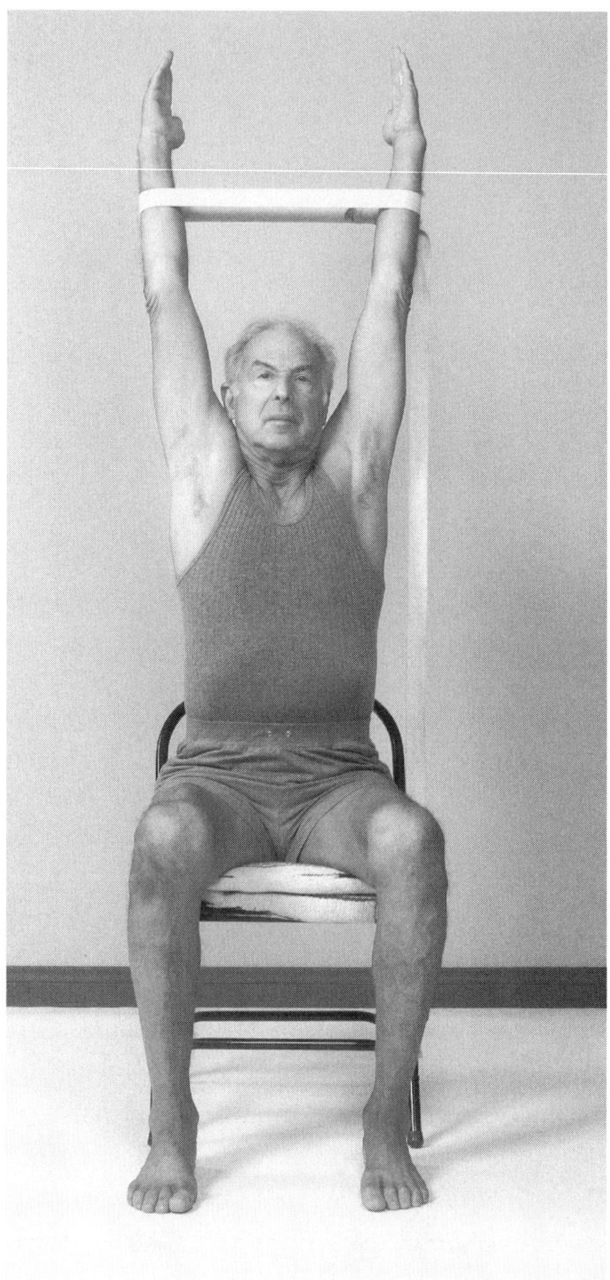

3. Stretch the arms forward with an inhalation; raise the arms in line with the center of the ears.

The chest and throat and essential parts of the breathing apparatus are already open considerably. By keeping the thumbs gently on the top of shoulder line, the instructor allows and helps the neck and cervical spine to rise with inhalation.

4. The student brings the arms out, so that the center of the biceps comes to the center of the ears.

5. Take in a breath in this position.

If this is not attainable, then any position, for example with the arms spread farther apart, or not quite totally overhead, is perfectly all right, as long as the arms are above the heart. This will still achieve part of the same purpose.

6. Bring the arms forward and down as you exhale. Rest the hands on top of the thighs.

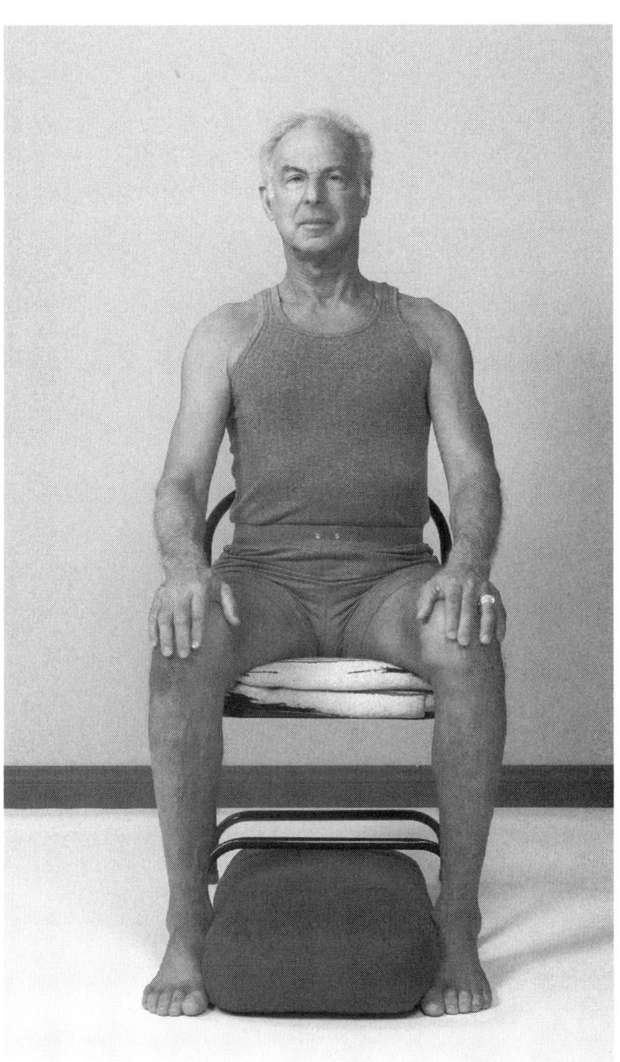

BENEFITS

This pose improves posture and maximizes the capacity of the lungs while extending the shoulders' range of motion.

Chair Uttanasana

Forward Bend Pose

It is important that in this energizing pose, a variation of Uttanasana, or extreme forward bending pose, that you adjust yourself to the chair. Each of us has a different body style. Some people need to place a folded blanket under their feet. If you are tall, then a folded blanket can be placed under the buttocks on the seat of the chair.

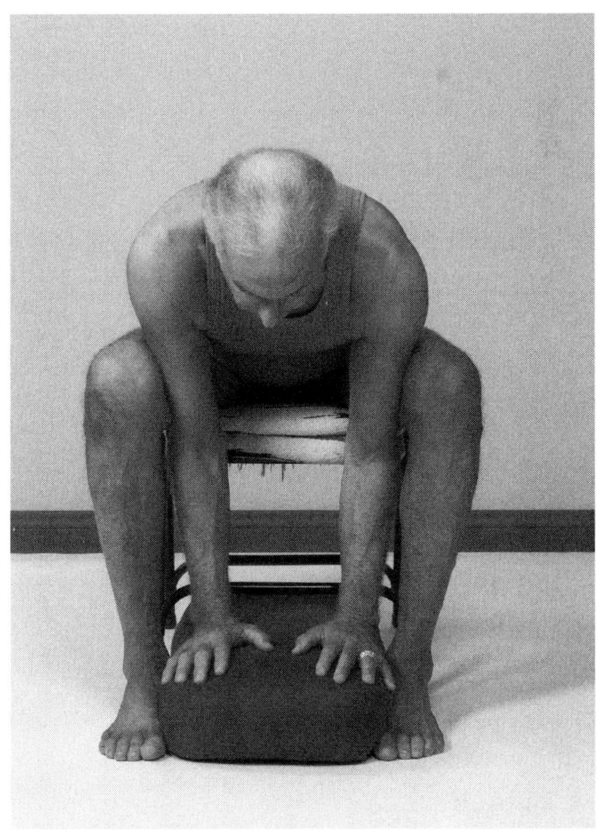

It is important that the knees are as close to parallel and in line with the hip joints as possible. Any position that you find yourself taking is perfectly all right, as long as it is close to the one pictured. It will begin to achieve the same purpose.

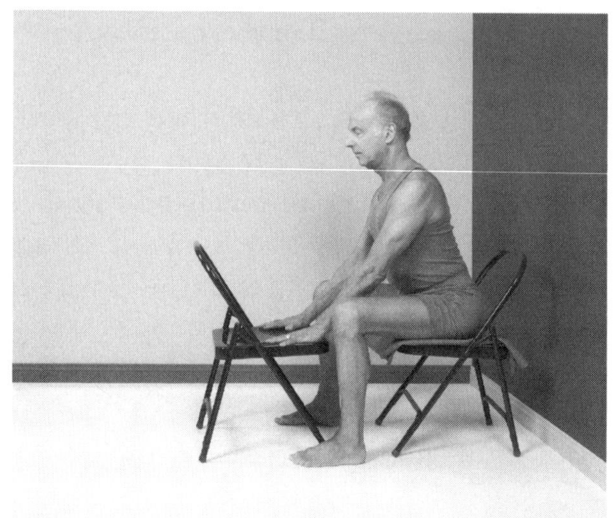

1. Sitting upright in the chair, place your hands over the knees to allow the spine and the central nervous system to be calm and relaxed.

2. Remove the hands from the knees, and with an exhalation, press the thumbs firmly into the hips joint. With an inhalation, stretch and extend the spine away from the hips.

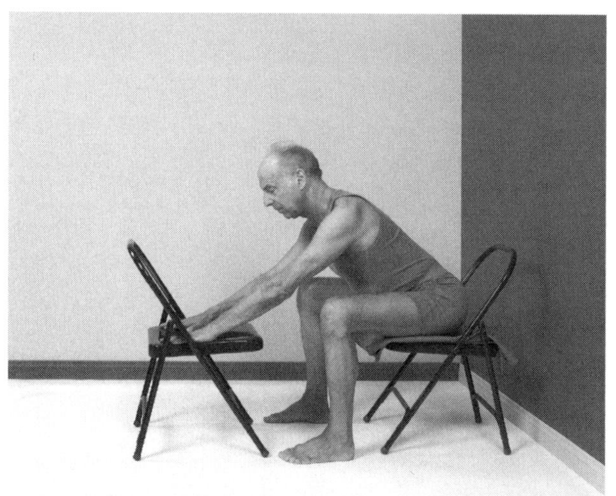

3. On an exhalation, place the hands either on the floor or on a bolster with the hands inside the legs.

4. Remain in this position for several breaths, attempting to initiate the breath from the lower back, moving it around the ribs to the chest.

5. To return to a sitting position, place your hands on the tops of your knees, press down, and with an inhalation press the torso up to an upright position. Sit quietly, and then move to the next asana.

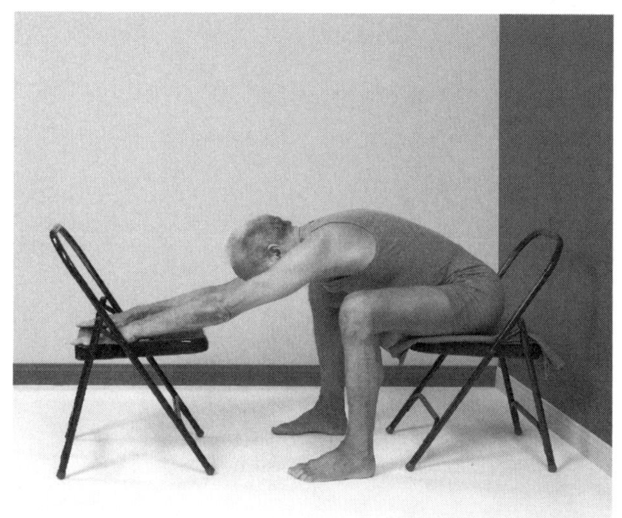

BENEFITS

This pose flushes and irrigates the kidneys, liver, and spleen and reduces stomach discomfort. The heartbeat slows, and the spinal nerves are rejuvenated. The pose often reduces depression, and students that are easily excited frequently become calm and cool, with a sense of well-being. Visual acuity often improves.

Chair Adho Mukha Svanasana

Downward-Facing Dog Pose

1. Place a chair securely against a wall. Be sure that it is in alignment.
2. Secure your safety belt, if you need one.
3. Put your feet directly under the knees, as you place your hands onto the seat of the second chair.
4. On the inhalation, raise the top of the head, keeping the chin parallel to the floor.
5. Release the shoulders away from the ears, and exhaling, push the chair forward and press the hips back.
6. On the next exhalation, push the chair farther forward, to bring the arms in line with the ears.
7. Continue to press the hips back, press the heels down, lift the inner elbows, and press the palms and fingers firmly into the chair seat.
8. Try to move the breath from the low back around the ribs, into the front of the sternum, allowing the abdomen to remain soft and free of pressure.
9. Upon taking 5 inhalations and exhalations, return to an upright position, place the hands on the top of the legs, and breathe evenly and slowly.

BENEFITS

This pose aids digestion, reduces gas, tones the lower back muscles, relieves discomfort from long periods of sitting, realigns the thoracic spine, and reduces tension in the shoulders and neck. It can be used to reduce stress and anxiety by calming the frontal brain

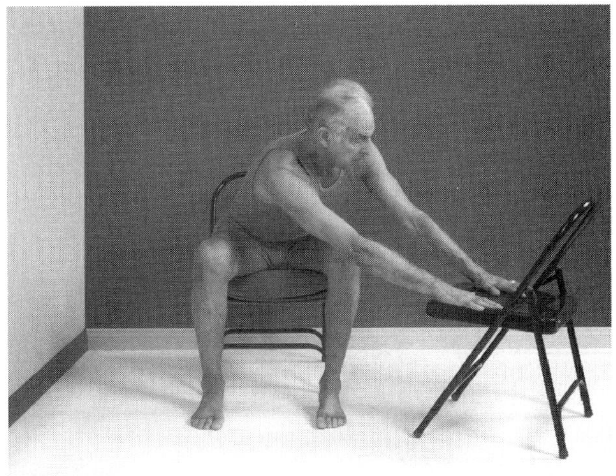

Chair Parsva Adho Virasana

Downward-Angled Hero Pose

1. Place a chair against a wall to insure that it is in alignment. Be sure the safety belt is in place if needed.
2. Move a folding chair to the left, to the side of the knee.
3. Place your hands on the seat of the chair, keep the knees in alignment with the hips, stretch the right arm slightly more than the left, and retain the right hip pressure into the chair seat.
4. On an exhalation, push the chair diagonally to the left. Hold the position and breathe smoothly and evenly for 5 breaths.
5. Return to the sitting position as you inhale.
6. Lift the crown of the head, sit quietly, and then repeat to the other side.

BENEFITS

This pose aids digestion, tones lower back muscles, and realigns the thoracic spine, neck, and shoulders. It also boosts circulation for the liver, kidneys, spleen, pancreas, intestines, heart, and lungs, allowing more oxygen to flow toward the brain. It stimulates the bowel to empty.

Chair Adho Mukha Svanasana at Wall

Downward-Facing Dog Pose

1. Place the chair facing the wall, so that the knees are near to it, with the feet directly under the knees.

2. Raise the arms either from directly in front of you or, if shoulder joint stiffness requires, bring the arms out to the side.

3. Turn the palms up and raise the arms vertically, in line to the ears, or as close to vertical as possible.

4. Place the hands up on the wall as high as possible, keeping the arms in line with the ear canals.

5. Open the outer edges of the armpits.

6. Rest the forehead on the wall, allowing the eyes to drop into the cheekbones.

7. Press the hips back into the chair seat, and lift the bottom edge of the sternum away from the pubis, to permit the diaphragm to drape softly out to the sides of the rib cage.

8. Extend the fingers away from the palm of the hand, breathing normally for 5 breaths.

9. Lift the head, move the arms out to the side of the torso, and turn the palms up to rotate the shoulder blades inward, supporting the back and ribs.

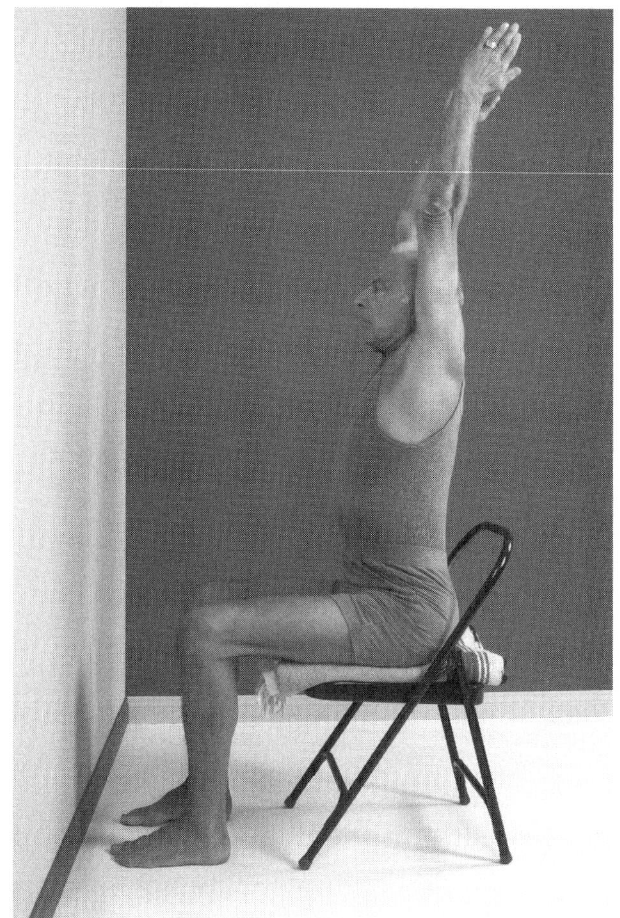

10. Rest the palms on the thighs and breathe evenly.

BENEFITS

This pose releases tension in the low back. It opens the chest and lungs so they take in more oxygen; tones the upper back, shoulders, and neck; relieves tightness in the muscles of the scalp; and continues to aid the digestive process. It increases flexibility in the hip joints, helps elimination of the bowels, and relieves pressure on the prostate gland. The pose also relieves pressure around and in the female reproductive organs. This is one of the essential asanas for those using a wheelchair or walker.

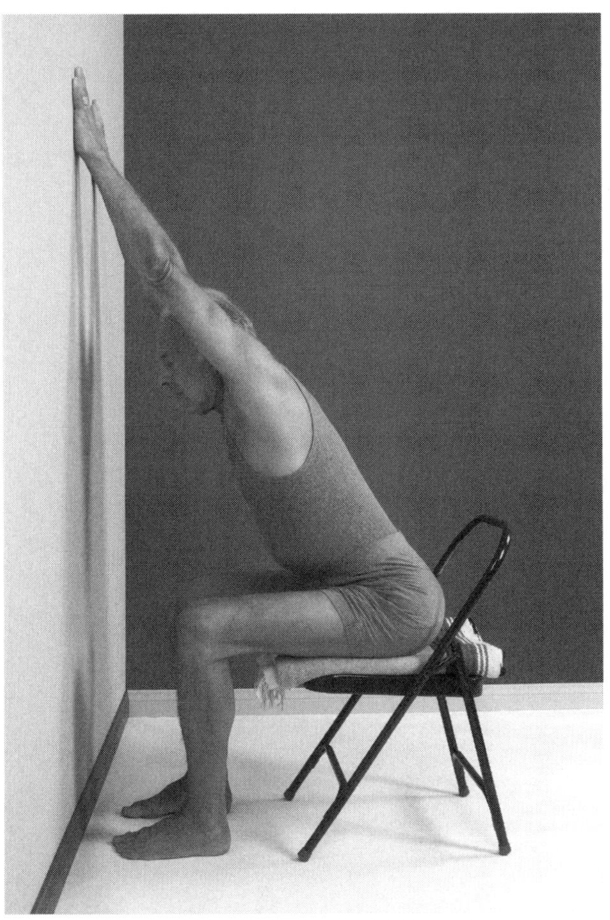

CHAIR SURYA NAMASKAR

Sun Salutation

This is an adaptation of the classic Sun Salutation, which effectively reaches into most areas of the physical body, providing an opportunity to develop coordination of the breath with a measured movement of the limbs and torso. This series of asanas is usually used as a warmup to a practice session.

Caution: Resist the temptation to press the tongue against either the roof of the mouth or the lower palate. Keep the breath even and without effort. Try to move smoothly from one position to the next without hesitation. Remember, practice is the key to success.

1. Begin by bringing your hands up to rest in front of the heart, with the upper arms lifted parallel to the floor. Press your fingers together firmly, pointing slightly away from the chest.
2. Bring your feet to rest under the knees. Distribute the weight from the balls of the big toes, across the sole of the foot, with the outer edge of the foot drawing back to the middle of the heel.
3. Keep the knees in line with the hip joints.
4. Extend the arms forward at the width of the shoulders, the palms facing each other. If there is a shoulder joint problem, extend the arms out to the side, with the palms facing up.
5. On the inhalation, bring the arms even with the center of the ears.
6. With the next inhalation, place the hands on the wall, stretch the arms up, retain your hips back, keeping the head parallel to the biceps.
7. Hold for 3 even breaths.
8. With an inhalation, slip the hands down to shoulder height, draw the wrists up and the shoulders down.
9. At the same time, move the right leg back outside the legs of the chair, and drop the right knee toward the floor. If the knee does not reach the floor use a folded blanket or bolster. If possible, pull the knee back into line with the hip joint.
10. As you advance the left leg forward, grip both hands under the knee, and with

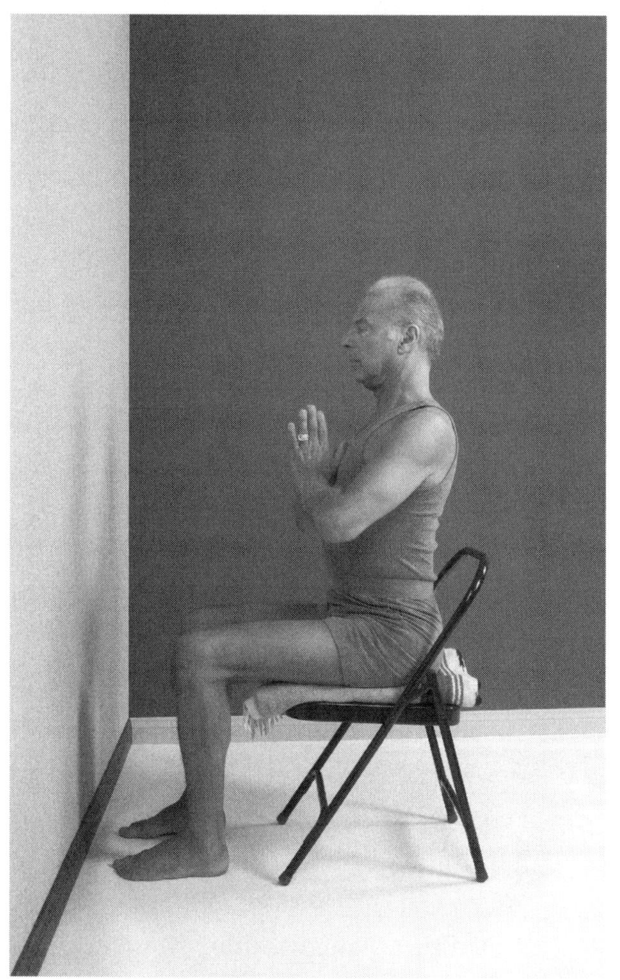

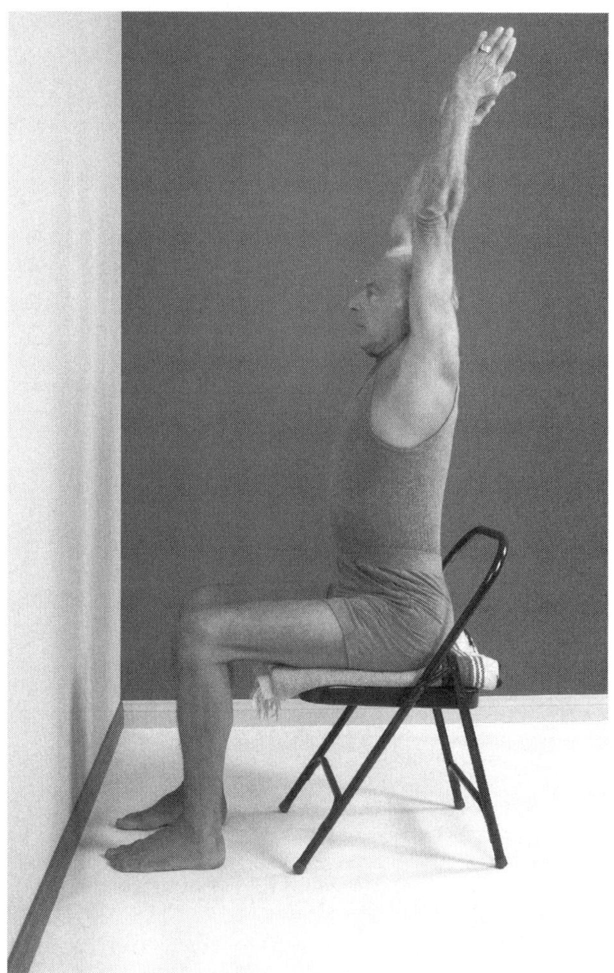

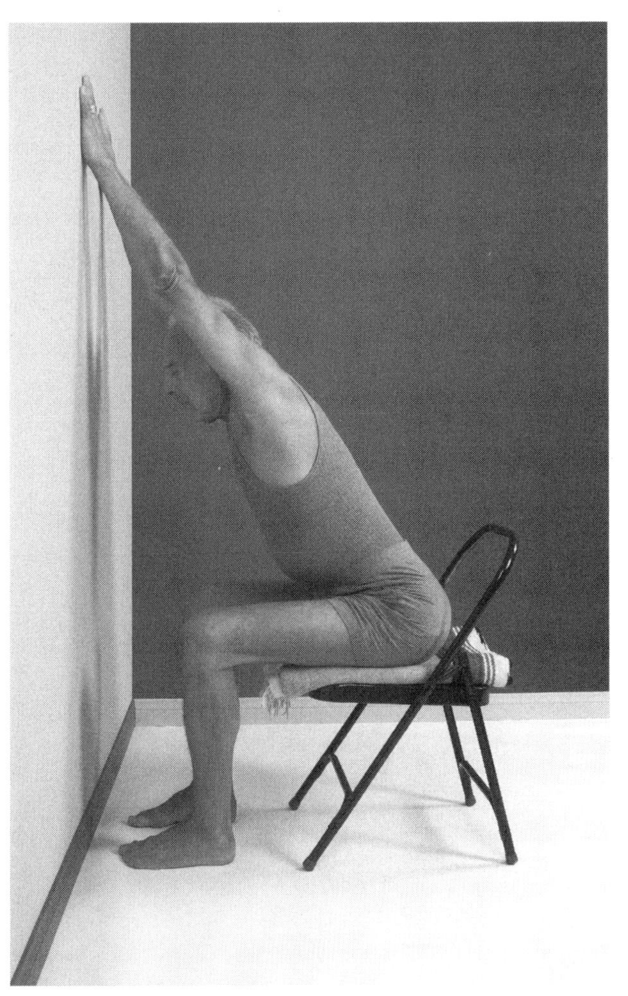

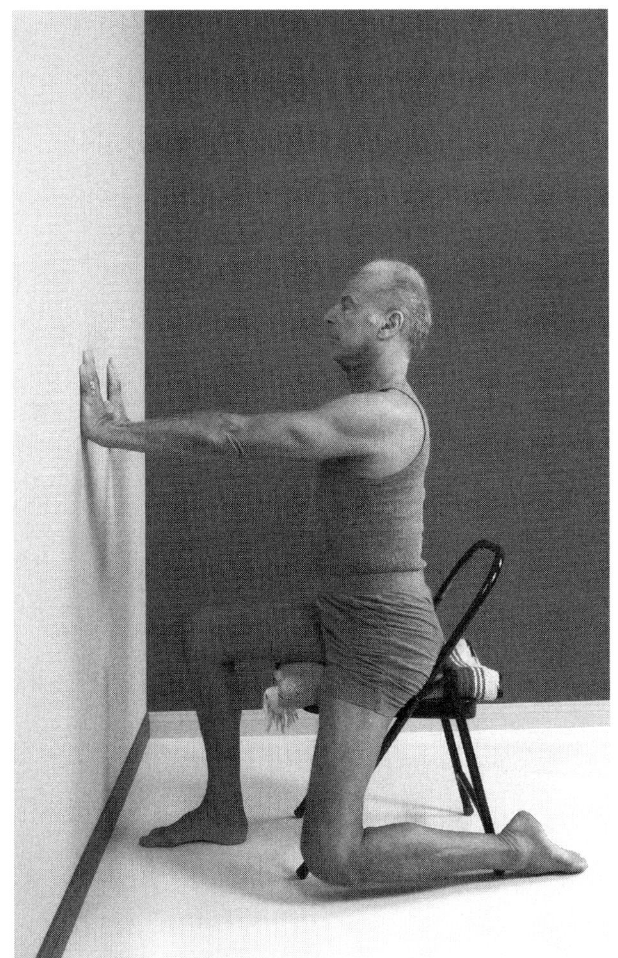

an exhalation pull the leg up sharply toward your chest.

11. With an inhalation, place the leg on the floor beside the other leg.

12. Lift the back waist, and try to bring the inhalation into the side chest.

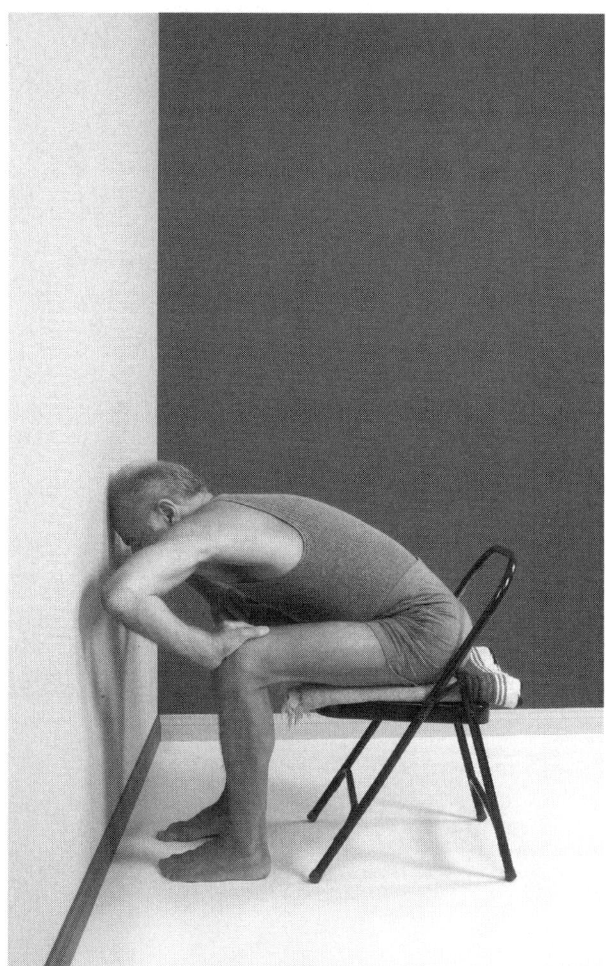

13. On the exhalation, place your hands on top of the knees and press the elbows forward, as you rest your forehead against the wall.

14. On the exhalation, drop the arms outside the legs, letting the entire area of the shoulder girdle drape downward.

15. Hold for 3 breaths.

16. With an inhalation, bring your arms up and press your hands on top of the knees. Press down to bring the torso and then the head to a vertical position.

17. Grip the sides of the seat of the chair and thrust the buttocks back. Push

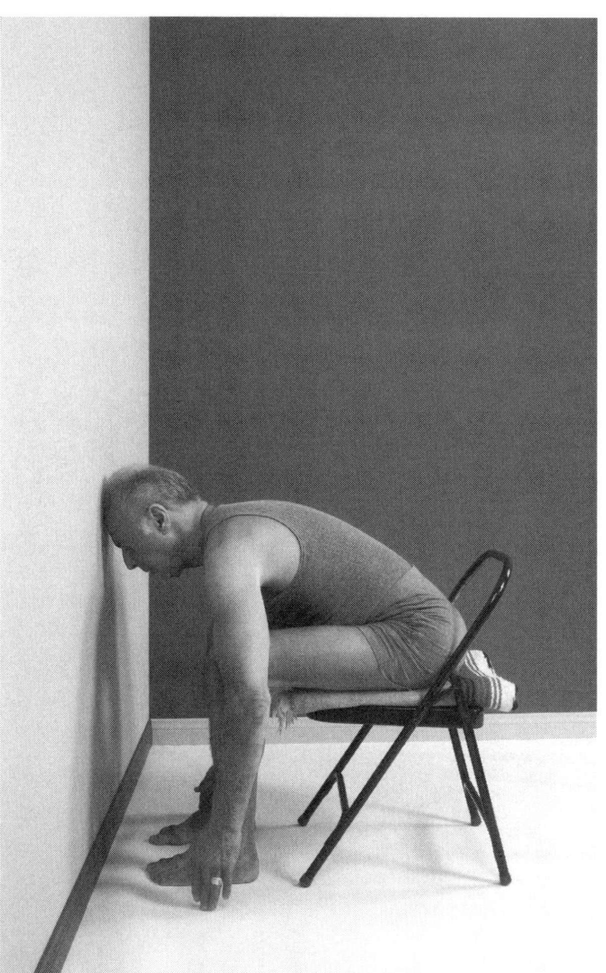

down firmly on your hands to lift the buttocks at least 3 inches from the seat of the chair.

18. Hold for 3 breaths. Then on an exhalation, sit down, swing the arms forward, and place the hands firmly against the wall at shoulder level again.

19. Set the right leg back, and drop the knee to the floor in line with the hip joint. If a prop is being used, continue to use it as before.

20. Draw the leg forward with both hands under the knee, pulling the knee sharply toward the chest with an exhalation. Then as you inhale, place the leg together with the other leg.

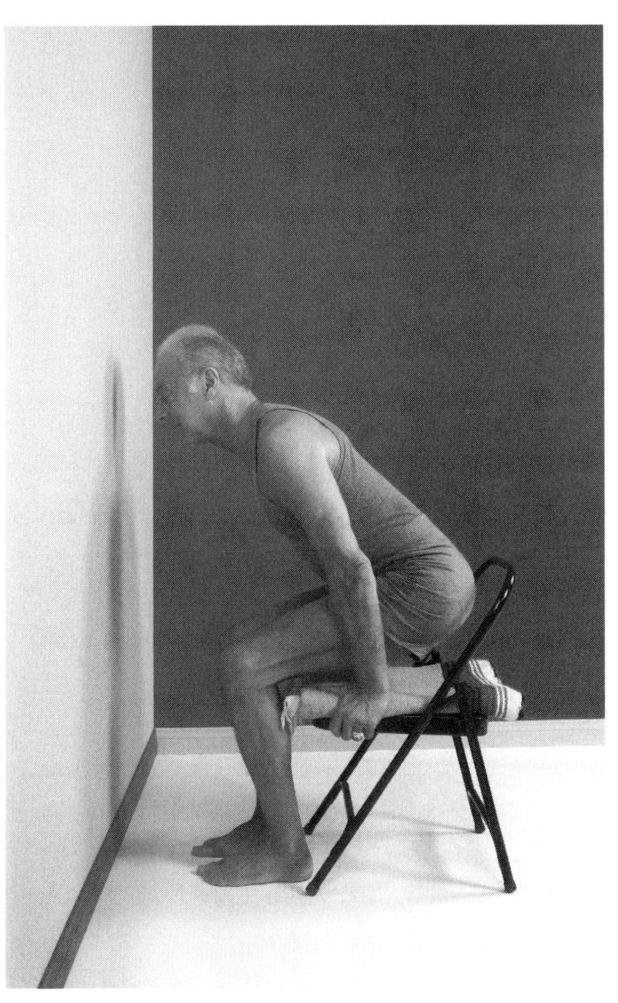

21. Raise the arms up again toward the ceiling, parallel to the ears.

22. Bring your arms down, and as your hands become even with the forehead, bring the palms together into Namaste at the heart.

23. Sit quietly. Breathe smoothly and evenly for at least 30 seconds. Observe your breath and the balance of the body. Observe any changes in the spinal column, chest position, and softness of the shoulder girdle, and allow the eyes to gaze forward. Release any tension in the forehead or temples. This series can be repeated several times, alternating from right to left.

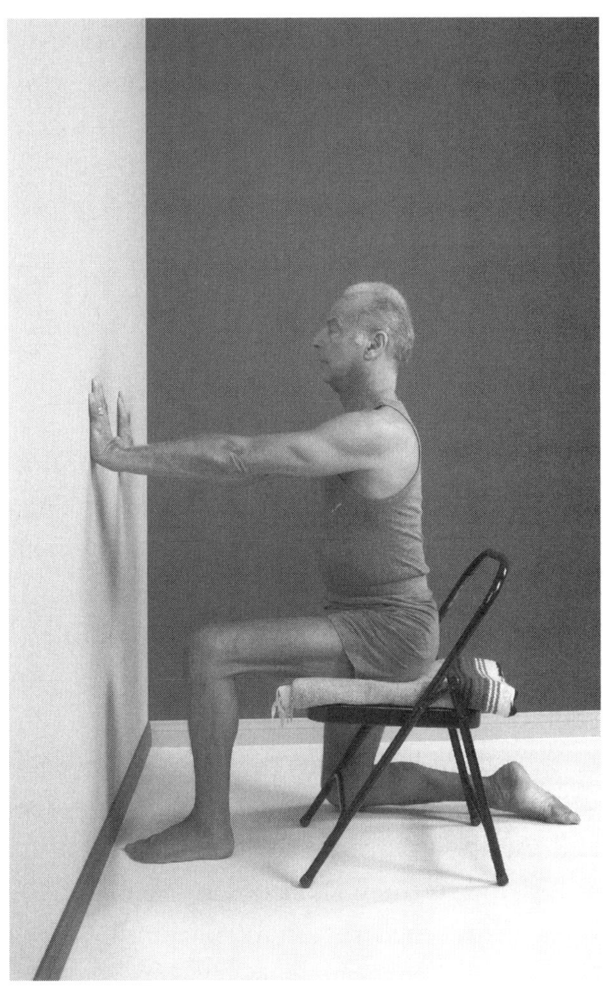

BENEFITS

This series can be used to energize and also to calm the nervous system, depending on the intent of the practice. It increases flexibility, range of motion, and circulation in the limbs, particularly the legs. When you sit for long periods of time with little or no movement, blood tends to pool in the lower limbs, causing edema and other conditions. This pose helps to reduce the swelling. Digestion improves, elimination can become regular, and breath improves in volume, timing, and placement. It contributes to a general feeling of contentment and accomplishment, all of which are positive feedback.

VIRABHADRASANA II

Warrior Pose II

1. Sit in the chair.
2. Move the hips to the left so the left buttock is slightly off the left of the chair. Then move the right leg as far as possible to the right, with knee bent at a right angle, as pictured.
3. Extend the left leg as far as possible.
4. Stretch the arms out to the sides, parallel to the floor.
5. Take a breath and stretch out to each side, until the pull connects the shoulders and the shoulder blades to the elbows to the wrists and to the insides of the fingers.
6. Proceed with the inhalation, bringing the belly closer to the spine and opening into the sternum.
7. Press firmly down into the seat of the chair and down in the heels with both feet.
8. Breathe into the chest, and if possible move the navel to the left.
9. Use more strength in the left arm and the left leg. Press the outer left foot to the floor, including the inner skin of the big toe.
10. Hold for 3 to 5 breaths, charging the chest with the inhalation and exhaling into the legs.
11. Bring the legs together.
12. Bring the arms down toward the hips and rest them, palms down, on top of the thighs. Sit erect and quietly for 3 breaths.
13. Now repeat the movement to the other side.

BENEFITS

This pose strengthens the leg muscles, relieves cramping in the calves and thighs, brings flexibility to leg and back muscles, and revitalizes the abdominal organs.

CHAIR VIRABHADRASANA I

Warrior Pose I

1. Sit upright in the hindmost of 2 chairs, with the back of the torso away from the support of the chair. Place both feet directly under the knees, feet facing straight ahead.
2. Place a blanket under your hips if you are tall and under your feet if you are short.
3. Draw the left leg back to bring it into alignment with the left hip. If the knee does not touch the floor, place a folded blanket under the knee to stabilize the posture.
4. Rest the outer edge of the right palm on the back of the forward folding chair, and lift the back waist, together with the sternum, on an inhalation.
5. Raise the left arm up, until it is even with the ear and in line with the bent knee, or whatever is possible. If there is a balance

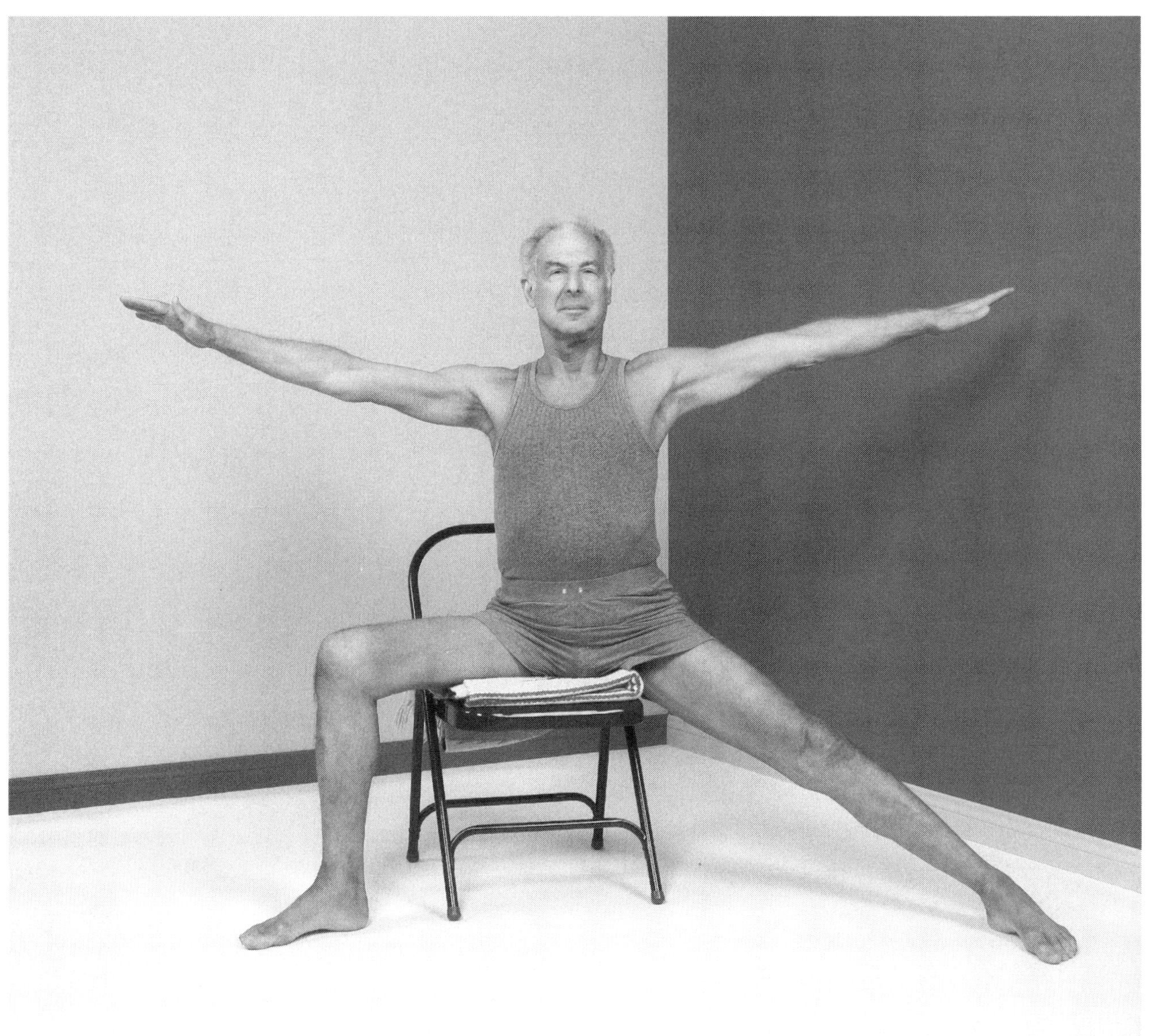

problem, keep one hand on top of chair, and when doing the pose on the other side, raise the same arm as the leg that is bent to the floor. If there is no balance problem, both arms can be raised on the inhalation.

6. Press the buttocks down into the chair seat. This tones the mid back muscles to counteract the effects of sitting for long periods of time in a soft, rounded back support.

The flexion of the bent leg on the folded blanket encourages additional blood flow into the pelvic cavity.

7. Return to the original sitting position with an exhalation, sit quietly for a few moments, and then repeat to the other side.

After completing both sides of the asana, remain sitting as much as possible away from the back of the chair.

BENEFITS

This pose helps to develop deeper breathing by expanding the chest. It relieves stiffness in shoulders, neck, and back and strengthens the ankles and knees. In most instances there is an improvement in the sense of balance and more stamina in the legs and arms.

Chair Utthita Trikonasana

Extended Triangle Pose

1. Sit upright in the chair, with a safety belt around the waist if necessary.

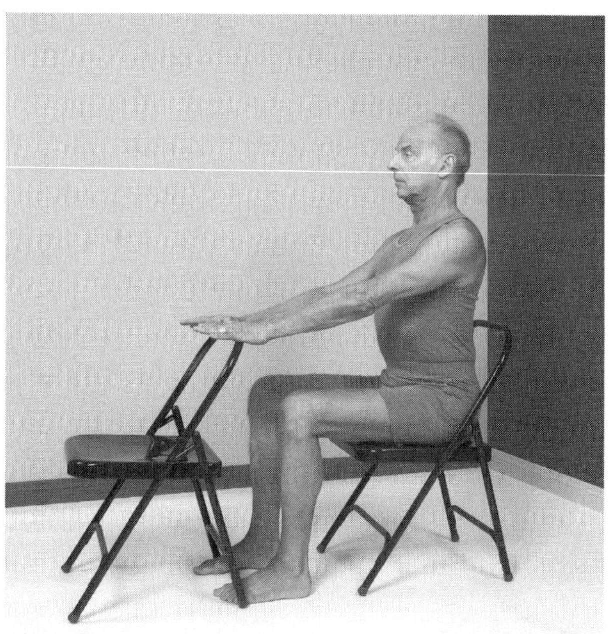

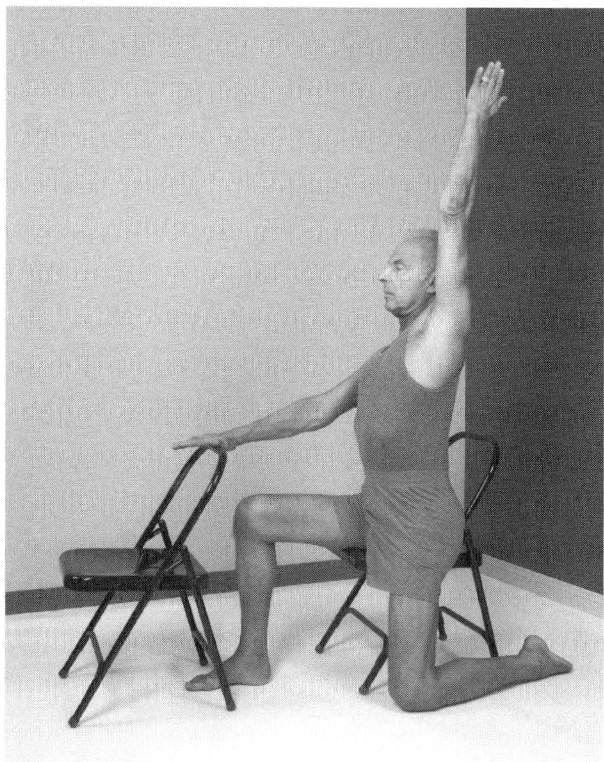

2. Bring a second folding chair to your right side.

3. Place a folded sticky mat with the folded edge even to the edge of the chair seat on the right.

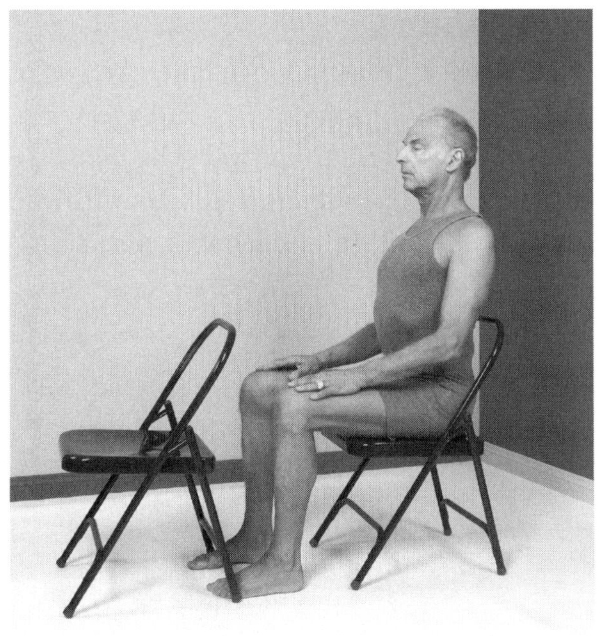

4. Bring your right leg to the right side of the chair as best you can, while keeping the foot flat to the floor.

5. Move your left leg to the left as much as the chair permits.

6. Move your hips to the left as much as possible, and lean over to place the right elbow on the sticky mat on the chair seat.

7. Take a few breaths, and then place your left hand on your left hip, dropping the elbow backward. This will enable you to open the chest and stimulate the abdominal organs.

8. Lean back against the chairs. They will support your shoulders, chest, and hips.

9. With an inhalation, stretch the left arm into the air in line with the right shoulder.

10. Take a few breaths. Then maximize the weight on the right hand and forearm, press down on the right elbow, and return to an upright sitting position. Breathe quietly.

After the pose to this point has become comfortable and can be done securely, then add a new level of challenge.

1. Using the same procedure as before, when you exhale and lean to the right, instead of resting the elbow on the chair seat, clasp the horizontal bar that supports the front of the chair.

2. Clasping the bar with the right hand, place your left hand on the hip and drop the elbow backward to open the chest cavity. Breathe into the upper ribs and chest area.

3. Do not distort the ribs in order to place the right hand on the bar. Instead, place the hand parallel to the seat of the chair in order to maintain the alignment of the spine and rib cage.

4. With an inhalation, raise the left arm in line with the right shoulder and the right arm.

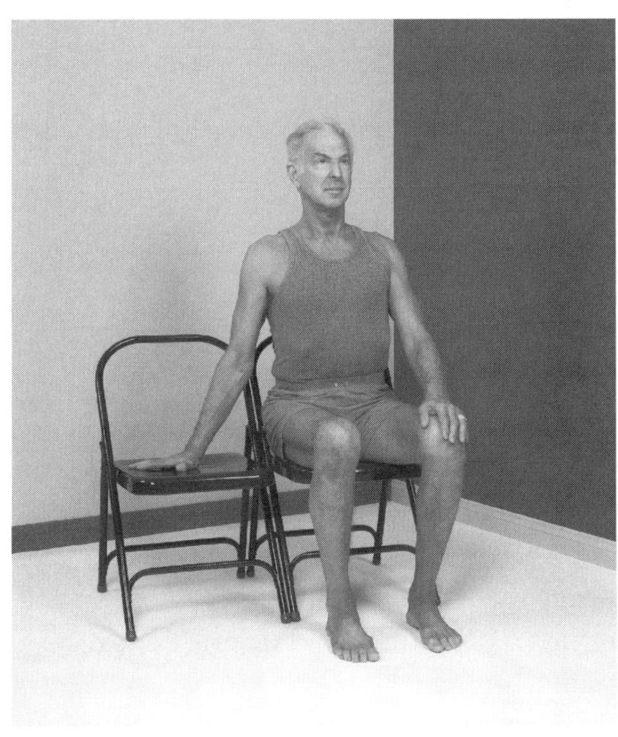

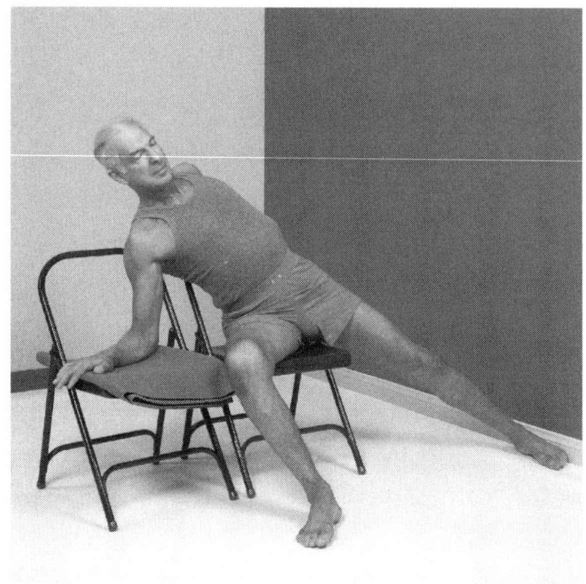

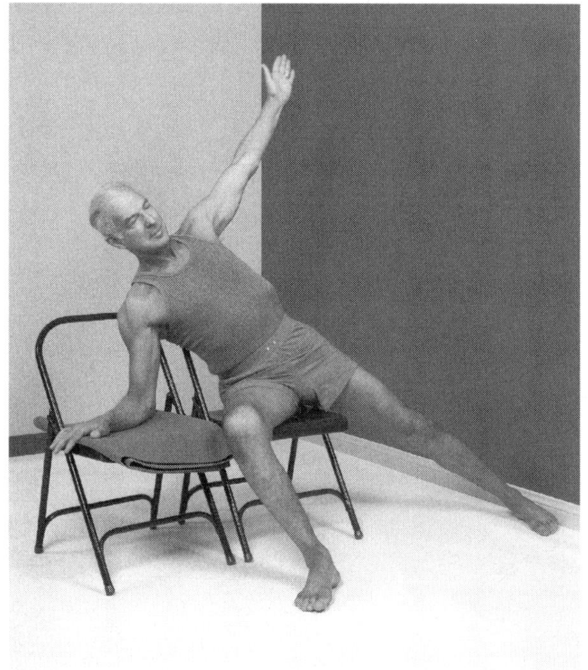

5. Hold the position for 3 to 5 breaths, and then reach out the left hand and arm firmly to the left, and press up into a sitting position. Remain seated quietly before continuing to the left.

BENEFITS

This pose creates a dynamic change in circulation in both the pelvis and the torso. Kidney function is stimulated. The digestive system is also stimulated, together with the elimination process. Tension in the spinal

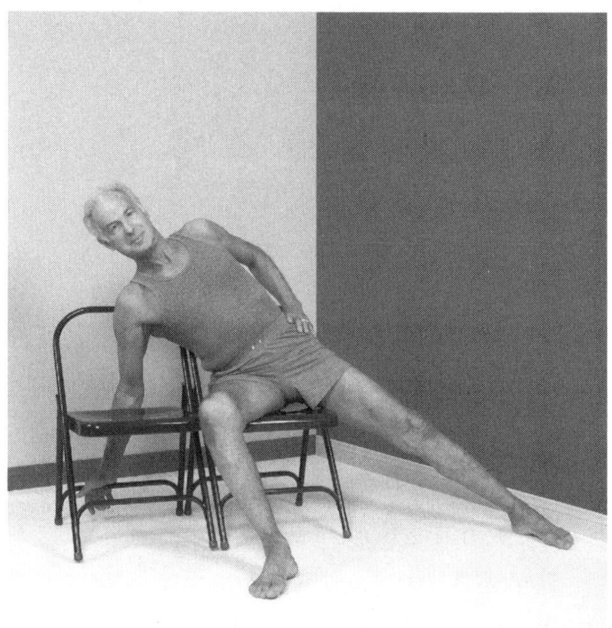

column and surrounding muscles is lessened. The lower back and pelvis are realigned, thereby counteracting the effects of long periods of sitting. The legs are toned, and the ligaments and tendons are revitalized.

VIPARITA DANDASANA

Chair Backbend

Pose I

1. To start, roll a sticky mat into a tight roll. This can be achieved by opening the

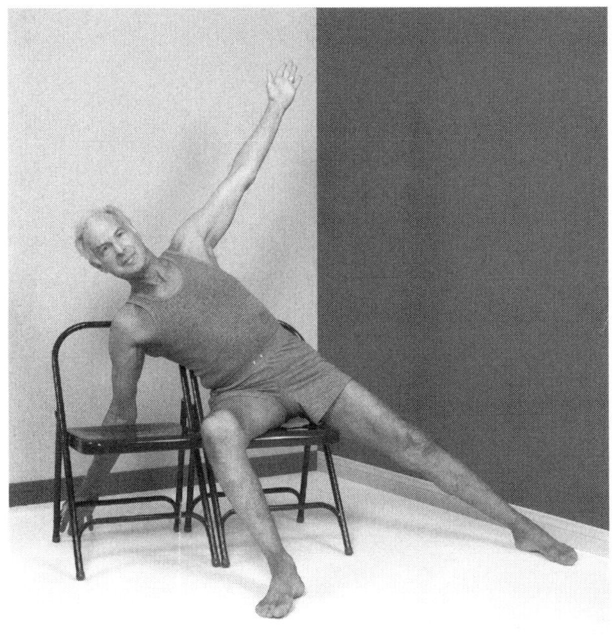

sticky mat and folding over one end about a foot.

2. Sit up as much as possible away from the back of the chair. The buttocks should be in the middle of the seat.

3. Lean back to make sure that the bottom edges of the shoulder blades are supported against the back of the chair.

4. Sit up and insert the rolled sticky mat behind you parallel to the spine and supporting the neck and the back of the head.

5. Press the feet into the wall, with heels 3 inches away from the wall and toes up on the wall, with knees slightly bent.

6. Firmly interlock your fingers in front of you. Then if possible place your hands behind your neck, with the little fingers on the occipital bone and the thumbs coming around to the side of the throat and resting on the collarbone.

7. Bring the elbows close to the ears and point them up to the ceiling.

8. Allow the head to rest in the palms, as you press your feet into the wall.

9. Gently release your head into your hands, with the sticky mat supporting the neck and back of the skull.

10. Gently rest your eyes into your cheekbones; do not press your tongue into the upper palate or the lower jaw.

11. Breathe gently, allowing the breath to move up into chest cavity. After 3 to 5 breaths, bring the head up first on inhalation, then stretch the arms up and forward.

13. Sit quietly, and allow the breath to rise into the chest again.

Notice that the assistant has braced one leg at the back edge of the seat of the chair,

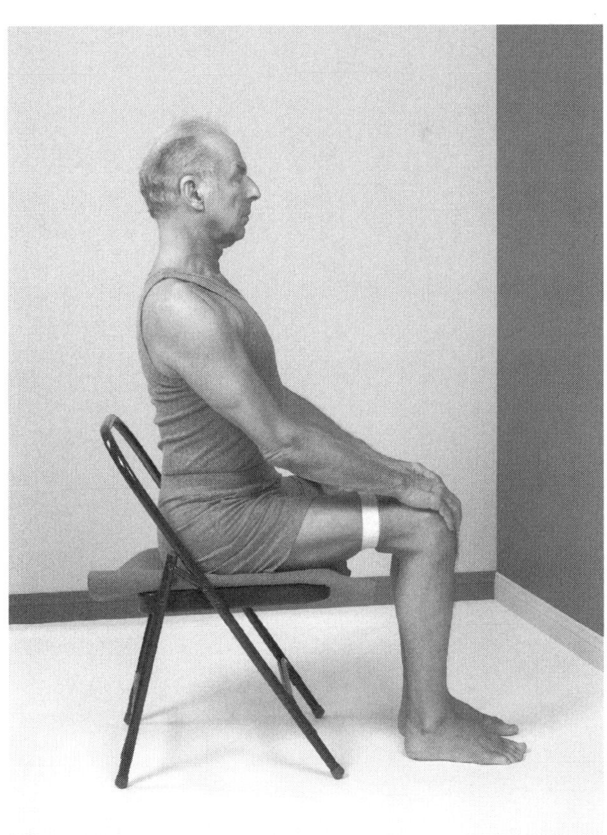

pressing the knee gently into the mid back. Hands are on the elbows, with the thumbs rotating the bicep outward and lightly lifting the arms up parallel to the ears. Caution: There should be no gripping or tightening of the throat.

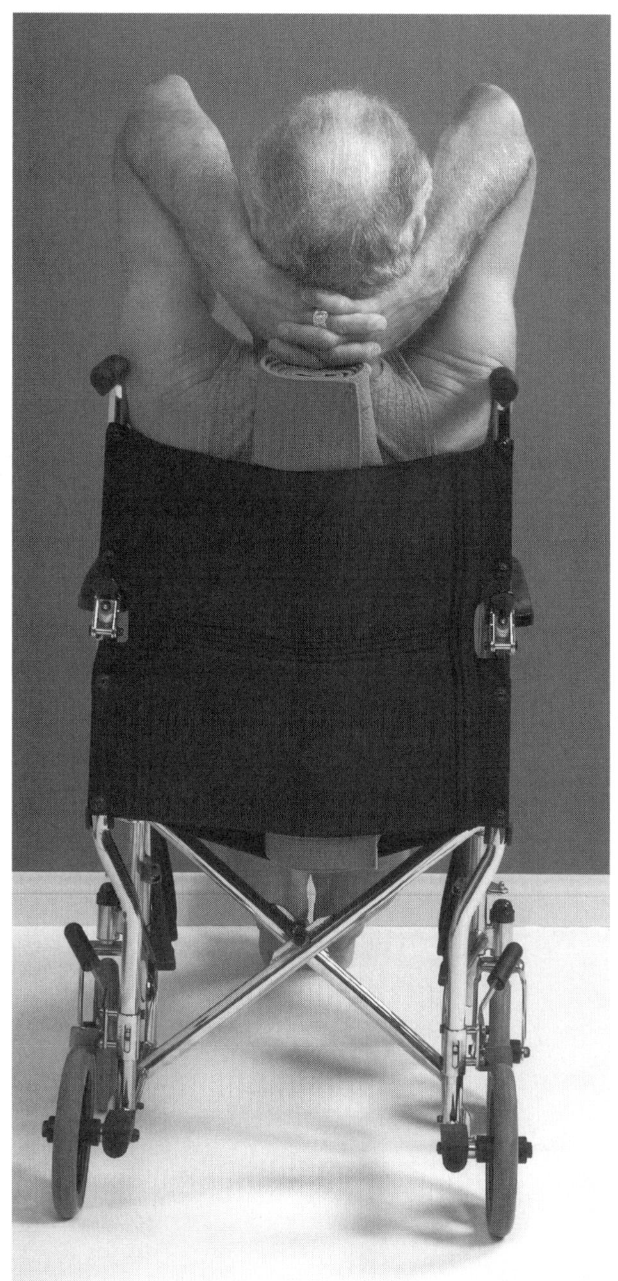

Pose shown in wheelchair

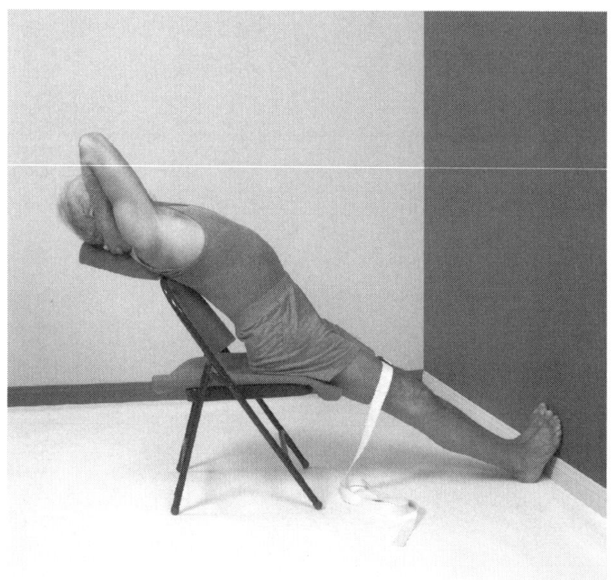

BENEFITS

This pose greatly relieves lower back issues. The diaphragm is released from the constant pressure of resting against the abdominal organs. Digestion is improved by realigning and stretching the intestinal tract. And as digestion improves, so does elimination. The chest area is enhanced by correcting the forward slump of the shoulders. Neck and shoulder discomfort is reduced.

Seated Urdhva Dhanurasana

Pose II

1. Sit in the first chair, your legs extended through the second chair toward a wall.
2. Slide forward but continue holding the first chair seat. Retract the elbows back away from the rib cage.
3. Place your sacrum at the edge of the second chair closest to the wall.
4. Put the heels close to the wall; rest your toes on the wall. Lie back with your

elbows on the seat of the first chair. Grip the sides of the seat of the chair and lower your torso.

5. Keep your head forward, until you are lying on both chair seats.

6. Adjust the first chair to fully support the head and the neck. If possible, bring your arms through the supports of the first chair back.

7. Keep the hands and arms parallel to the ears.

8. Press the top of your thighs firmly toward the floor, and stretch your arms and legs any amount. If the shoulders are too wide,

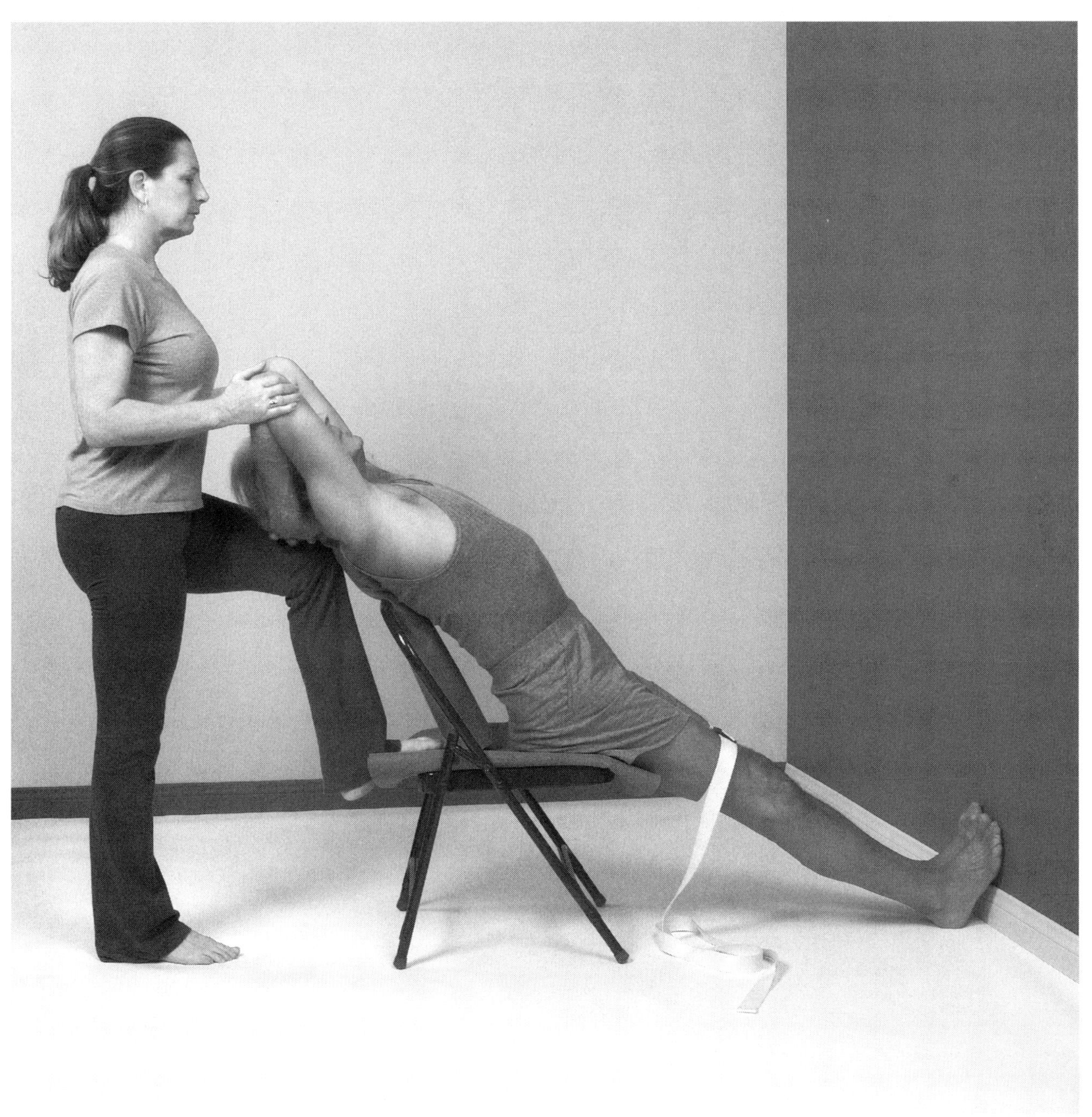

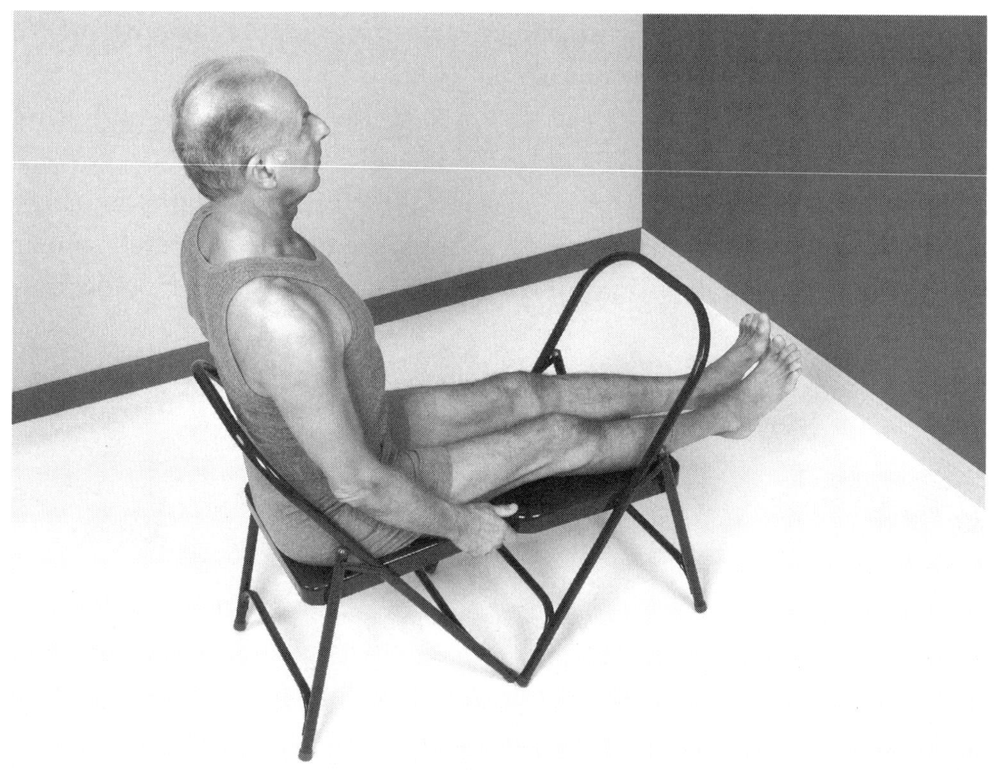

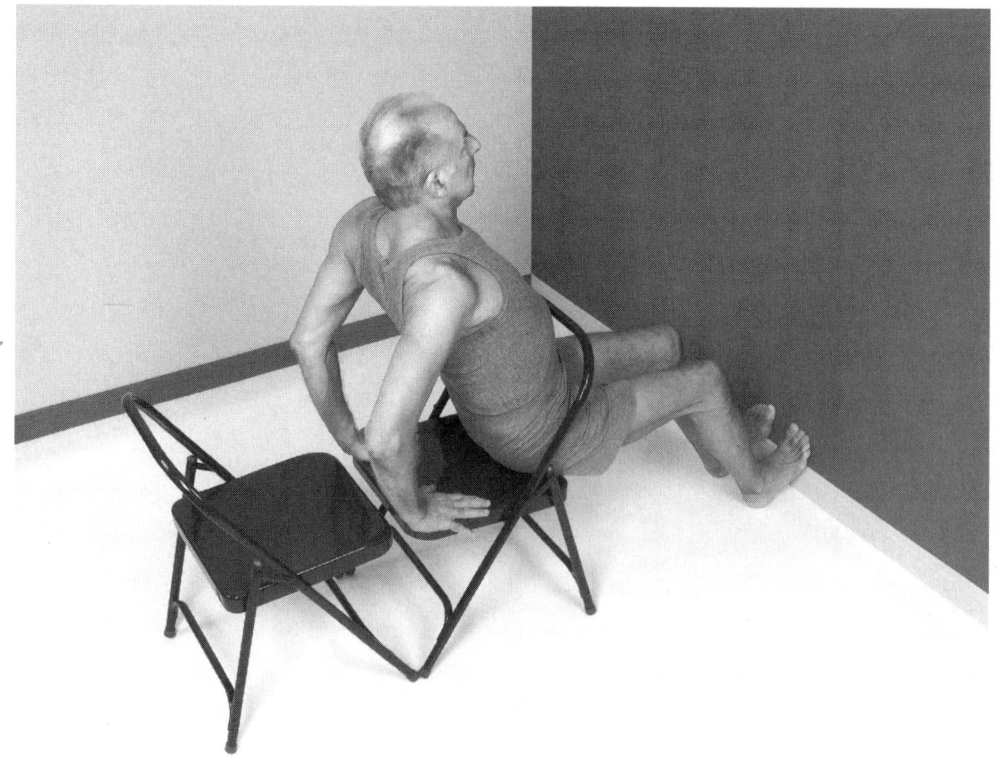

the arms can be extended outside the chair back supports.

9. Keep the weight of the eyes resting lightly under closed lids in the cheekbones.

10. Hold for 5 to 10 breaths. Bend the knees. Withdraw the buttocks to the middle of the second chair.

11. Move the first chair away from the hips. Lower your hands as close as possible to the buttocks.

12. Press down firmly and sit up reasonably quickly.

13. Cross your arms on the top of the second chair.

14. Sit up straight and breathe evenly and quietly. It is recommended that seated twists follow the backbends.

BENEFITS

This pose releases any tension in the spine, completely revitalizes the muscles of the upper torso, stimulates additional circulation to many organs, tones and strengthens the arms and legs, and creates additional flexibility in the shoulder and pelvic girdles. It brings joy and lightness to the body and spirit and is stunningly effective in lifting the weight of depression and anger.

SEATED JATHARA PARIVARTANASANA

Chair Lateral Twist

1. For a variation on this pose, take the strap and again make a small loop and lace it into the right thumb, with the instructor stabilizing the arms by supporting the wrist bones.

2. The practitioner turns the abdomen first then the sternum and then the shoulders.

3. Keep your nose in line with the sternum, so there is no tightening of the clavicle, shoulder blade, ears, face, or eyes.

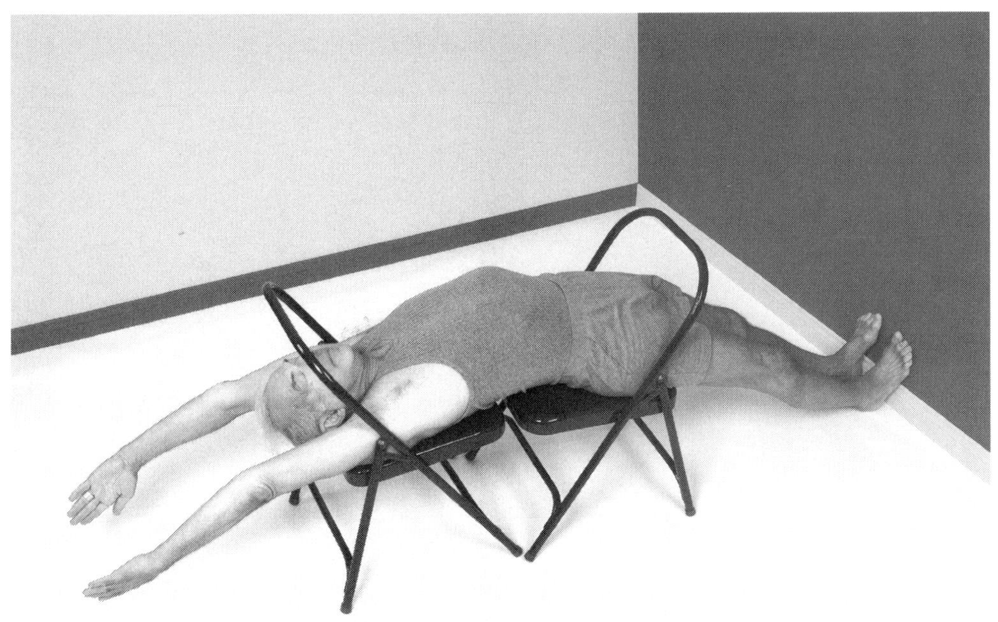

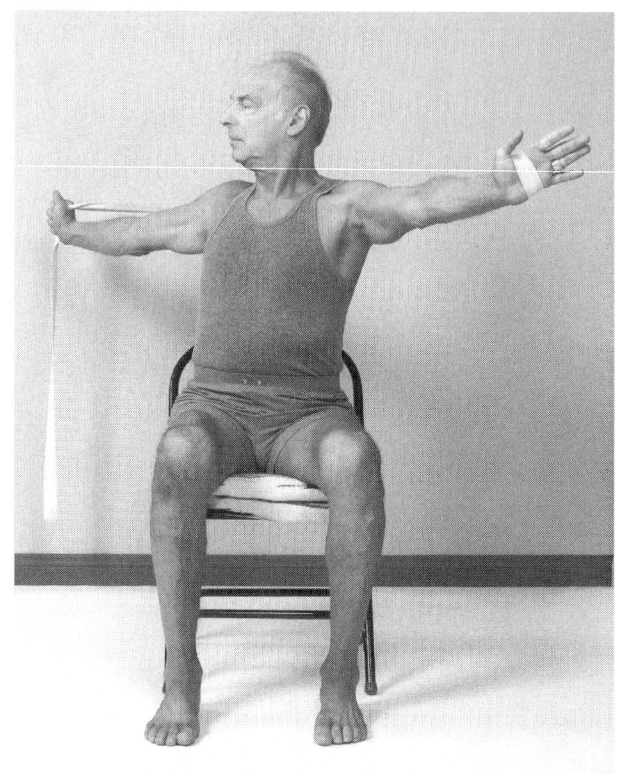

4. The inhalation comes as you untwist back to the center and then turn again to the other side, starting at the navel or the center of the abdomen.

5. Keep the legs firm, turn the chest with the shoulders, hold the arms horizontally, and breathe comfortably. Again the breath comes in from the base of the nostrils and out of the tip of the nose, reaching into your center with the force of each breath.

BENEFITS

Upper extremity strength and thoraco-lumbar muscular and joint mobility are improved with this posture. It simultaneously calms and ivigorates.

Seated Poses

These poses stimulate digestion and elimination; improve flexibility in the shoulders, spine, hips and legs; and encourage deeper and smoother breathing.

Marichyasana III Variation

Twisting Seated Pose

1. Put three chairs side-by-side, turn the end chair to face the other two, and sit on it so the back is supported. Lift the chest and press the sit bones onto the seat of the chair.

2. Take your legs one at a time up onto the other chairs by lifting them with your hands behind each knee. This allows the groin to stay loose and soft.

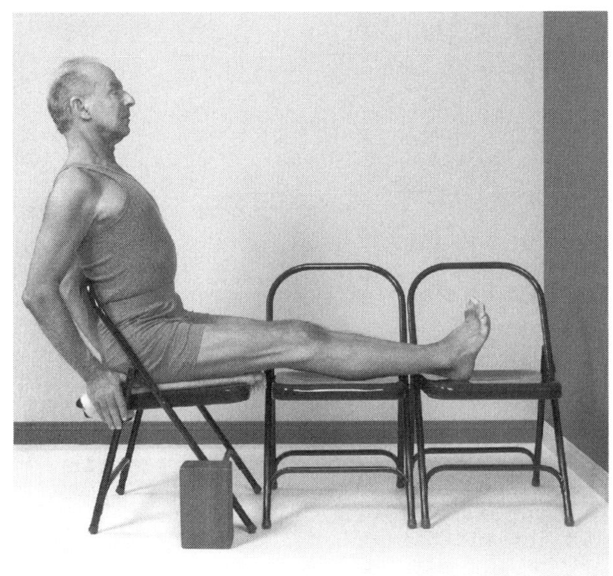

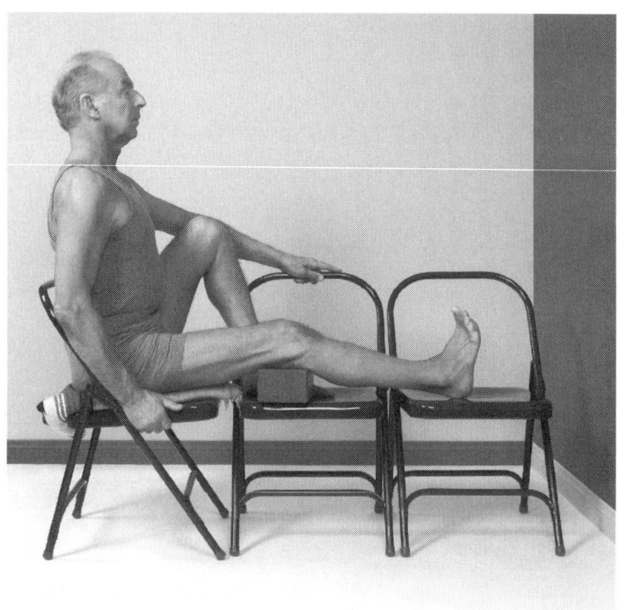

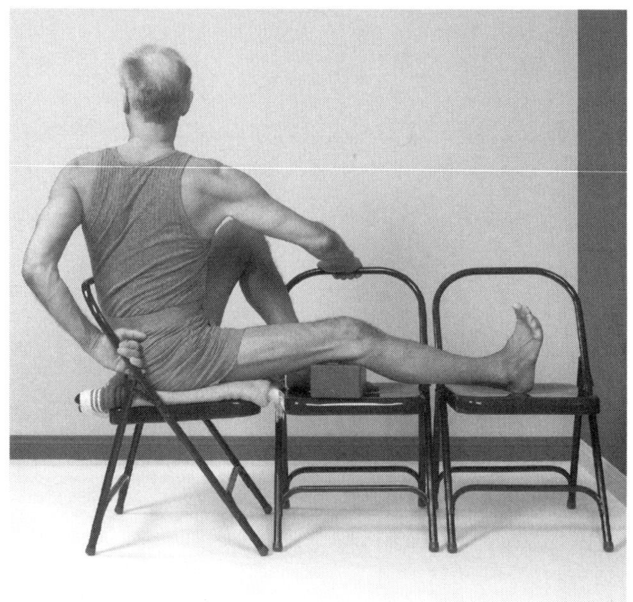

3. Turn and squarely face the feet. Raise up the left knee with your hands; brace the leg against the back of the chair.

4. Position your torso parallel to the chair backs, then extend the right leg. Now reach around with your right hand and hold onto the back of the chair against which the left leg is resting.

5. Now inhale smoothly and lift the chest. An instructor can encourage and support your lifting the spine by placing their right knee against the right mid thoracic spine.

6. Now inhale and turn the abdomen toward the left leg. As you do so, turn the chest and the shoulders, slipping your right elbow, if possible, around the left knee.

7. Reach with the left hand around the back of the chair to hold the seat as close to the spine as is comfortable.

8. Let the back of the chair you are sitting on to support the rib cage from the hips to the armpit. Lower the shoulders evenly.

9. Turn your head to face the right foot, and lower the inside of the right knee to the seat of the chair. Bring the left knee closer to the body.

10. Inhale slowly. Remain in this posture for 15 to 30 seconds. While you do this, continue to draw the bottom right ribs down and to the left.

11. Simultaneously press the left heel into the seat of the chair in order to lift the sternum. The instructor may guide the right shoulder blade down and toward the hip. The idea is to turn the torso, not the shoulder itself. Therefore the instructor might also encourage the left ribs to come back and around to the right. Make space by lifting the entire torso while it is in rotation.

12. Release the pose by first releasing the abdomen, then the right arm, and then the left arm.

13. Return your body to the right. Then bring your right leg to the floor with your

hands. Do the same with your left leg and turn to face forward while sitting in the chair.

14. Rest a moment, then spread your feet by turning the toes slightly in and heels slightly outward. Lower your hands to rest gently on your thighs, and continue with slow and even breaths. Then repeat the pose on the other side by changing the position of the chairs.

BENEFITS

This pose stimulates all the organs in the torso to improve function. Sitting posture is improved. It enhances flexibility in the flanks, hips, and legs and reduces leg cramps. Tension in shoulders and neck is lessened, resulting in fewer headaches.

Pasasana Variation

Chair Twist with Bolster

1. Begin by securing the safety belt. Bring the feet under the knees. If the leg is long, place a folded blanket under the buttocks. If the leg is short, place a folded blanket under the feet. Put a bolster or folded blankets on the thighs. This is important if the student is full-figured, so as to not cramp or pinch the organs in the torso or pelvis, or if there is a limited range of motion.

2. Sit up, turn toward the bolster, and grasp the back leg of the chair with the right hand in order to maintain balance.

3. Raise the left arm up even with the ear, pressing the sit bones down into the chair seat.

4. Lift the rib cage and turn the navel toward the bolster to bring the left elbow to the top of the bolster on the right side.

5. Keep the head in line with the spine, and try not to tighten the throat.

6. Extend the fingers of the left hand as if pressing against a wall and breathe smoothly and evenly for 3 to 5 breaths.

7. Return the arm up in line with the left ear on the inhalation. Bring the arm down on the exhalation and sit quietly.

Please note that the left ear is more in line with the left leg, rather than leaning to the right or looking down or back. This assures that the muscles of the mid and lower back are not put to any undue strain. After

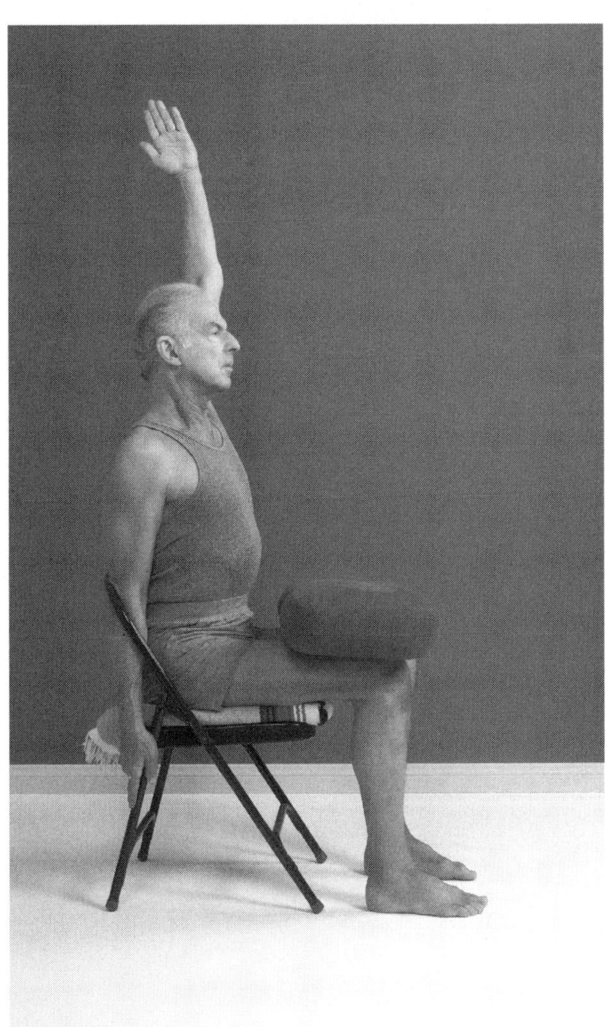

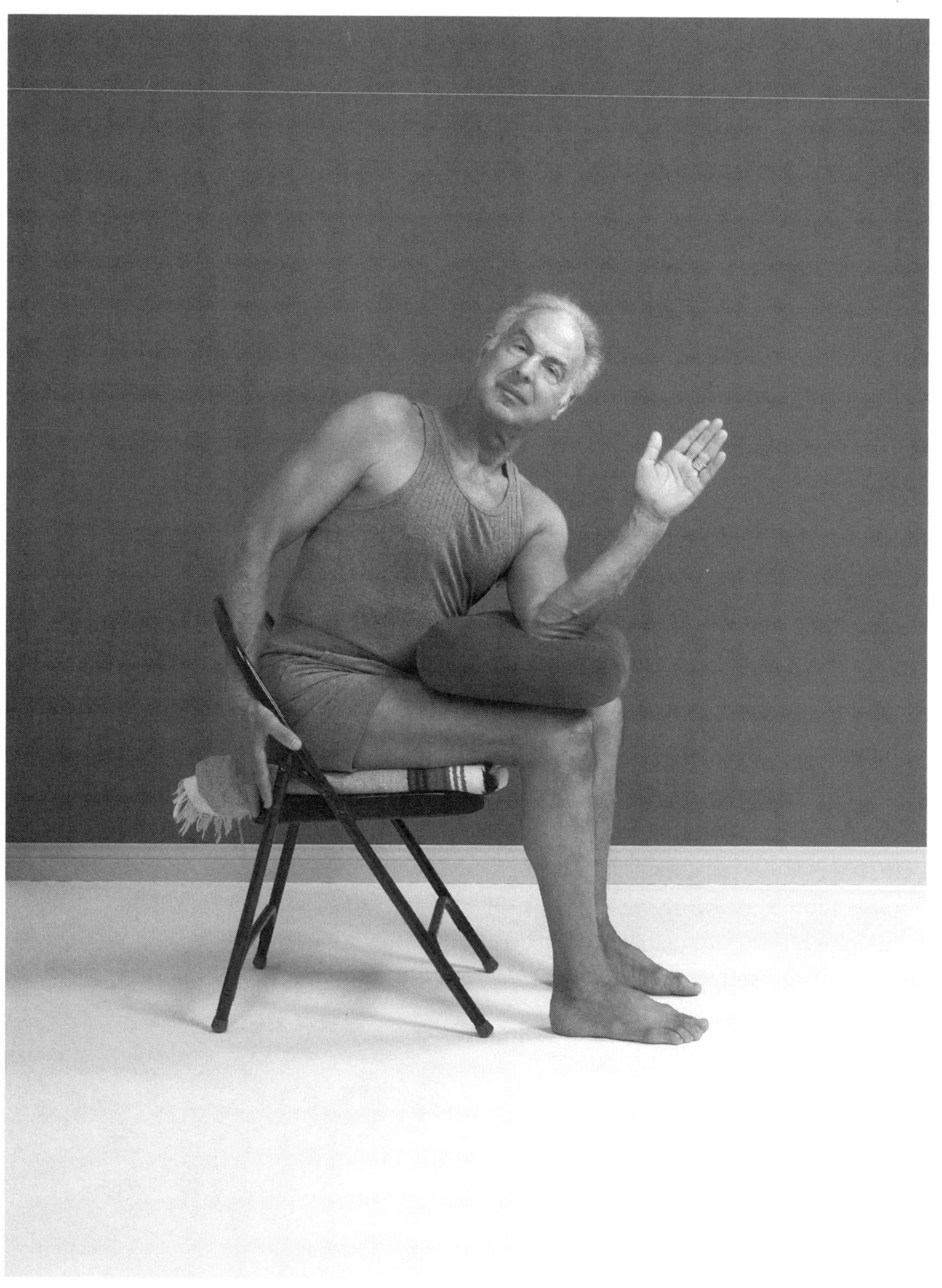

returning to center, sit for 10 to 20 seconds and then repeat to the other side.

BENEFITS

This pose is excellent for the digestion. It relieves lower back discomfort from sitting for extended periods of time. It aids elimination and reduces flatulence and the frequency of constipation. It increases flexibility in the hip joints and increases circulation in the torso, pelvis, and limbs.

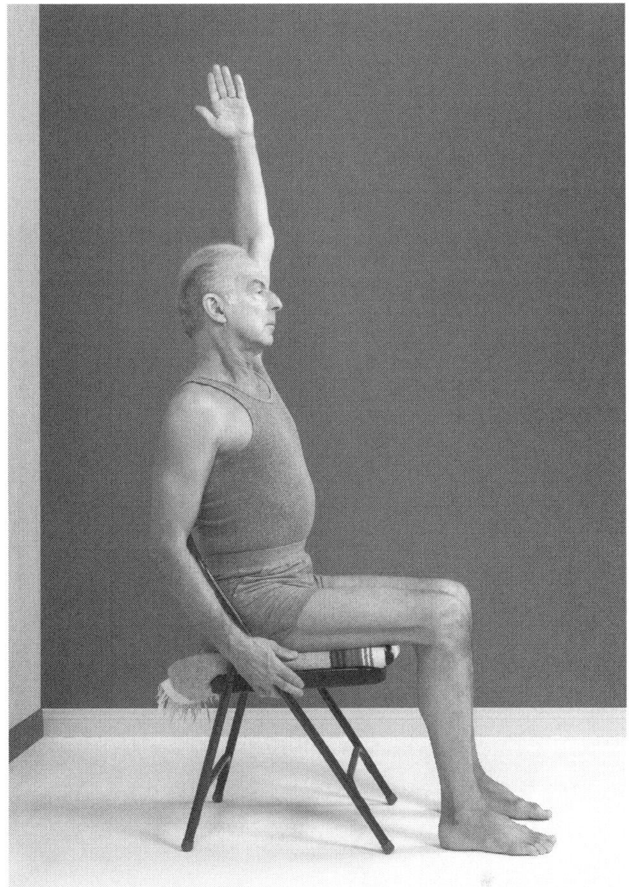

MALASANA VARIATION

Seated Chair Twist Without Bolster

1. To begin, sit erect in the chair, feet directly under the knees. If tall, place a folded blanket under the buttocks. If short, place a folded blanket under the feet. With an inhalation, lift the left hand parallel to the left ear.

2. Grasp the seat near your right hip with your right hand. With an exhalation, turn the navel toward the right leg.

3. With an inhalation, stretch the left arm up past the ear, and with a sharp exhalation, bring the left elbow to the outside of the right knee as shown in the photograph.

4. Bring the head back so the left ear is in line with the left knee, and open the palm of the left hand and fingers, as if they are pressing against a wall.

5. Each exhalation should bring the back of the left upper arm closer to the floor. Look straight ahead. Hold the position for 5 to 7 breaths.

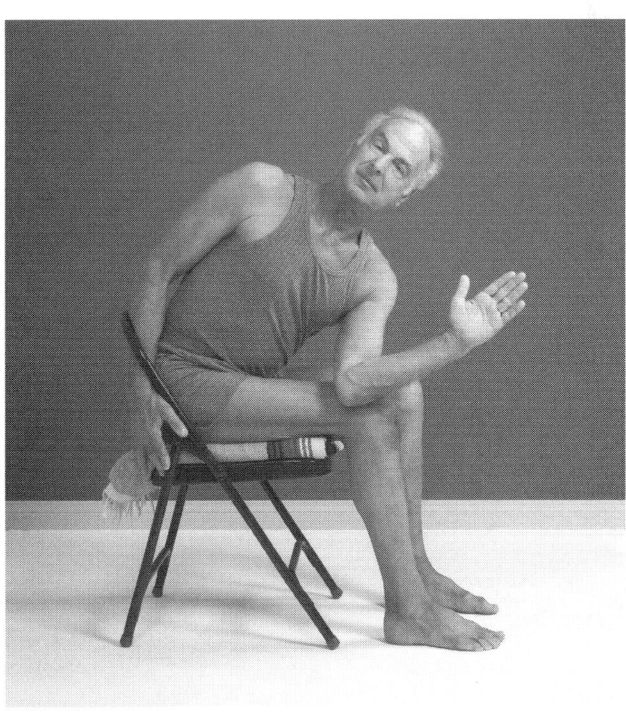

6. Continue to revolve the right side of the navel toward the right rib cage. If possible, the left hand can be moved inside the strut of the chair back to further stabilize the position.

7. To release the pose, return to the position of the picture shown for step 1 as you inhale.

8. Then with the next inhalation, place your hands back on the top of your thighs. Sit quietly, then repeat on the other side.

BENEFITS

This pose is excellent for the digestion. It relieves lower back discomfort from sitting for extended periods of time. It aids elimination and reduces flatulence and the occurrence of constipation. It increases flexibility in the hip joints and increases circulation in the torso, pelvis, and limbs.

Chair Baddha Konasana

Cobbler's Pose

1. Place a folding chair with the seat facing you. Secure the safety belt.

If the range of movement is limited, turn the chair around so the back of the chair can act as a support. Place a folded sticky mat on the seat.

2. Raise the legs by holding behind the knee to release the hamstrings and tendons. Place the feet together: toes and heels

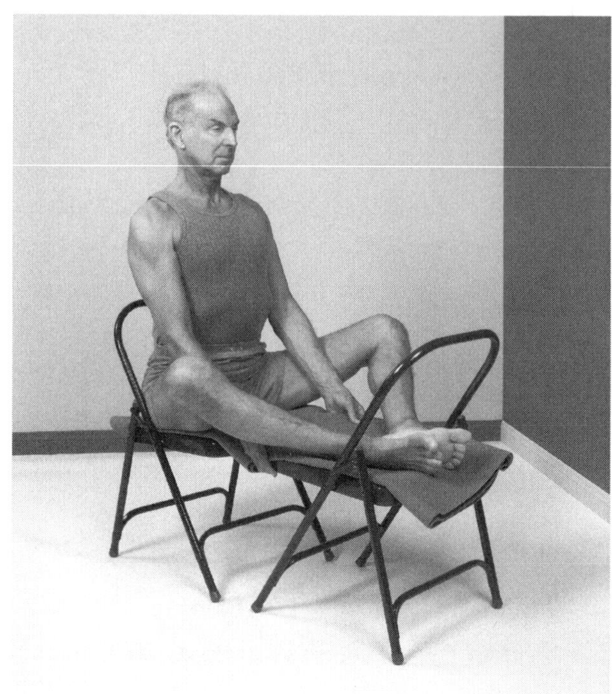

touching if possible. If there is undue pressure in the groins, then support the outer knee with the backs of chairs placed under the legs or a strap passed around the outside of the knees.

3. Sit up away from the back of the chair. If this presents a problem, then place a rolled sticky mat, or a folded blanket, or a foam block between the chair back and the mid back behind the heart area.

4. Inhale and lift the rib cage and side chest. Exhale behind the navel. Hold the position for 10 breaths or whatever is comfortable.

5. If maintaining an erect torso is difficult, place your hands behind you, holding onto the arms of the chair and pressing down.

6. The second phase of the pose starts by holding the back of the second chair either on the side or at the top. Then draw the second chair closer to the first, thereby further opening the legs.

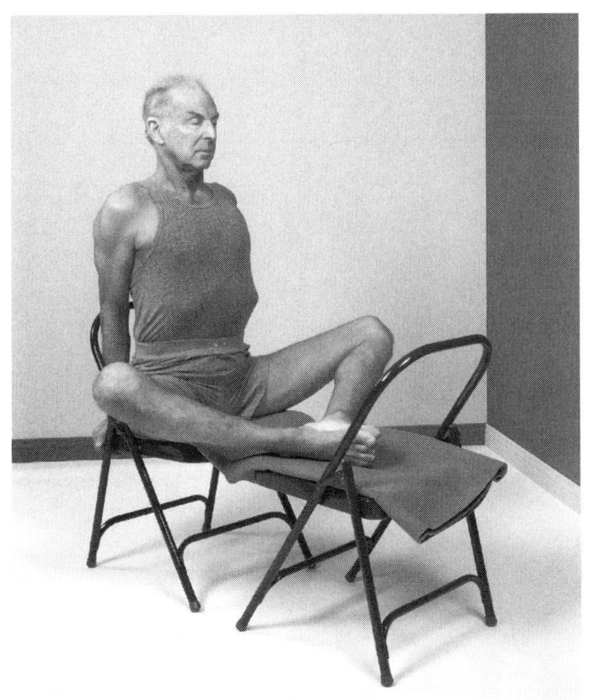

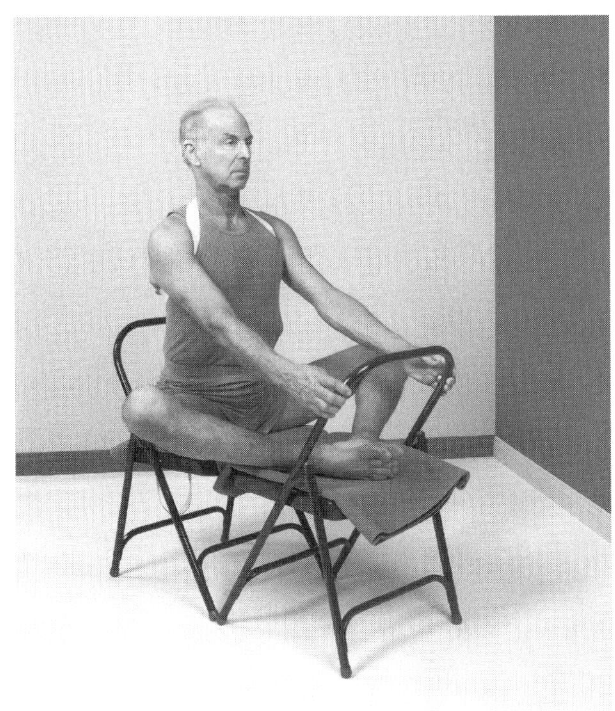

A shoulder strap can also be used to facilitate the proper alignment of the torso.

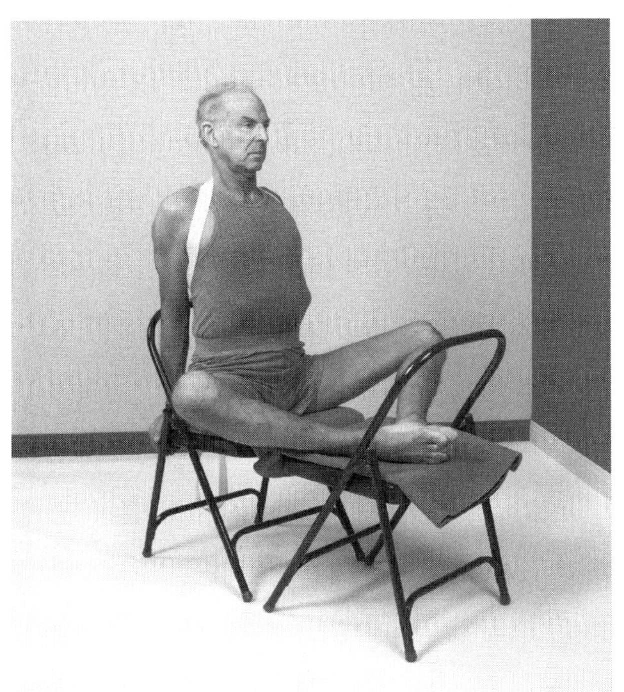

Hands grasping upper arm of chair.

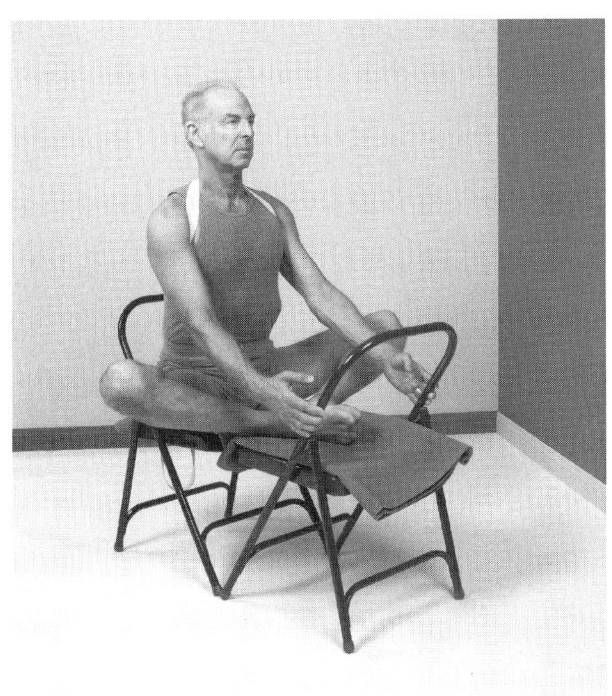

Clasping lower on the arm of the chair.

7. To exit the pose, use your hands on the outer side of the knees, and raise the knees up and together slowly and carefully.

8. Then place the hands behind the knees, and draw the back flesh of the knee toward the hips, as the legs stretch forward and rest on the seat of the chair.

9. Turn to sit squarely in the chair, lowering one foot at a time gently to the floor. Sit quietly with both feet on the floor.

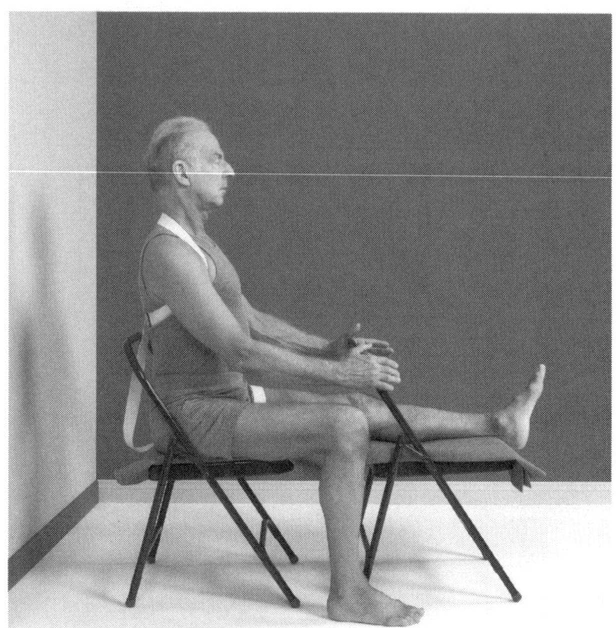

Chair Preparation for Janu Sirsasana

Head-to-the-Knee Pose

1. Sit up away from the back of the chair, using a prop if necessary to support the torso. Place another folding chair in front, with the seat facing away from your chair. Please note that a strap has been placed around the shoulders and over the back of the neck, like a harness. The buckle is in the middle of the back; the tail can be used to tighten the strap to hold the shoulders back. This will improve the posture and strengthen the torso. This device can be used in many asanas throughout the book to enhance posture and develop an awareness of alignment.

2. Lift the left leg and put the foot through the back of the second chair. If the leg is long, support the foot with a third chair.

3. Let the right foot rest fully on the floor, parallel to the thigh, perpendicular to the calf.

4. Sit up, breath into the side chest, and extend the left heel away from the left hip.

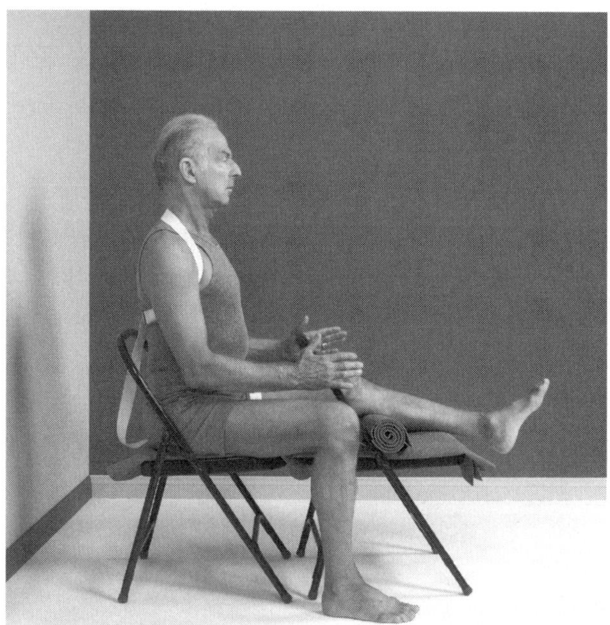

With roll.

5. Hold the position for 5 to 10 breaths. Bend the knee by placing the left hand on the inside of the knee and lifting it up quickly.

6. Return both feet to the floor. Sit quietly for 3 to 5 breaths and repeat on the other side.

If there is increased pressure behind the knee, use a rolled towel or sticky mat to reduce any tension on the hamstrings.

Chair Janu Sirsasana

1. Face two folding chairs toward each other. Place a folded blanket on the seat of one chair. Bring a third folding chair to the right side. Bend the right leg and place the right foot against the left thigh. Support the right leg with additional folded blankets on the third chair.

2. Raise the rib cage away from the back of the chair, lift the bottom edge of the sternum, and press the buttocks back and down into your seat

3. Gently turn the navel toward the inner left leg without distorting the neck or head.

4. Hold the position for at least 5 even breaths and then release.

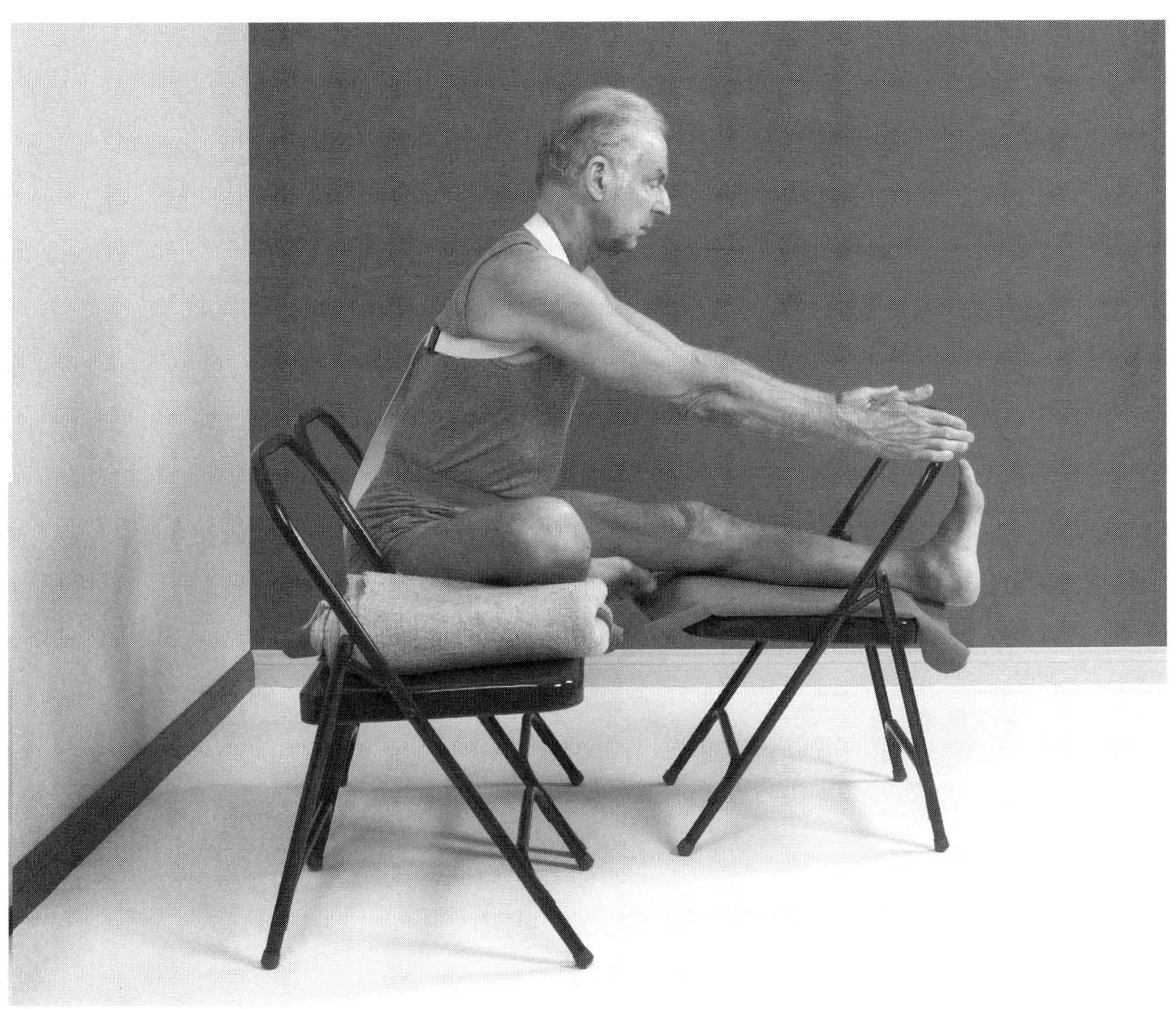

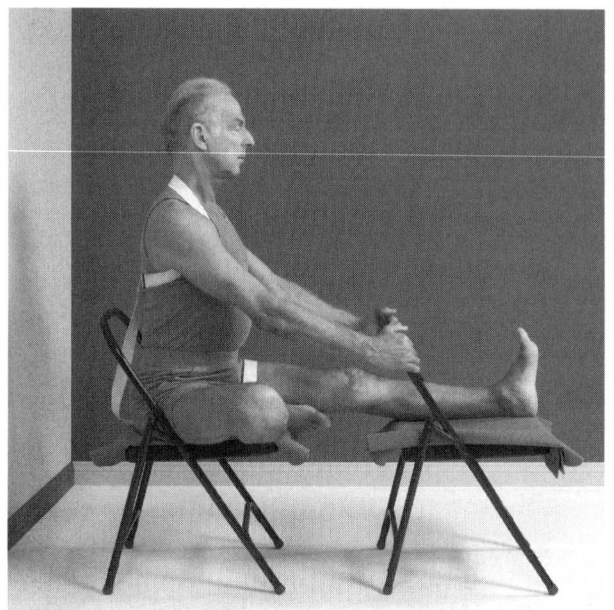

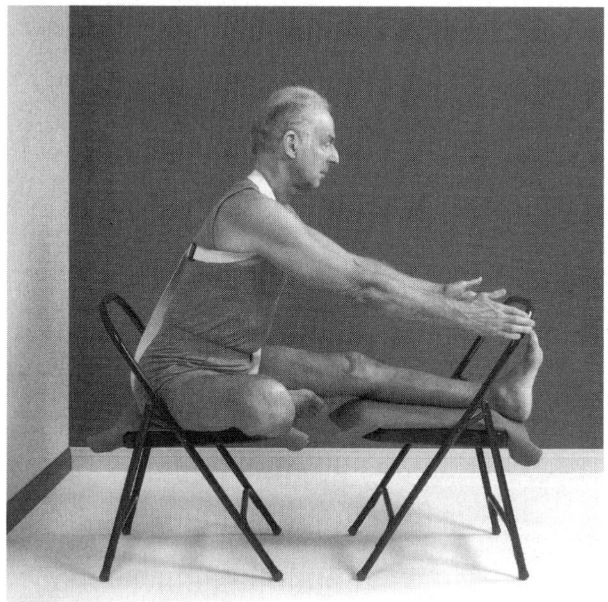

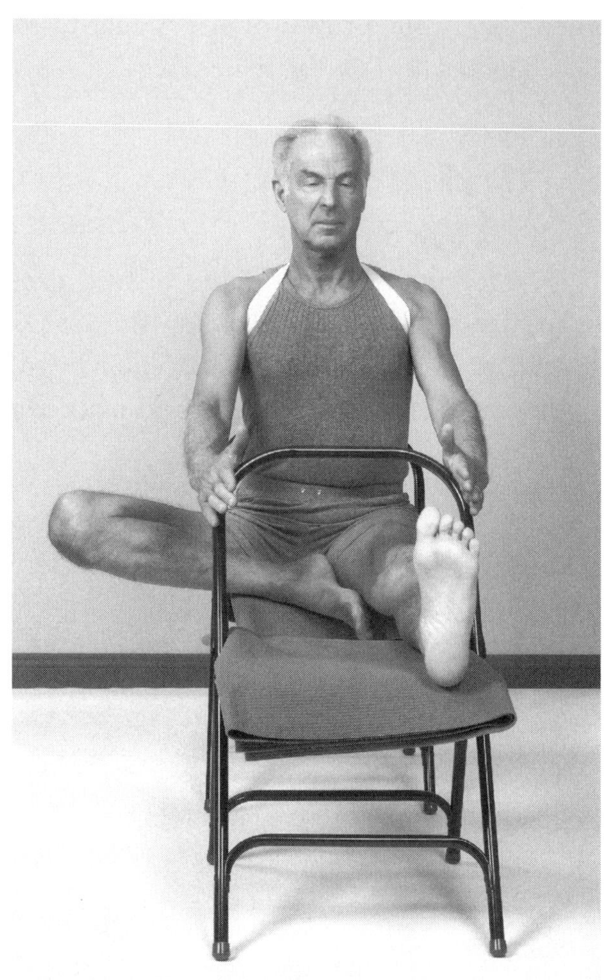

5. Use your right hand to bring the right knee up, and using the hands behind the right knee, stretch the leg forward next to the left leg. Bring the third chair with the folded blankets to the other side and repeat the asana.

BENEFITS

This asana is a combination of Baddha Konasana (Cobbler's Pose) and the seated twists. It greatly enhances digestion, elimination, flexibility of legs and arms, and relaxation of the shoulders, neck, and spine. It tones the legs and arms and lengthens the hamstrings.

If blankets are not necessary you will only need two chairs, as shown above.

Chair Upavistha Konasana

Seated Wide-Angle Pose

Pose I

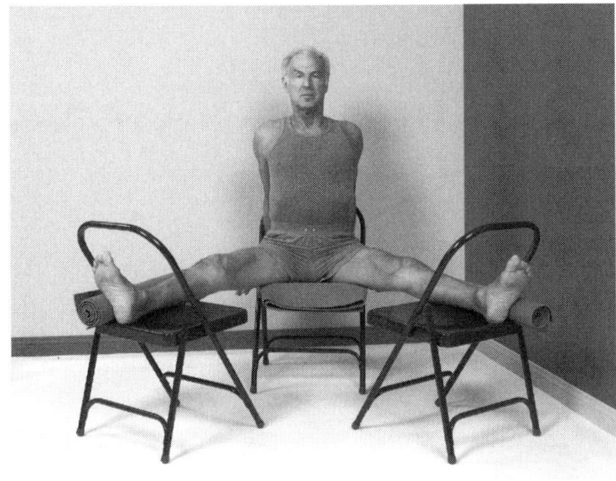

1. Begin by securing the safety belt. Bring two folding chairs in front and to either side of your chair, with the seats facing you.

2. Place your legs on the chair, with the back supports of the chair bracing the legs.

3. Place a rolled sticky mat between the chair and your legs to keep the legs and feet in alignment. Please note that it is a moderate opening of the legs only. Notice that the feet point up as much as possible, and the inner knees are turned toward the seats of the chairs.

4. Bring the torso away from the back of the chair, using props if necessary. Sit on the tips of the sit bones, bracing your hands behind you.

5. Bring the breath into the sides of the chest, press down on the hands, and lift the sides of the chest as much as possible.

6. Remain in the posture for 5 to 10 breaths. Return to center by bringing the chairs together slowly and carefully. Remain seated with the legs stretched forward, supported on the chairs. Sit quietly and breathe.

BENEFIT

This pose opens the groins, increases circulation in the lower pelvis, and increases flexibility in the hips. There is a reduction of tension in the mid and lower spine and a general overall toning of the legs and arms. A sense of peaceful quiet becomes readily apparent.

Pose II

Bring the hands to rest on top of the shins. Hold for five to ten breaths.

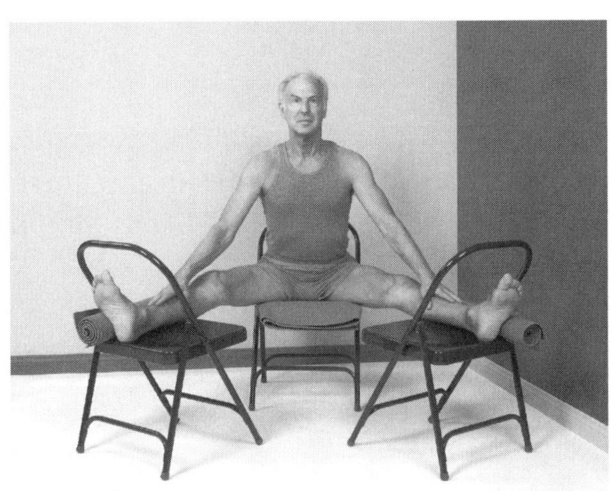

Pose III

1. For extended forward movement, place your hands on top of the chairs and press the hips and sit bones back firmly.

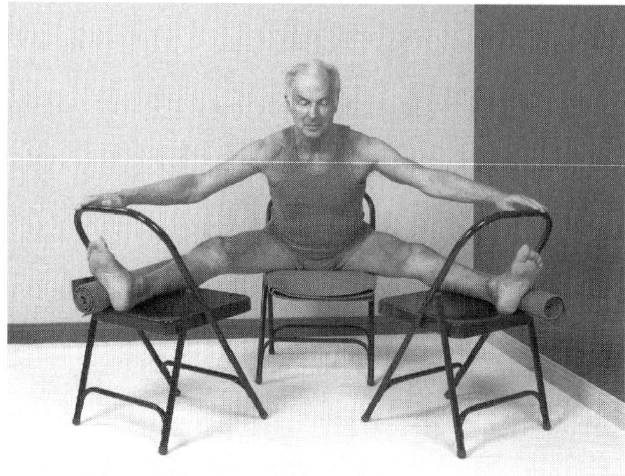

2. Keep the bottom of the sternum lifted away from the pubis.

3. Hold for 5 to 10 breaths.

4. To release the pose, place the hands on the shins. Hold for 5 breaths. Then place your hands behind your hips and hold for 5 breaths.

Pose IV

For the advanced pose, spread the chairs farther apart. Bring the head and torso parallel to the hips. Keep the hands on top of the chairs.

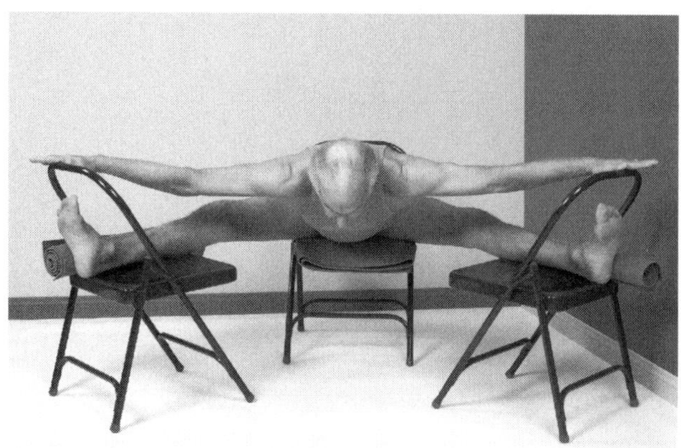

To complete the pose, rest the palms on top of the toes, and stretch the arms any amount. If there is concern regarding balance, a fourth chair can be placed under the head, with the forehead resting on a folded blanket.

Chair Uttanasana

Forward Bend Pose

1. Begin by securing the seat belt with enough slack to be able to bend forward. If necessary, use a shoulder harness. Place a bolster between the feet, toes forward, ankles braced by the sides of the bolster.

2. Sit up, and with a few breaths align the head with the center of the pelvis.

3. On an exhalation, place the hands palms down on top of the knees and lean forward 30 degrees.

4. Then slip the hands down the inside of the legs to the mid calf, and lean forward 60 degrees.

5. Keep the head in line with the spine. With an exhalation, place the palms down onto the bolster, between the legs if possible.

6. Then gently press the knees against the outer upper arm and the arms against the inner knees. This action will release tension in the lower spine and hips.

7. If there is any difficulty maintaining the head in line with the spine, a second chair can be placed under the head, with folded blankets or bolsters on the seat to support the head.

8. Only the forehead rests on the support so that the nose is free from pressure. Rest the eyes against the cheekbones. Hold

for at least 30 seconds to 1 minute at the start. Build up to 2 minutes.

9. Return to a sitting position by keeping your head down and placing your hands on your knees.

10. Hold for several breaths, then use the hands to push up slowly on the count of 10 to a sitting position. Sit quietly for 10 to 20 breaths.

BENEFITS

This pose tones the kidneys, liver, and spleen and reduces discomfort in the stomach. The heartbeat is slowed and the spinal nerves rejuvenated. Depression in many instances is reduced, and students that are easily excited often become calm and cool. Vision often improves, and there is a general sense of well-being.

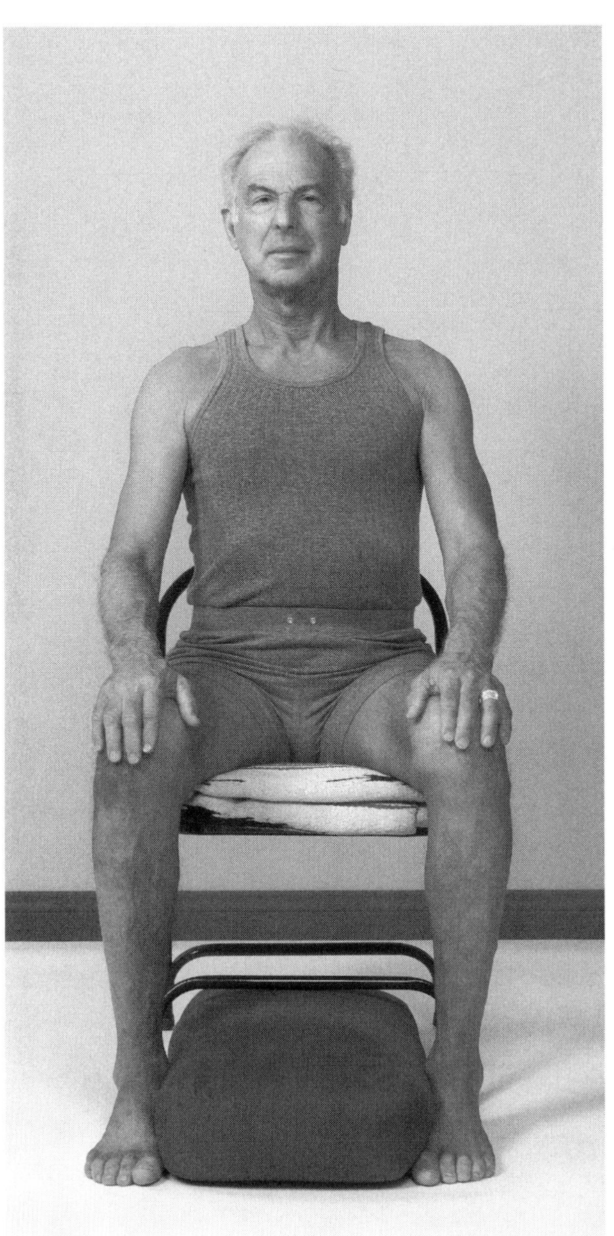

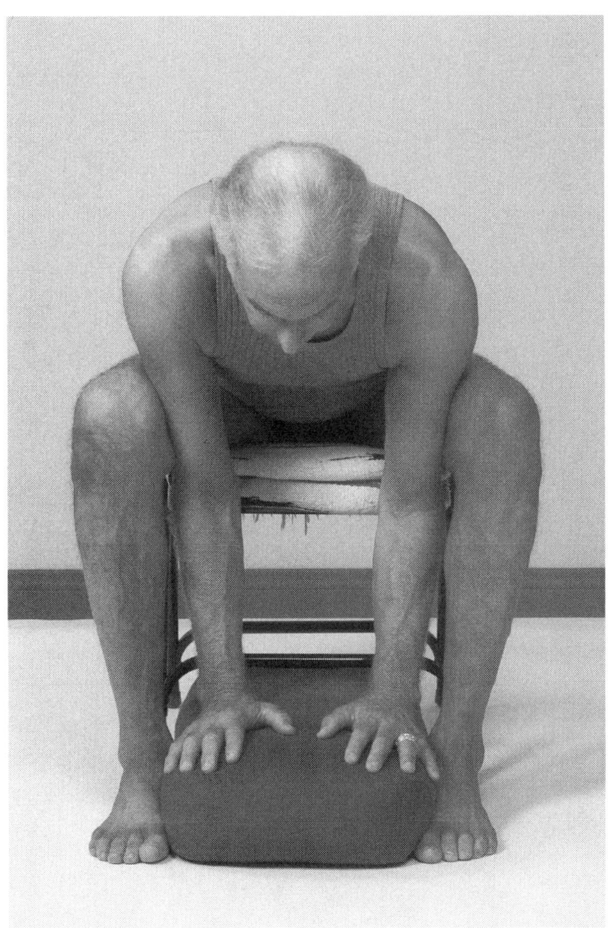

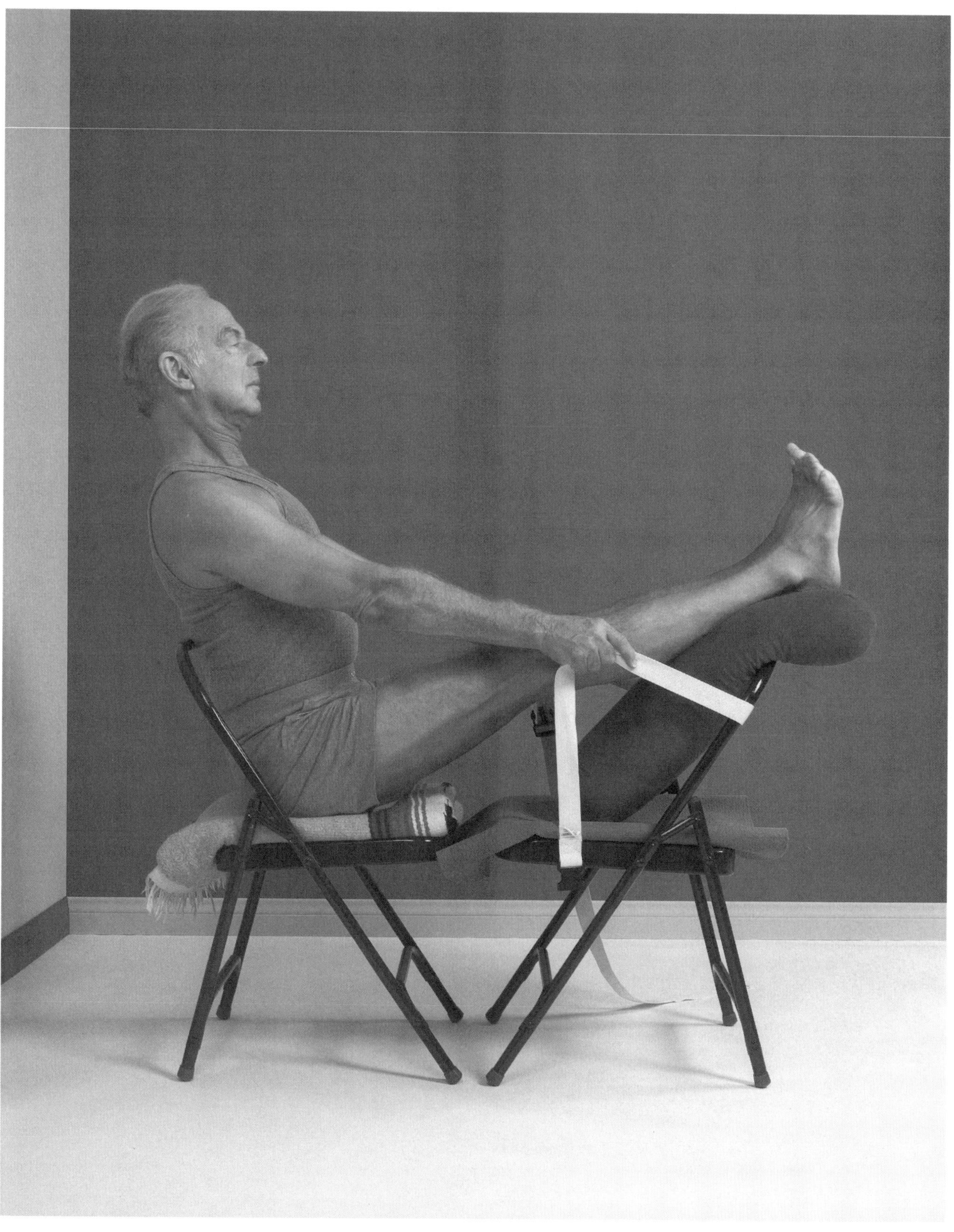

Chair Ardha Navasana

Supported Boat Pose

Note: This asana is not to be done before at least three months of practice. Then it is usually performed toward the end of a practice or class session.

1. Secure a safety belt after facing two folding chairs toward each other.

2. Position a folded sticky mat on the seat of the second chair. A blanket can be folded over the back of the first chair for comfort.

3. Lift both feet onto the edge of the folding chair, and arrange the bolster at the angle illustrated.

4. Extend the legs up toward the back of the folding chair, grasping a strap in each hand that is placed midway on the back of the second chair around the bolster.

5. The bolster can be placed flat on the seat to accommodate those who are tight in the hamstrings or have a balance problem.

6. Raise the chest and side ribs. Keep the head in line with the spine and breathe easily. Try not to hold the breath. If there is undue stiffness in the neck and shoulders, the chair can be moved next to a wall to support the head. Hold the posture for at least 5 to 10 breaths.

7. Release the strap. Bend the knees; rest the feet on the edge of the second chair seat. Push the chair away and lower the legs to the ground, using the hands to keep the groins soft, and return to a sitting position.

BENEFITS

This pose is very beneficial for the liver, spleen, and gall bladder. The back muscles, which become flaccid due to the shape of the chair and prolonged sitting, are strengthened. This pose works against osteoporosis.

Chair Savasana

Relaxation Pose

1. Place a folding chair in front of your chair, with the seat facing forward. Put a folded sticky mat on the seat.

2. Place a bolster so that one end rests against the back of the second chair and the other end rests on your mid thighs (similar to the position of the bolster on the facing page). Additional blankets can be used to accommodate a stiff spine and hips.

3. Lean forward to rest the head face down on the bolster, with a towel or blanket supporting the forehead.

4. Keep the nose free from any pressure. If possible cross the arms over the head resting on the bolster.

5. If it is difficult to rest your head on the bolster, then use folded blankets or another bolster to provide greater comfort.

6. The arms can also rest on the seat of the chair if it is difficult to raise them over the head.

7. Allow the eyes to rest into the cheekbones, and position the tongue away from the upper and the lower palate. Make the breath to be smooth and even. Try to stay focused on the breath. It is natural to let your thoughts wander into the past, into

the future, or to take in the events of the day. Part of savasana is to learn to be in the moment. It is also the time that the effects of the day's yoga practice have a chance to be absorbed into the conscious mind.

8. When it becomes difficult to remain in the rhythm of the breath, then it's time to slowly rise up from the support of the bolster. Lift your head from your chest. Open your eyes on an inhalation.

Seated/Floor Series

This series is appropriate for the student who is able to sit on the floor unassisted.

Supta Padangusthasana

Reclining Big-Toe Pose

Stage I

1. To begin, lie down on the floor and place a folded blanket under your head, a rolled sticky mat under the left knee, and a block under the left heel, with the left foot pressed firmly and evenly into the wall. Bring the shoulder blades toward the spine and lift the chest.

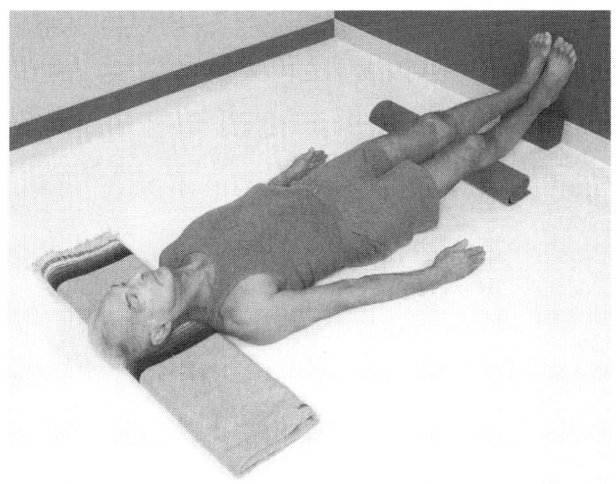

2. Exhale and bend the right knee toward the chest in line with the right shoulder. Bring both hands behind the knee, elbows toward the floor.

3. On an inhalation, bring the knee slightly away from the chest.

4. On an exhalation, press the knee toward the shoulder. Keep the hips and shoulders level, and continue to extend the left leg as much as possible toward the wall.

5. Turn the inner left knee firmly toward the floor or the sticky mat.

6. With an inhalation, stretch the right leg to the wall, resting the heel on the block. Move the sticky mat to support the back of the right knee. With an exhalation, repeat the flexion process to the left. Repeat the process 3 or 4 times each on the right and the left.

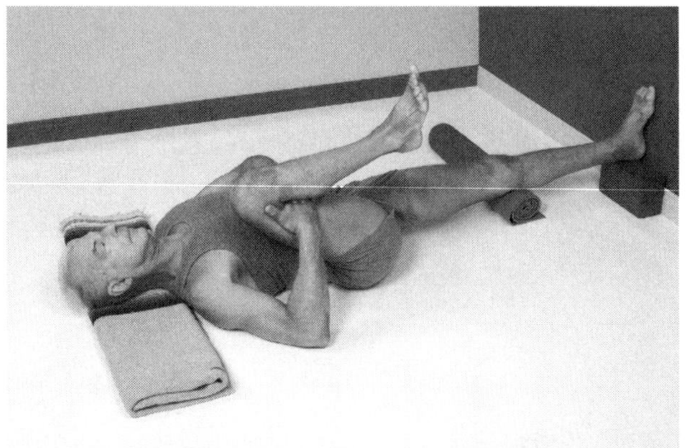

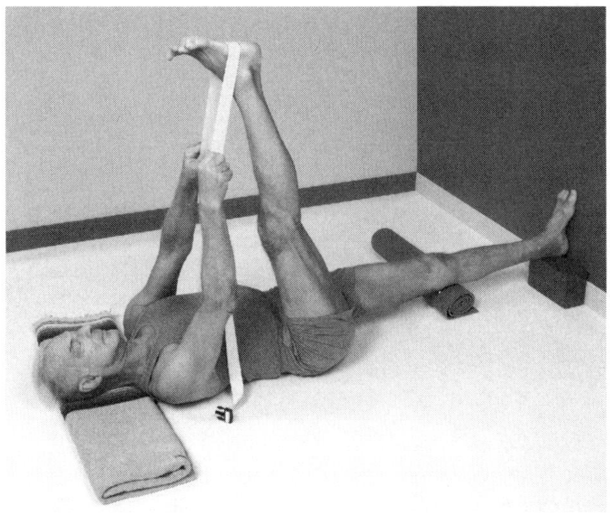

Stage II

1. Return the sticky mat and block to the left leg. Bend your right knee toward the right shoulder. Place a strap around the right foot at the bottom of the arch and top of the heel. Hold one end of the strap in each hand. Keep the knee soft

2. As you inhale, extend the right leg either 90 degrees to the hip or slightly toward the head.

3. Straighten the arms, still holding one end of the strap in each hand.

4. Draw the shoulders away from the ears, lift the chest and side ribs, and keep a firm but not an aggressive grip on the strap.

5. Lift the leg up and away from the floor. Hold the position for 5 to 10 breaths, consistently moving the right hip and sit bones down toward the wall. Be sure that the right and the left waist are equidistant from the top of the pelvis.

6. To release the pose, lower the right leg toward the wall, letting the strap slip slowly through your hands until the right heel is resting on the block.

Stage III

1. Return to the beginning posture

2. Either place a strap around the foot as instructed before, or grasp the right big toe with the first and second fingers of the right hand on the inside of the toe and the thumb on the outside.

3. Extend the leg at 90 degrees to the right hip, keeping the knees soft.

4. Press the left hip firmly to the floor with the left hand. Then slowly, while straightening

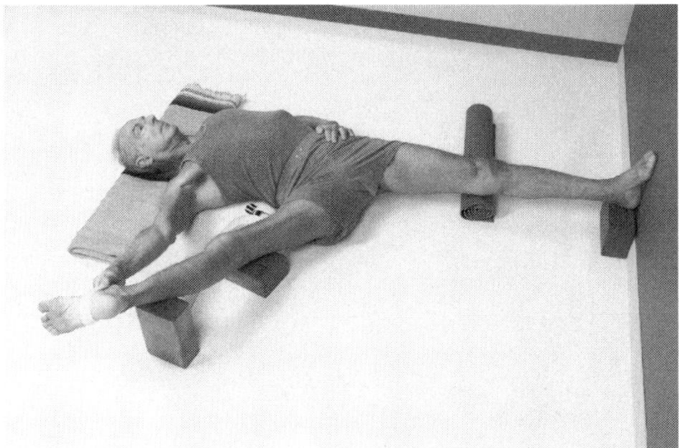

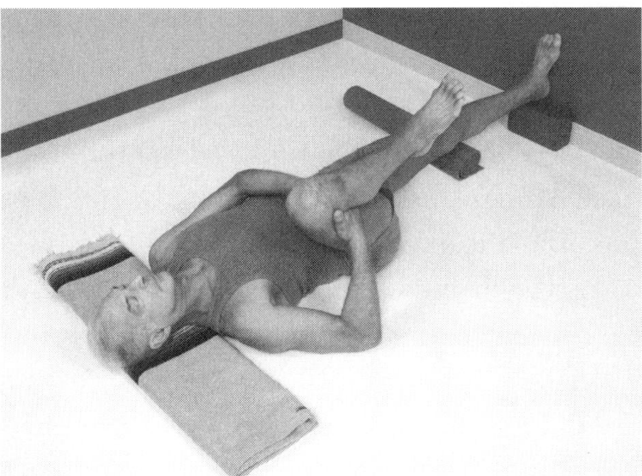

the right leg, drop the leg to the right, extending it 90 degrees to the right hip. If necessary, support the right leg with a block at the knee and at the ankle. Please note that the left hip does not rise from the floor. The right leg and arm are as straight as possible and the right chest is lifted toward the ceiling.

5. Continue to press into the left foot and leg, and with each exhalation draw the navel toward the left. Hold the pose for 5 to 10 breaths.

6. Then draw the leg back up to 90 degrees and return to the original position.

BENEFITS

This pose tones the arms and legs, elongates the sciatic nerve, and in some cases improves paralysis of the legs. Increased circulation in legs and hips improves neural response. Stiffness in the hip joints is reduced. Supta Padangusthasana prevents hernias from developing.

DANDASANA

Staff Pose

1. Sit on a folded blanket. Use as many folded blankets as necessary to elevate the spine. Extent the legs forward, with the inner knee rotating downward to the floor.

2. Rotate the top of the thighs inward (from the outside to the inside).

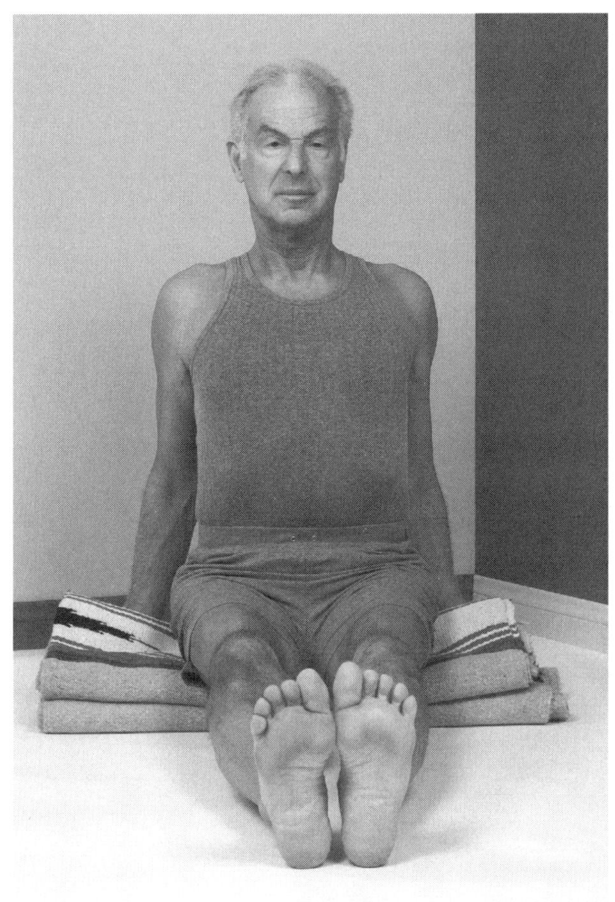

3. Place the hands on the blanket, fingers forward. Soften the elbows, bringing them back parallel to the rib cage.

4. Extend the heels away from the hips, pressing the balls of the feet forward. Lift the chest and bring the bottom of the sternum up and away from the pubis.

5. Lift the back waist. Remain in this posture for 5 to 10 breaths. If there is tension in the hamstrings or backs of the knees, place a folded blanket or rolled sticky mat under the knees.

6. To release from the pose, bend your knees and lie back on the floor, with the hips supported on one folded blanket. If necessary, the rolled sticky mat can remain under the knees. Lie quietly and breathe smoothly and evenly.

BENEFITS

Dandasana stretches adductors and strengthens quadriceps, reducing scissor-gait.

PASCHIMOTTANASANA

Seated Forward Bend Pose

1. Sit as you did in Dandasana. Sit on blankets to accommodate stiff hamstrings You may need to place a rolled sticky mat or folded blanket under the knees if the knees are not touching the floor. This depends upon the ability of the student and how many blankets are used underneath the buttocks.

2. Place a chair over your legs, between the feet and the knees. Put your palms face down on the seat of the chair (not pictured).

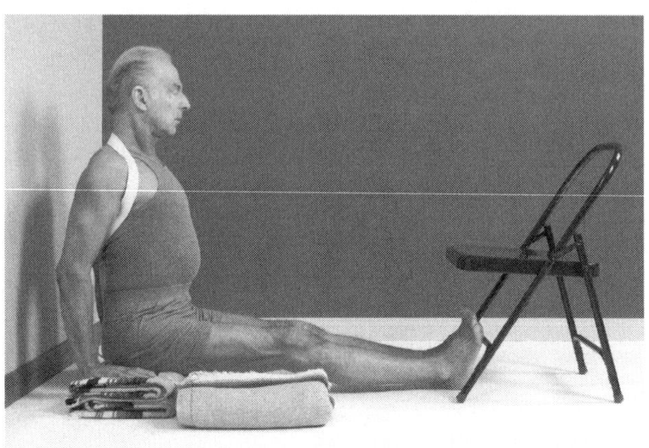

Please note that a shoulder brace is used. Inhale.

3. With an exhalation, press the hips back and push the chair forward as much as possible but to where it is still comfortable.

4. Each inhalation lifts the torso. With each exhalation press the chair further forward.

5. Hold the position for 5 to 10 breaths and slowly, with each inhalation, return to an upright sitting position. This pose can be repeated 2 or 3 times.

BENEFITS

This pose gently moves the abdominal organs and stretches the hamstring. It also tones the kidneys and rejuvenates the whole spine. It improves digestion. By supporting the hands on the seat of the chair, this asana creates a sense of peaceful quiet.

SEATED BADDHA KONASANA

Bound-Angle Pose

1. Begin by sitting in Dandasana. Be sure that the centers of the heels are resting on

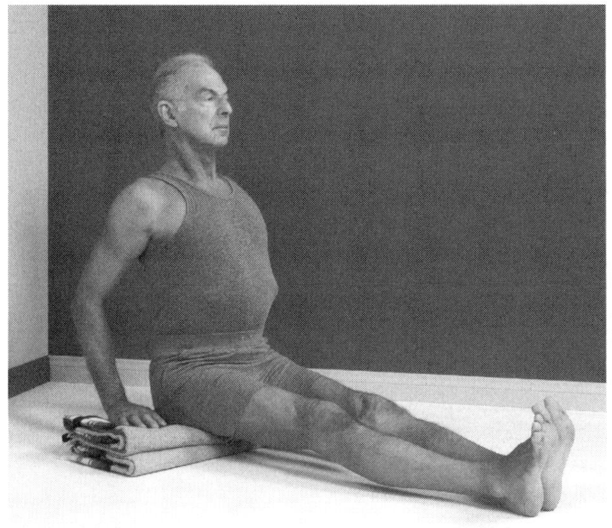

the floor. Press the balls of the feet forward and take a few breaths.

2. Then drop the legs open, resting the little toe on the floor.

Place the right hand on the inside of the right knee. Draw it back quickly, with the knee moving out and the foot in line with the pubis. Do the same with the left leg, bringing the soles of the feet together in front of the pubis. The pressure at the heels and the soles of the feet should be equal.

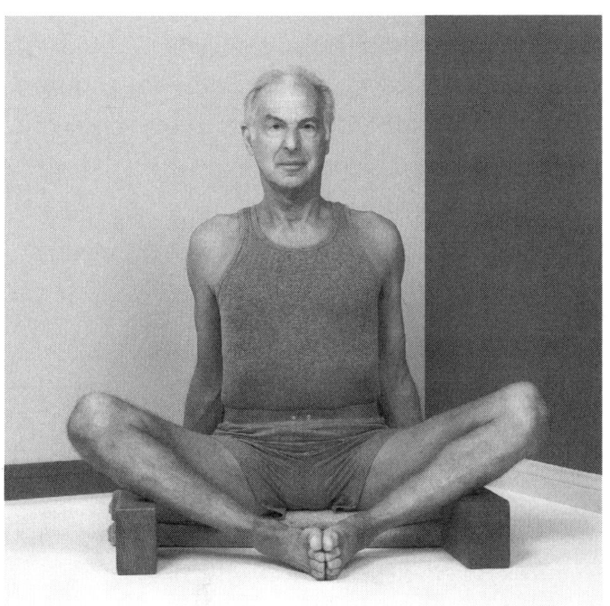

4. Place the hands behind the hips with fingers pointed forward and the elbow joints soft. Raise the side chest; move the shoulders away from the ears.

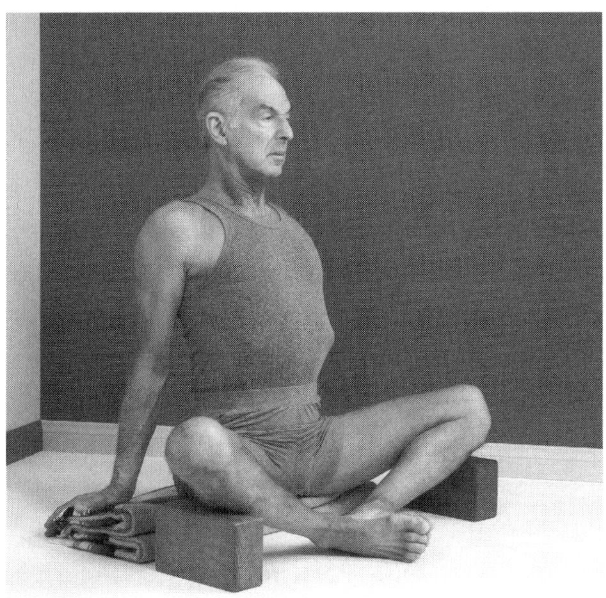

If there is undue pressure or strain in the groins or legs, support the outer knees with blocks or blankets.

5. Maintain the position for 1 or 2 minutes.

6. Charge the chest with an inhalation and direct your exhalation into the legs. There is a tendency to try and push the knees to the floor, which can cause discomfort at the groins and inner thighs. Instead

it is suggested that the inner thigh and knee press outward, away from the hips, and that supports be used under the knees to eliminate any chance of damage. Therefore encourage the groins to be soft. It is also very important that the torso lift, using the arms to press against the blanket or floor. Note that the chest is open, without sticking the ribs out, thus tightening the diaphragm. The torso is balanced over the pelvis. The breath is steady, rising from behind the navel into the side chest.

BENEFITS

This pose can be an effective tool to control urinary disorders. The pelvis, abdomen, and lower back receive additional circulation. The kidneys, prostate, and bladder are kept healthy, and the occurrence of sciatica and hernia is reduced.

Adho Mukha Baddha Konasana

Downward Bound-Angle Pose

This variation enables the student to increase hip flexibility and strengthen the lower back muscles. Begin with the same setup as in the previous asana.

1. Place a chair in front, with the seat facing toward you. Place a folded blanket or bolster on the seat of the chair.
2. Use your hands on the seat of the chair to bring the shoulders away from the ears.
3. Lift the chest and rib cage by pressing down firmly with the hands on the chair seat.
4. With an exhalation, push the chair forward. As the torso extends forward, the hips must press back deeply into the blanket or bolster.
5. Be sure that you do not push the chair beyond your capacity. Then if it is comfortable, rest your forehead on the support.

Note that the hands are placed half way between the seat and the top of the chair.

Note that the nose is free, and the skin of the forehead is pressing gently toward the eyebrows.

6. If it is too difficult to push the chair in this position, the asana can be performed by crossing the legs, with the right leg in front, knees supported (simple cross-leg posture). You will experience the same results.

BENEFITS

This pose can be an effective tool to control urinary disorders. The pelvis, abdomen, and lower back receive additional circulation. The kidneys, prostate, and bladder are kept healthy, and sciatica and hernia are reduced. There is the added benefit here of permitting the brain to relax. Tension in the neck and shoulders is reduced. The pose reduces agitation and nervousness, thereby lowering stress.

Janu Sirsasana

Head-to-the-Knee Pose

1. Begin with Dandasana seated on a blanket or bolster, depending on the degree of flexibility and comfort.

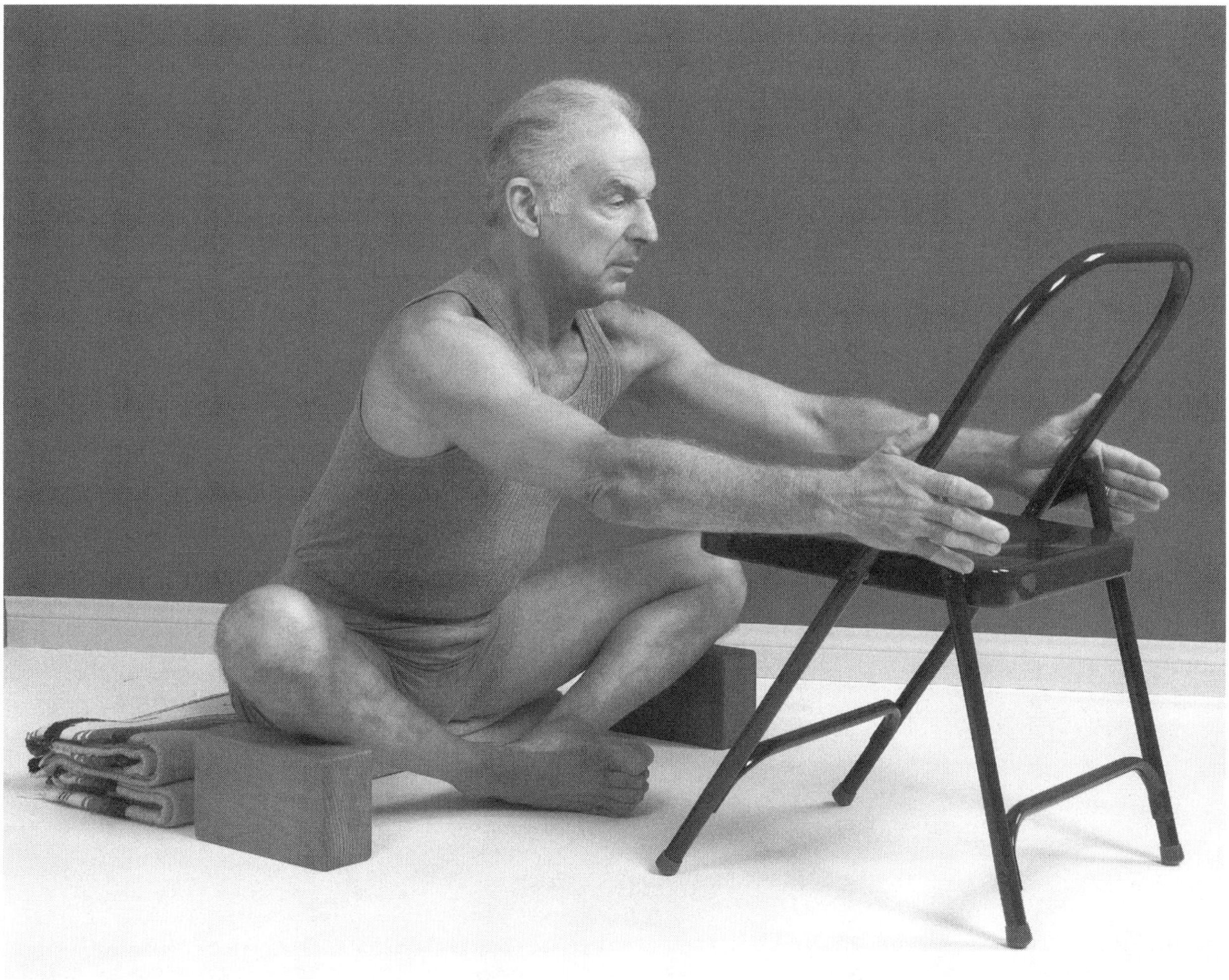

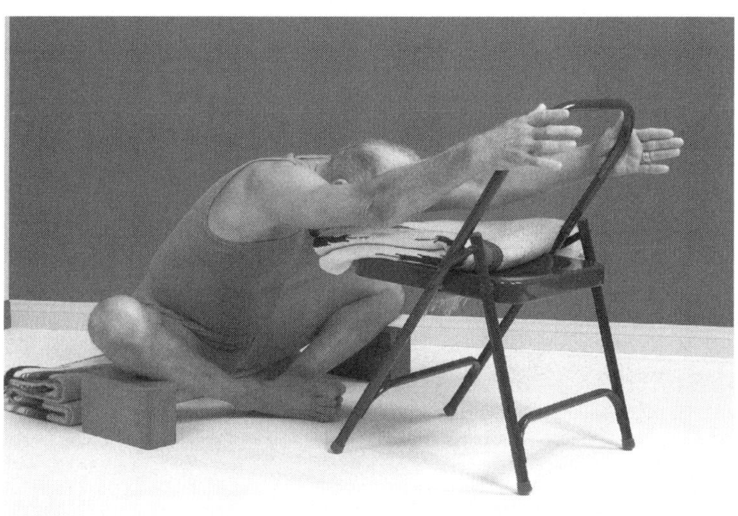

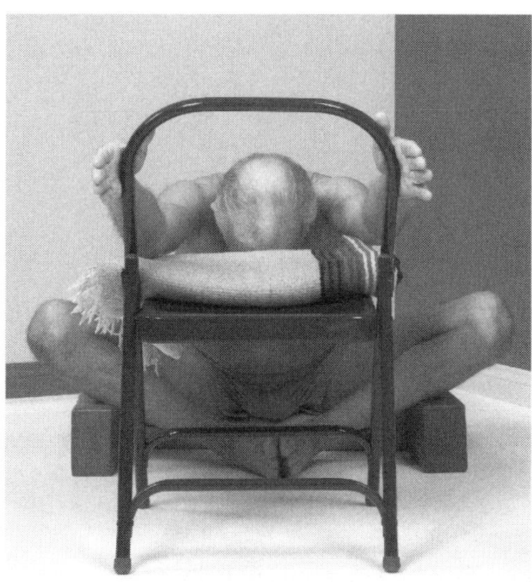

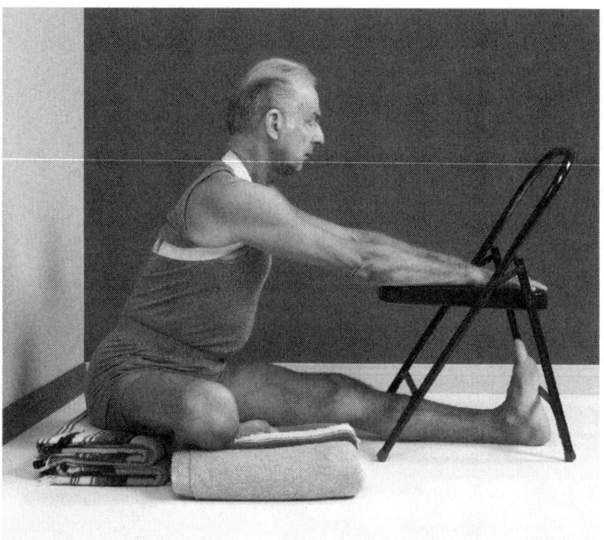

2. Use the arms and hands placed by the hips to lift the chest and rib cage. Note that the shoulder harness is used to facilitate the proper posture.

3. Place a folded blanket at the right. Place a chair over the legs near the ankles, with the bar near the shinbone.

4. Then with an exhalation use the right hand behind the right knee to quickly lift the leg out to the side and bring the right heel close to the right groin or the middle of the left thigh.

5. Press the right heel firmly against the inner left thigh.

6. Release the right knee, to rest the thigh on the folded blanket.

7. Bring the chair closer to the hips, so the leg of the chair can support the inner knee, and the seat of the chair is extending to the left.

8. With an exhalation, turn the navel firmly toward the inner left thigh, moving away from the dome of the right knee.

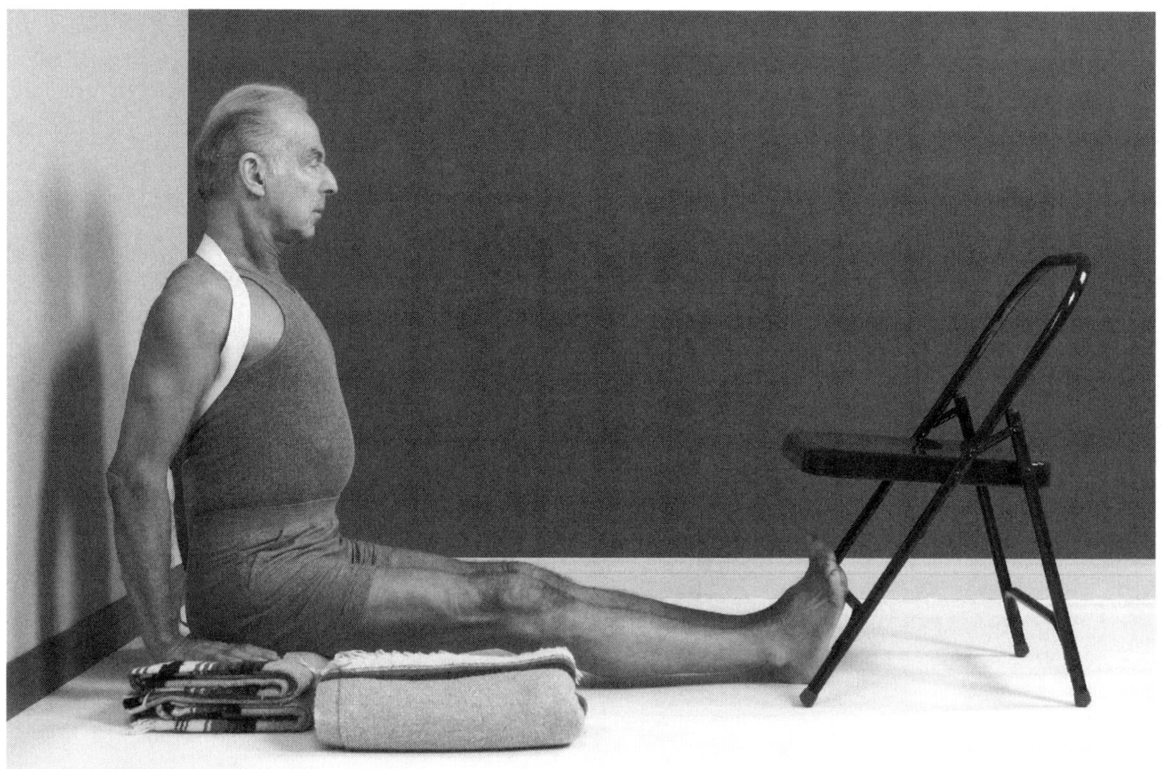

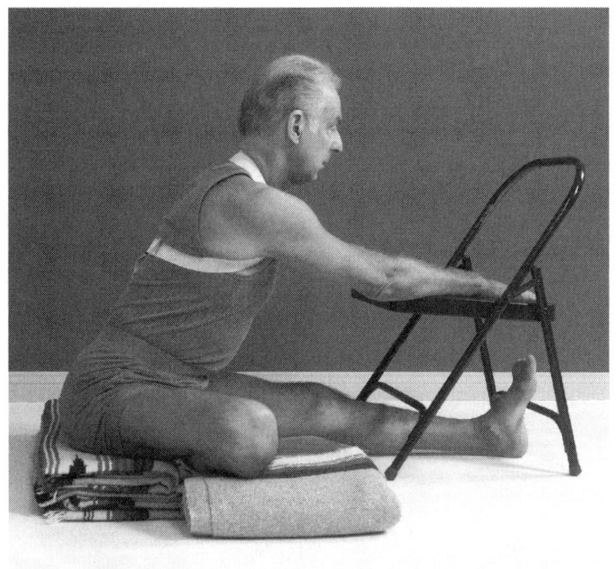

9. Press the hips back firmly into the blanket or bolster.

10. Reach across the seat of the chair more with the right hand, to increase the turning of the mid spine. Move the chair forward with each exhalation; pause with each inhalation. Try to keep the head in line with the spinal column, with the eyes resting into the cheekbones.

11. As the range of motion increases with practice, the hands can be brought up to grasp the arms of the chair. As this happens the chair can be pushed farther forward over the extended left leg. It is also possible to rest the head on a folded blanket or bolster on the seat of the chair in order to move deeper into the asana.

12. Breathe evenly, bringing the breath from the back around the ribs to the sternum. Hold the asana as long as it is comfortable.

13. Then use the hands to press down on the chair seat and raise the torso, keeping the head in line with the spine. Use the right hand on the outside of the right knee to bring it up.

14. Then place both hands behind the knee to draw the hamstring muscles and tendons back toward the hips, as if putting on a long stocking. Place the legs together and sit in Dandasana for several breaths. Then repeat on the other side.

BENEFITS

This pose aids digestion by flushing the liver and spleen. The kidneys are toned. By remaining in the pose, distress from an enlarged prostate gland can be reduced. The legs and arms are strengthened, and the hamstring muscles are stretched, improving flexibility and cutting down spasticity.

SUPPORTED SARVAGASANA

Shoulder Stand

A word of caution: Inverting the body is important for those of us who have MS. But please take into consideration what is appropriate and safe. In many cases simply putting your feet and legs up on the seat of a chair, with a lift under the pelvis, is a sufficient inversion.

Lying on a sofa, with several pillows under the legs so that the feet are above the heart, is also considered a safe inversion. In many cases, lying on a bed with pillows under the legs to raise the legs slightly above the heart, or putting the legs up on the wall with pillow support, is also very effective.

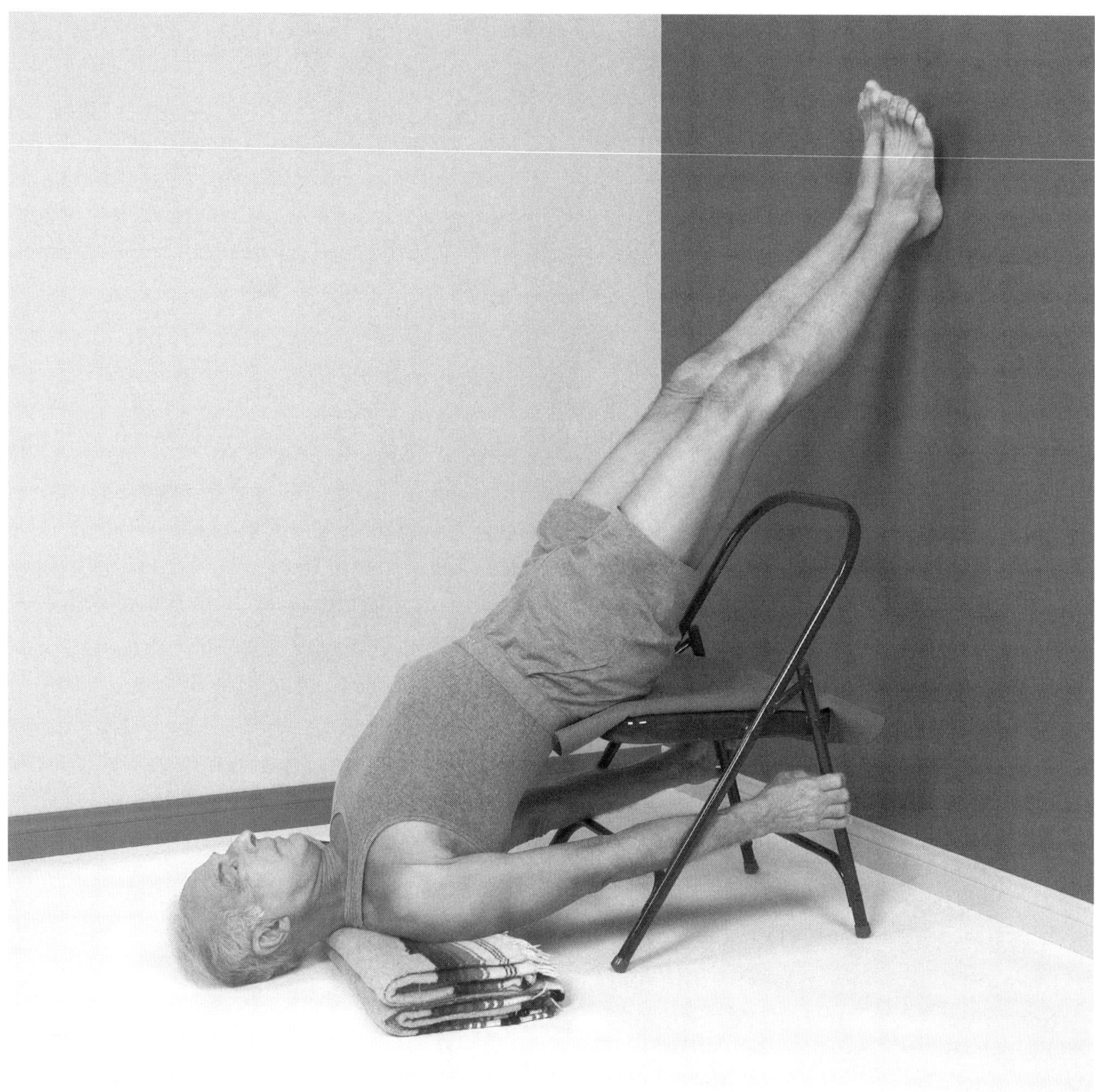

It is recommended two months be spent putting the feet slightly above the heart level before attempting Supported Sarvangasana or any other inversion. That would include Viparita Karani, as illustrated in the beginning chapters and shown here with the legs at 30 degrees, working up to 60 degrees, and then with the buttocks close to the wall to achieve a 90-degree angle.

If you have any blood pressure condition or eye pressure condition, obtain a doctor's permission before attempting this asana. I would also recommend that a Certified Iyengar instructor with an Intermediate Junior 2

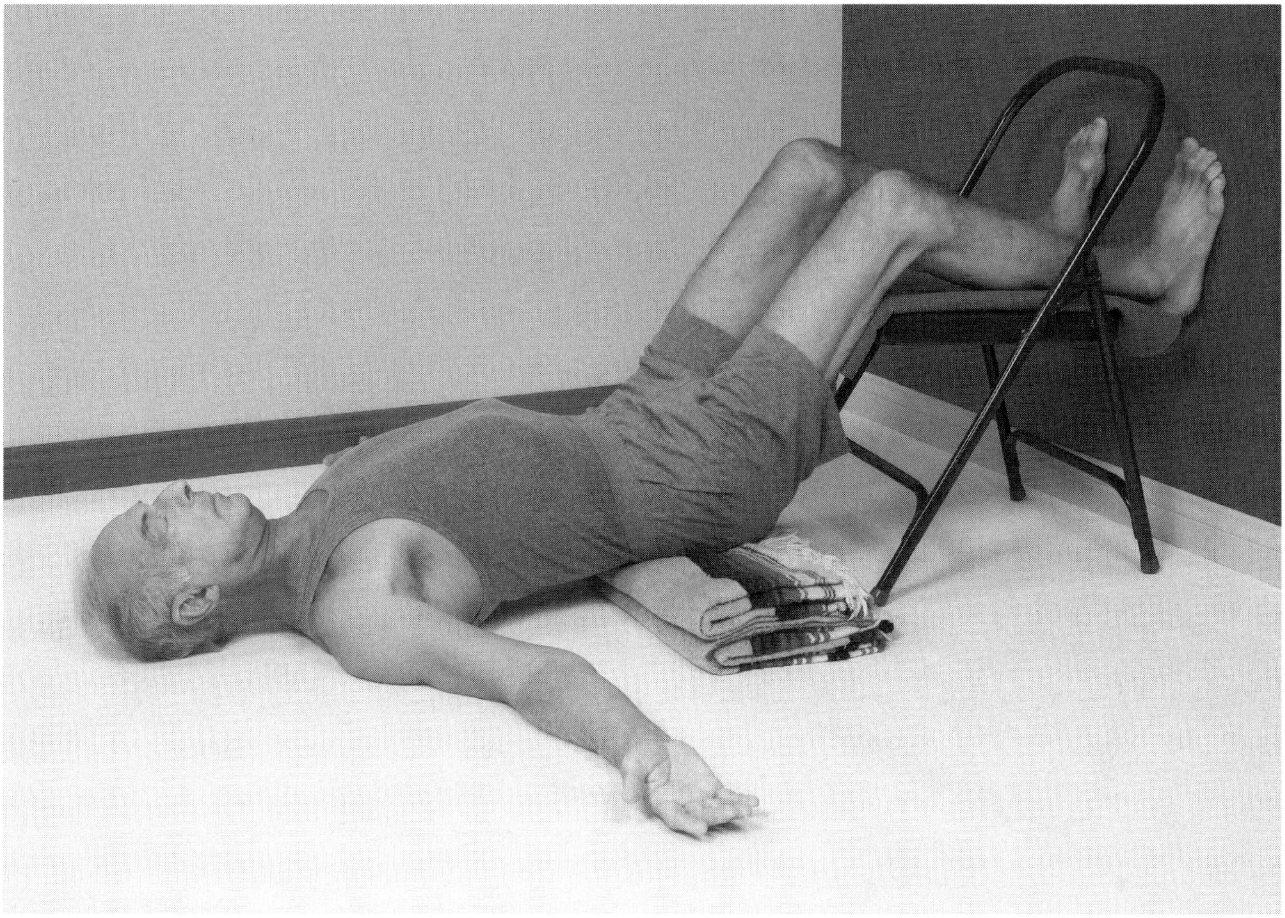

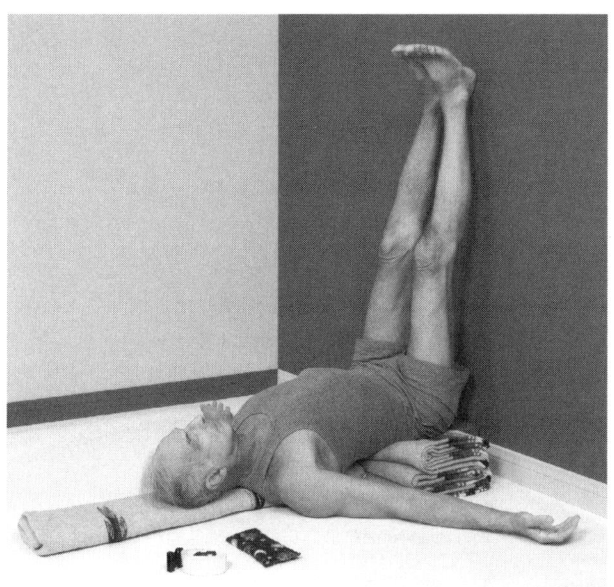

Viparita Karani

or above certificate be consulted and present when this asana is attempted.

1. Begin with a bolster, a chair, and a sticky mat. If tall, put one or two sticky mats on the seat of the chair.

2. Be sure that the folded edges of the sticky mats are in line with the edges of the seat of the chair.

3. Do not allow the sticky mats to extend beyond the edge of the chair seat. Two blankets folded into thirds may be placed under the shoulders. The length and width of the neck has to be considered in determining how much lift is needed.

4. If the torso is short, then a bolster can be placed under the shoulders and only one sticky mat on the seat of the chair. Lie down on the floor, with the chair near the wall.

5. Place the props under the shoulders, with the blanket positioned so that the shoulders are at least 1 or 2 inches from the edge.

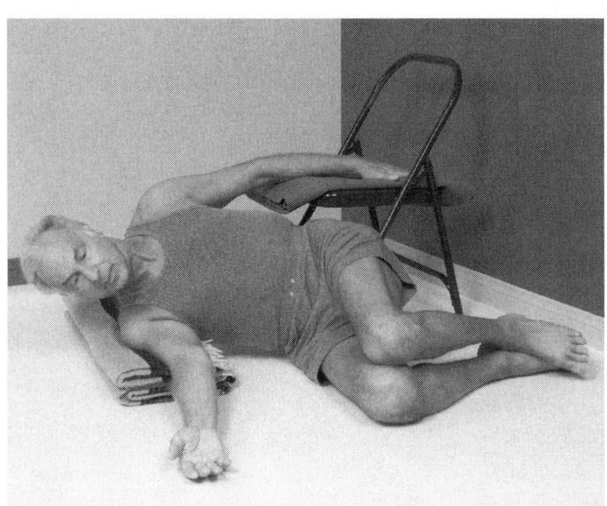

6. Extending the right arm forward, lie down with the hips close to the chair, legs bent. Roll slowly over on your back.

7. Then lift your feet onto the edge of the chair seat.

8. Take hold of the front legs of the chair and raise the hips and pull the chair quickly toward you in order to place the edge of the seat of the chair at the sacrum.

9. When the chair is secure and in the proper position, put your feet on the top of the back of the chair.

10. The hands and arms can be drawn through the legs of the chair, either to grasp the front legs or the back legs, depending upon your ability.

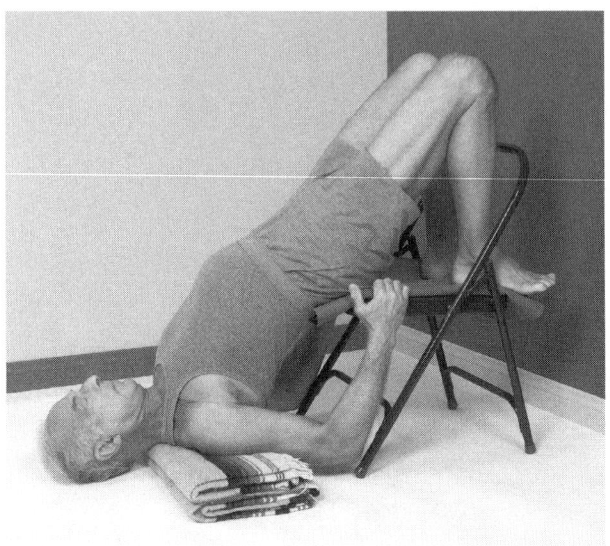

11. Then with an inhalation, lift the legs up and rest them against the wall with firm pressure on the large toe and heel.

12. If possible, turn the inner knees to the wall and rotate the upper thighs inward through the front groins to the back of the thigh.

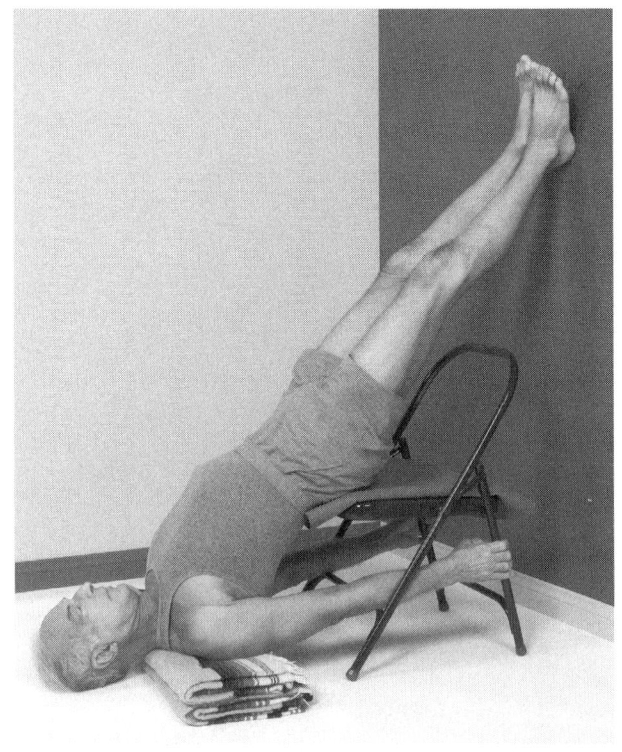

13. Bring the outer edge of the shoulders toward the floor. Draw the shoulder blades away from the ears and upward to support the ribs and lungs beneath them.

14. The center of the throat remains soft, and the head is balanced between the two points of the occipital bone as it moves gently away from the shoulders.

15. The eyes are resting in the cheekbones with the lids closed.

16. If it is difficult to hold the legs in this position, a strap can be placed around the mid thigh with a medium grip.

17. If it is necessary to open the chest, grip the seat of the chair with the hands, and press the elbows down firmly toward the floor.

18. The legs can be lifted away from the wall into a 90-degree angle with the hip joint, if a more intense inversion is desired.

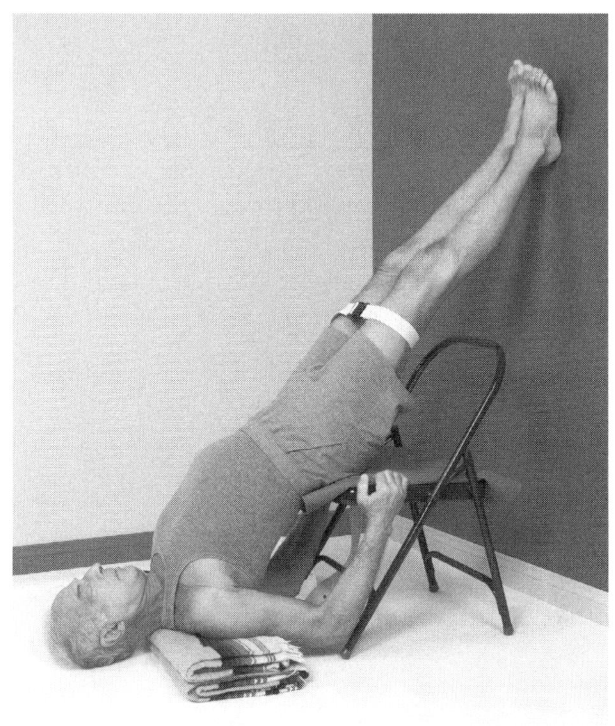

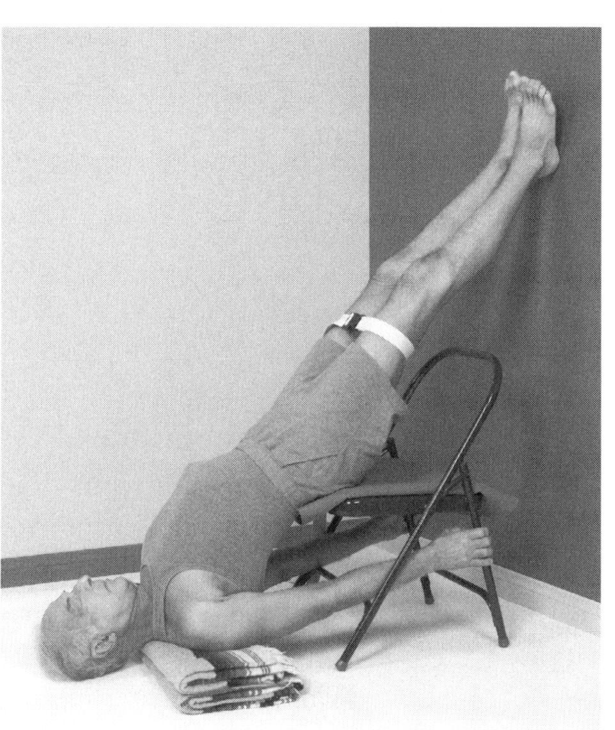

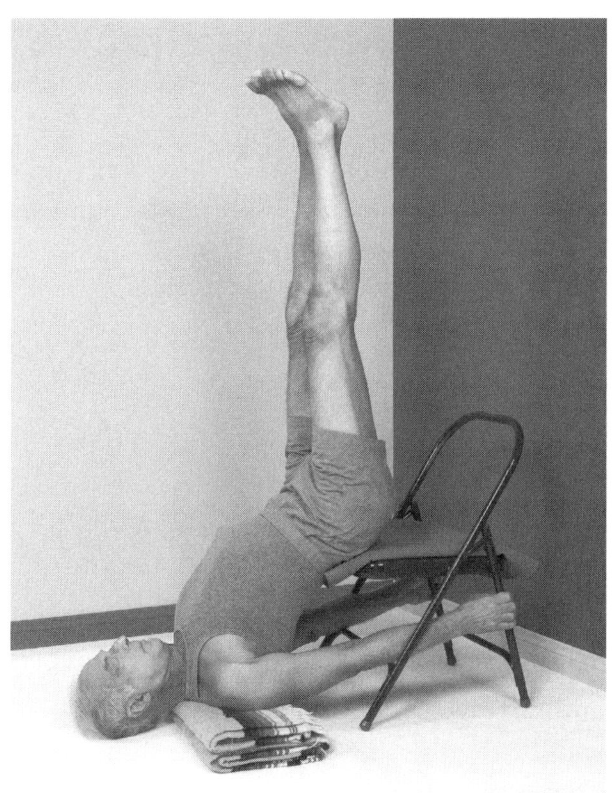

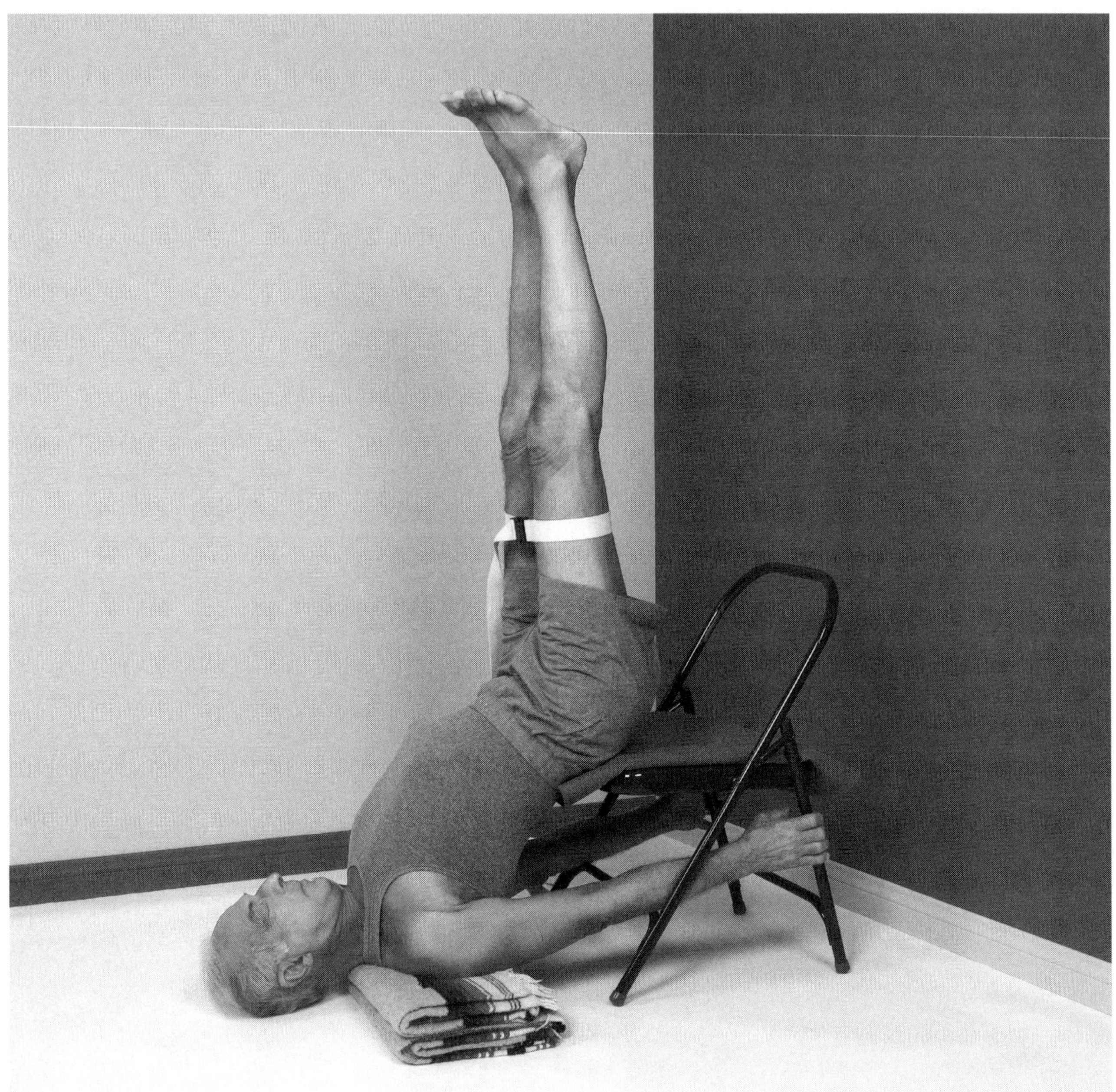

19. A strap can be added to help stabilize the posture.

20. After a period of practice, the pelvis can be opened further by bending the knees and resting the feet on the seat of the chair, supporting the shins on the back supports or seat of the chair.

21. To release from the pose, move the seat of the chair away from the sacrum toward the feet. Bring your feet to the center of the chair seat, keeping the hips slightly elevated.

22. Move the blankets or bolster toward the front legs of the chair, and rest the hips

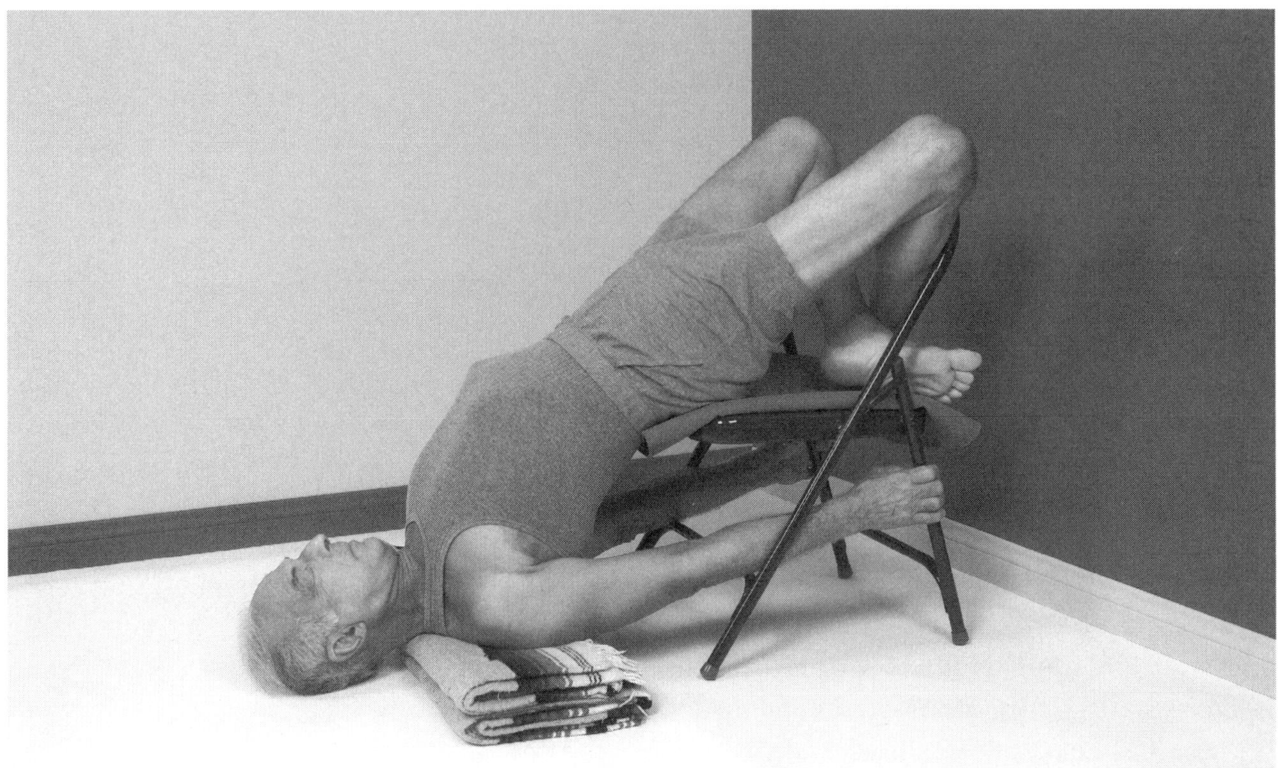

on the seat for support, allowing the legs to remain on the seat of the chair.

23. Remain in this pose for twice the time that was spent in the asana. Eyes are closed with the eyeballs resting toward the cheekbones. Do not force the eyes down. Let them float down with the breath.

24. The tongue is relaxed between the upper and lower palate. Breathe evenly. Then roll to the right.

25. Rest the head on the right arm, keep the knees soft, and relax the left arm in front of you.

26. Slowly push the chair toward the wall until your sacrum softly reaches the floor.

27. An alternative recovery would be to bring the right arm under your head, stretch the right leg toward the wall, and if possible ground the right foot onto the wall.

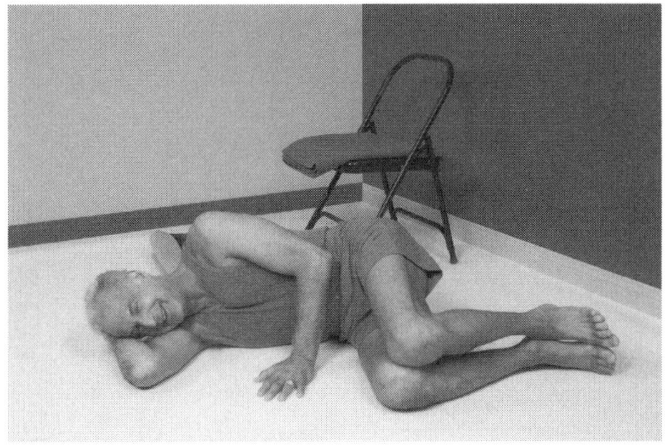

28. Bring the back of the head into line with the right heel, and lie in a straight line from head to toe.

29. It is important that the recovery from the asana be unhurried. The blood circulation should be allowed to return to normal, reestablishing the normal relationships between the heart, lungs, liver, and brain.

BENEFITS

This asana is one of the most important elements of the practice for those of us with Multiple Sclerosis. It brings harmony and balance and the sense of happiness to the mind, body, and the nervous system. In Sirsasana you are always looking outward, experiencing the strength and balance of the pose. In Saravangasana you are supported and gazing at the full body in all its beauty and power. With this reaffirmation, you are encouraged to allow the benefits of Saravangasana to become part of your daily life. The thyroid, pituitary, and pineal glands receive blood and additional nutrients. As a result, there is increased functioning due to a balanced body and brain. While there are many other benefits cited in *Light of Yoga*, the emphasis here is on the effect of the asana on the nervous and endcrine systems.

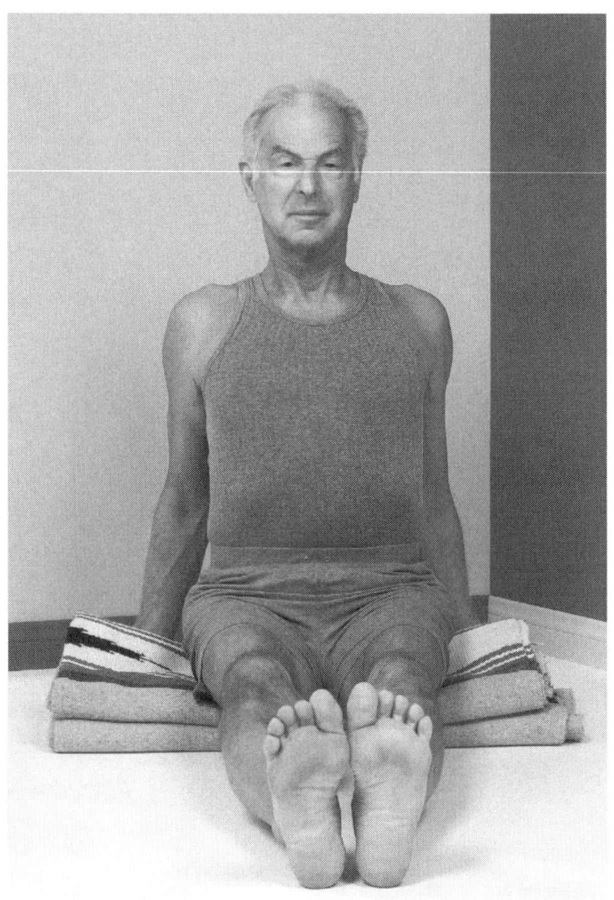

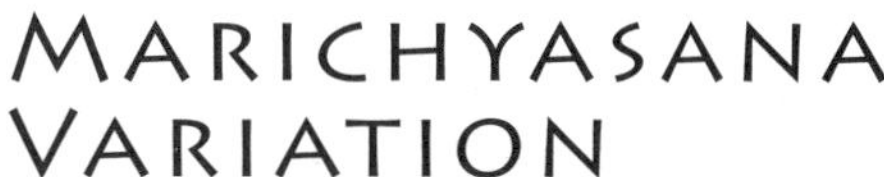

MARICHYASANA VARIATION

Grandfather of the Sun Pose

1. Start by sitting in Dandasana, with 1 or 2 folded blankets, depending on height, under the buttocks.

2. Lift the chest and side ribs, and press the heels away from the hips. Place blocks under the left knee and under the left heel and a folded blanket or block behind the right buttock against the wall.

3. With an exhalation, flex the right knee. Use the right hand on the inside of the right knee to draw the leg back, resting the heel against the blankets and under the knee. Inhale and raise the left hand in the air parallel to the left ear.

4. On an exhalation, begin to turn the navel to the right, moving the left elbow toward the right knee.

5. Hook the inside of the elbow around the right knee. Extend the palms and fingers parallel to the chest.

6. Keep the nose in line with the heart and the back of the head in line with the left hip.

7. Place your right hand on the block to bring both shoulders away from the ears.

8. The right ribs move back, coordinating with the left ribs moving forward.

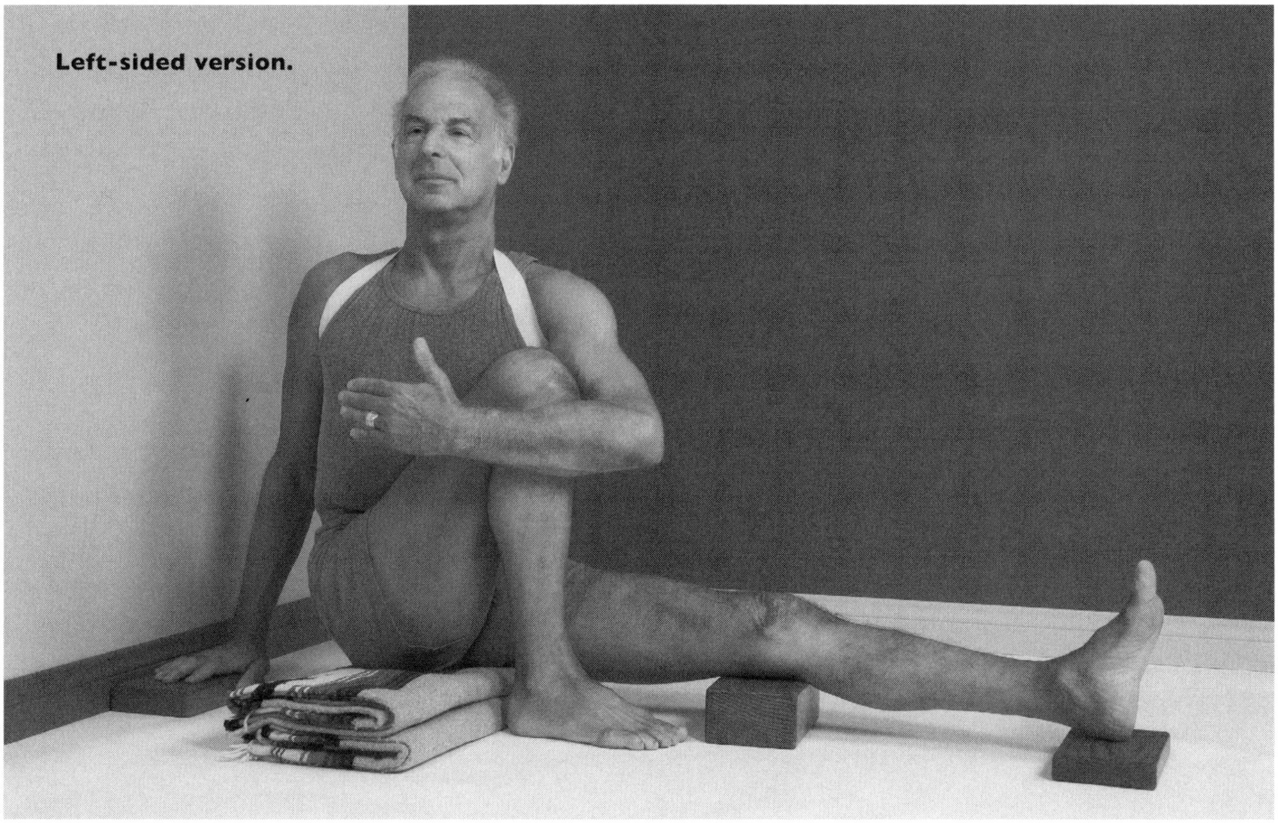

Left-sided version.

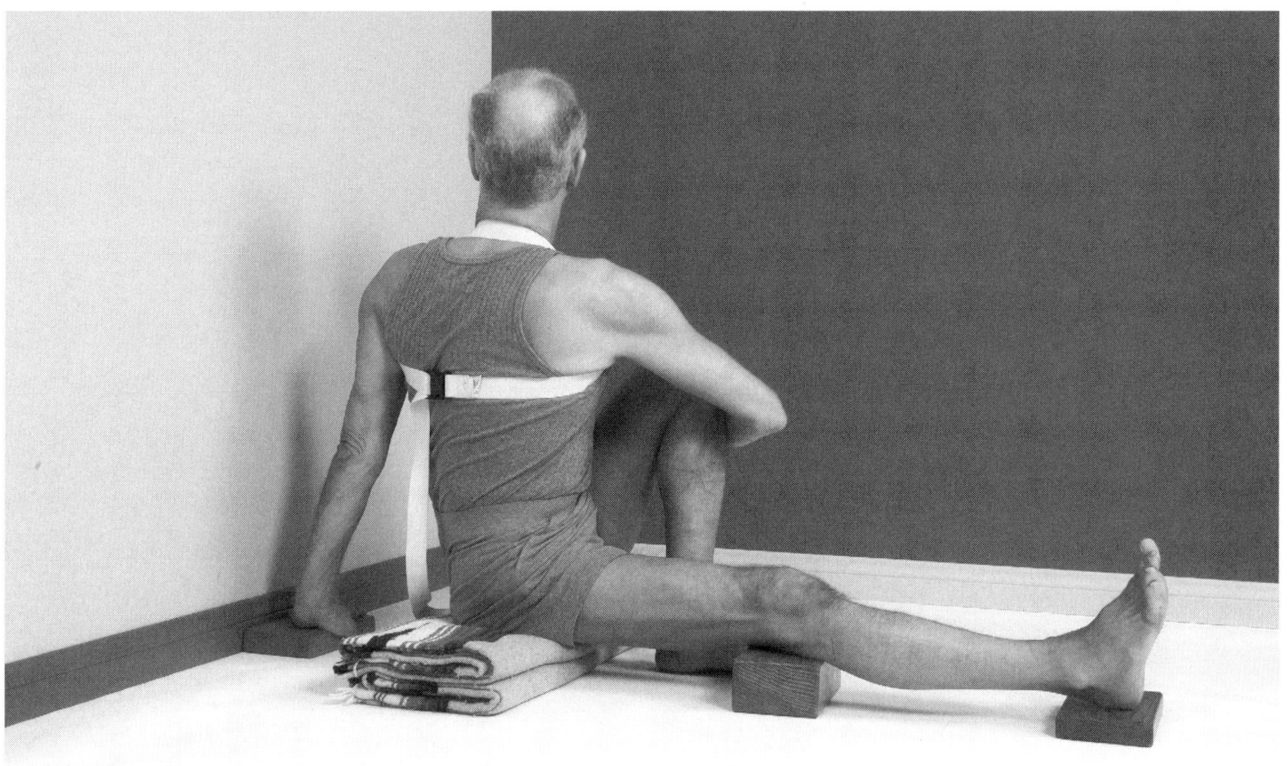

This movement strengthens and tones the mid back and abdominal muscles. If possible stand into the right foot and press the right hip forward to avoid any strain on the sacrum.

9. Breathe evenly, directing the breath into the right lung.

10. Please note that the height and placement of the blocks under the left leg may vary according to the length of the legs.

11. It is also recommended not to turn the head or neck in this asana because there is always the possibility that plaques could be present in the cervical spine. Any unwarranted pressure in this area could be detrimental to the student.

This picture illustrates the asana to the left, with the right leg supported. It is important that the back waist be lifted. The area between the lower ribs and the top of the pelvis should be even on both sides. The right arm extends from the center of the right shoulder blade to the elbow. The shoulder blades are parallel to the chest.

BENEFITS

This asana is recommended after Sarvangasana and before any forward bending postures. It reduces backache and discomfort in the hips. Lumbar mobility is increased. This stimulation of the liver, kidneys, heart, lungs, and digestive and elimination systems is dynamic and essential.

Pranayama and Relaxation

The breath is the metronome to the music of the soul.

—Eric Small

A Brief Explanation

The study and practice of pranayama is an essential and important factor in developing a sustained hatha yoga practice. (Prana means the life force, and yama means discipline.) If you are interested in pursuing the full and dynamic investigation into pranayama, then it is suggested that you read Light on Pranayama by B. K. S Iyengar. For pranayama to be utilized by those of us with multiple sclerosis, Mr. Iyengar recommends that only four of the pranayama disciplines be used.

Some cautions and suggestions that should be mentioned: Bowels and bladder should be empty. It is best if the stomach is empty, but a cup of milk tea or cocoa may be ingested. Allow at least 6 hours after a meal; a light meal can be taken after the practice. The practice should be done in a clean and airy place that is as quiet as possible.

The best results from pranayama will be achieved when a steady and regular practice is performed at the same time of day, if possible. The best time is early in the morning or late afternoon. If a class session is the only time to practice, then the instructor will create the best possible atmosphere. The classic posture is sitting with folded legs in various positions. If you have a limited ability to maintain an erect posture, Mr. Iyengar suggests that the prone position be used.

It is also suggested that if a wheelchair or chair is necessary, that a rolled sticky mat or blanket be placed parallel to the seat of the chair, behind the shoulder blades, to help open the chest.

an effective tool to reduce this overheating. Trembling and perspiration will occur when beginning this practice. It will disappear after a short period of time.

The head normally hangs down, with the chin near the raised chest. Some of us with MS have a condition known as L'hermitte's syndrome. In order to avoid any possibility of it occurring, permit the head to drop only a short distance. Draw up the mastoid bone

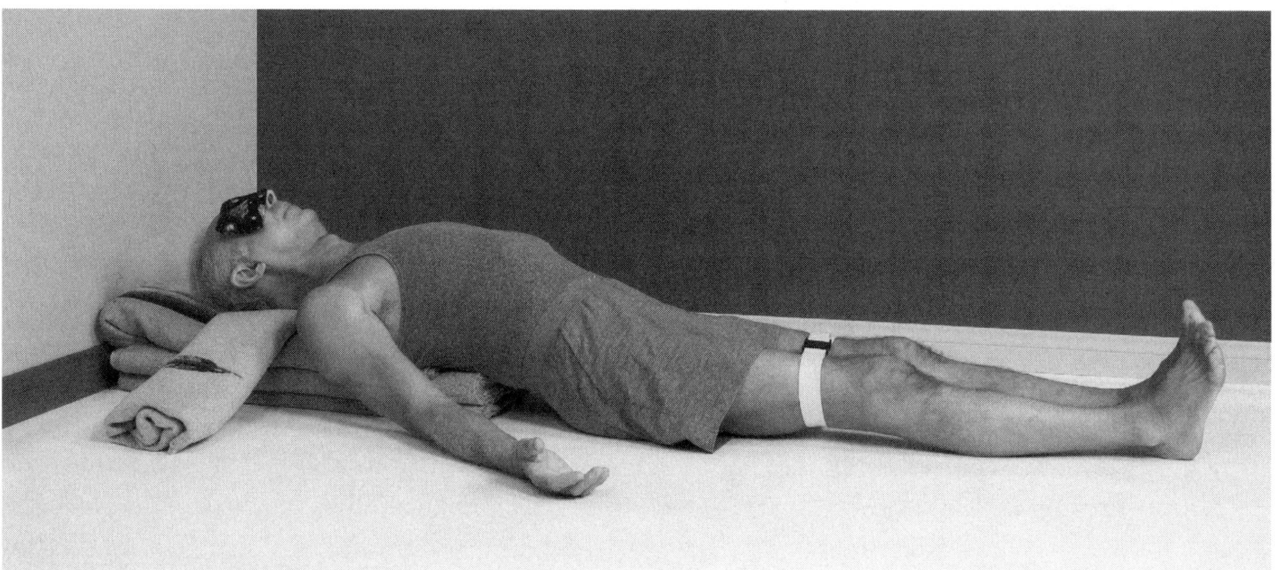

behind the ears, and concentrate on bringing the eyes down into the cheek bones. This will create the same effect as pressing the chin toward the chest.

Allow the tongue to rest away from the top and bottom palates and the throat and neck to be relaxed and soft. Keeping the breath even will lead to healthy nerves and an evenness of mind and temper. Do not force the breath or harden the body. If the

There should be no strain in the face, eyes, ears, neck, shoulders, arms, thighs, or feet. Please note that a strap is used around the thighs to release tension. Rolled sticky mats can also be used, by placing them parallel and tightly against the legs to help maintain relaxed legs and feet.

The nervous system of MS students has a tendency to become overheated due to the stress of everyday life. Pranayama is

practice is harsh and aggressive, the respiration process and the nervous system will be adversely affected.

Allow the hands to rest on the thighs if sitting, and on the floor with the palms up and the fingers completely relaxed if in a prone position. (The hand position known as Janu Mudra, which is the tip of the thumb touching the tip of the index finger, and the description of the chakras, is not dealt with in this book. That material is best investigated under the personal guidance of an experienced certified instructor.)

When it is no longer possible to concentrate on the breath and keep the pace of the breathing smooth, then stop. It is not recommended that you continue the practice of the breath when it is no longer positive and comfortable. In the beginning, your practice may only last 5 minutes. That's all right. The next day start again. You may then be able to practice only a few minutes more. Do not be discouraged. It will take time and practice to develop the ability to maintain and accomplish the full practice. Regardless of the apparent lack of progress, you are moving forward. Mr. Iyengar has often said that the practice of yoga is like a fine meal. If you eat quickly and gorge on the food, you miss out on the subtleties and nuances of the experience. If instead you take small bites and savor the different flavors and textures, the experience becomes memorable. Yoga is absorbed into the consciousness in tiny incre-

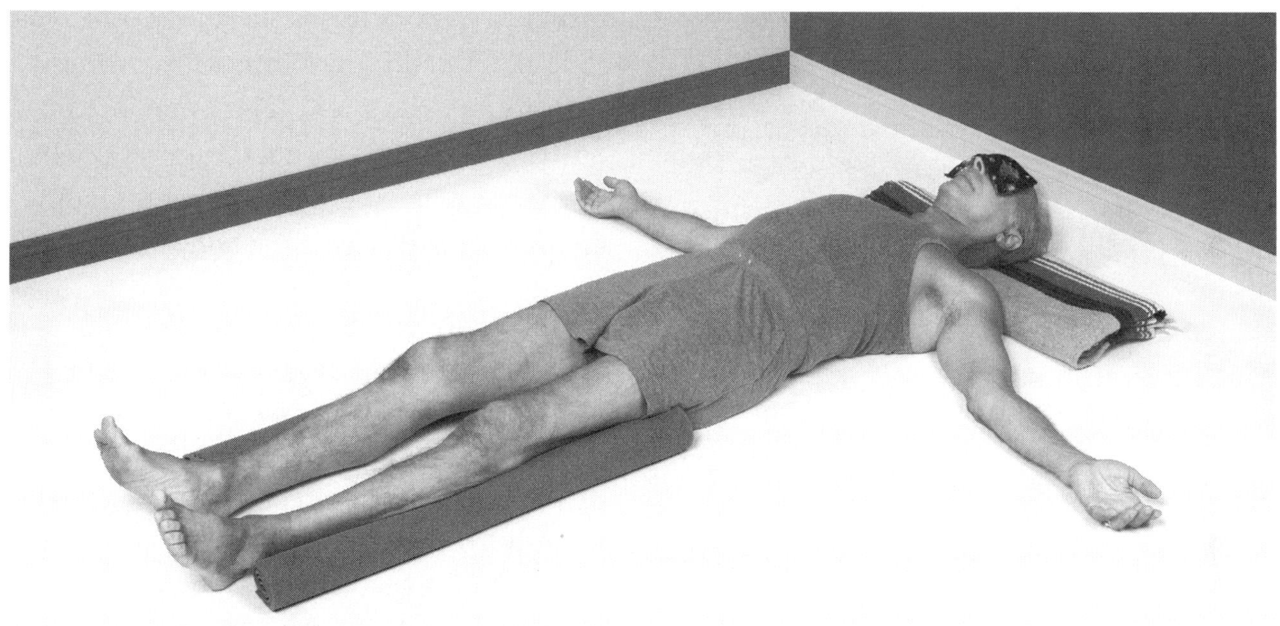

ments, penetrating into the infinite structures of the body, becoming part and parcel of the whole being.

After performing your pranayama practice, lie or sit in Savasana. Spend at least 5 minutes allowing the mind to become very quiet and the body to be completely relaxed. As a result of the Savasana, the body and the mind are refreshed.

With these suggestions it is hoped that you will experience the wonder and enjoyment of this part of your hatha yoga practice. Remember, for best results the one-on-one instruction and guidance of a qualified teacher is invaluable.

Prone Position

1. Start first of all with arranging the blankets. Fold the blankets into quarters, remembering that each person has a different body. Your teacher, trainer, or therapist will be able to adjust these poses to adapt them particularly for you.

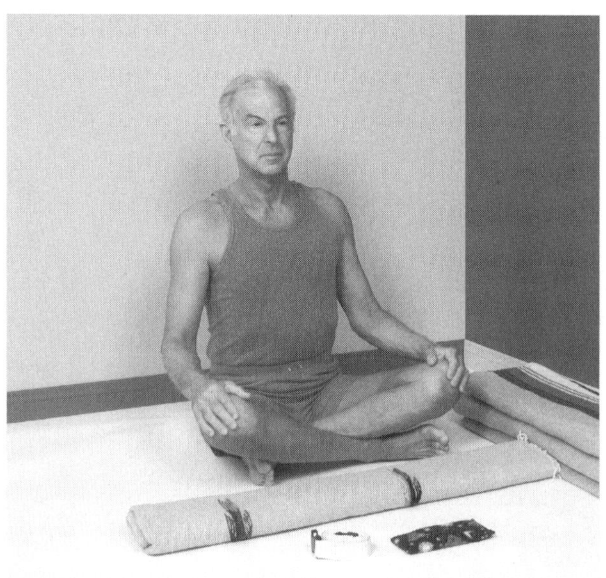

Blanket folded into quarters.

2. Place a strap on your thighs, then lower your hands to the floor, slightly behind the hips, fingers pointed forward. Raise the chest, keeping the chin tucked toward the collarbone. Begin to bend the elbows toward the floor as you slowly lower your torso onto the blankets. As your hands slip toward the hips, slide them under the buttocks, pressing the flesh toward the knees. This is important in order to place the sacrum, the spinal column, and the head into proper alignment. This promotes full relaxation of the body and brain.

When women lie prone on the floor it is important that the blanket does not lie beneath the lower back, but for men it is perfectly all right.

Women's organs are arranged a little differently than men's. Women need to avoid any pressures against the kidneys, colon, or reproductive organs. So when a woman lies back, the blankets (2 or 3) are positioned just at the bottom of the ribs, and the lower back is free from any pressure

The head, from the shoulders (not from the ears but from the shoulders) upward, is supported by the blankets. In some cases it is difficult for the legs to be relaxed, and you will want to use a strap at the middle of the thighs to hold the legs firmly into the pelvis and allow the weight of the leg and pelvis to descend.

3. You can enhance this even more by putting a bolster or a blanket under the knees, depending on your size.

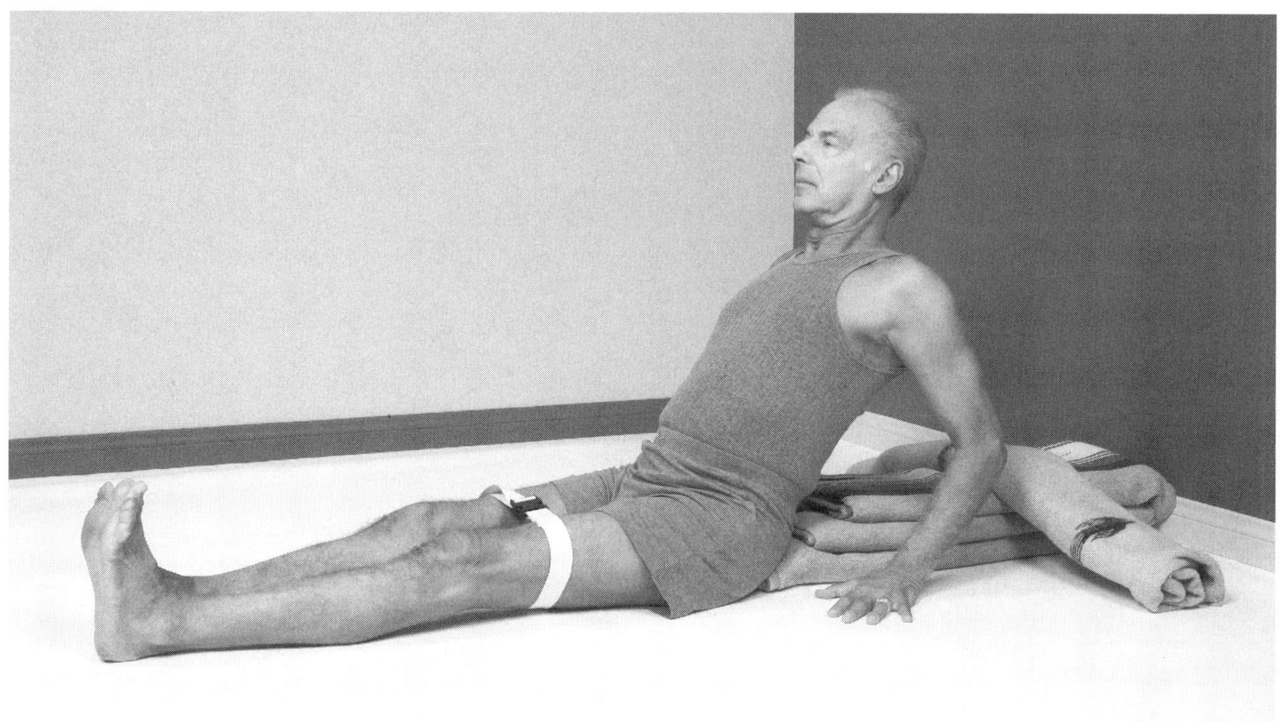

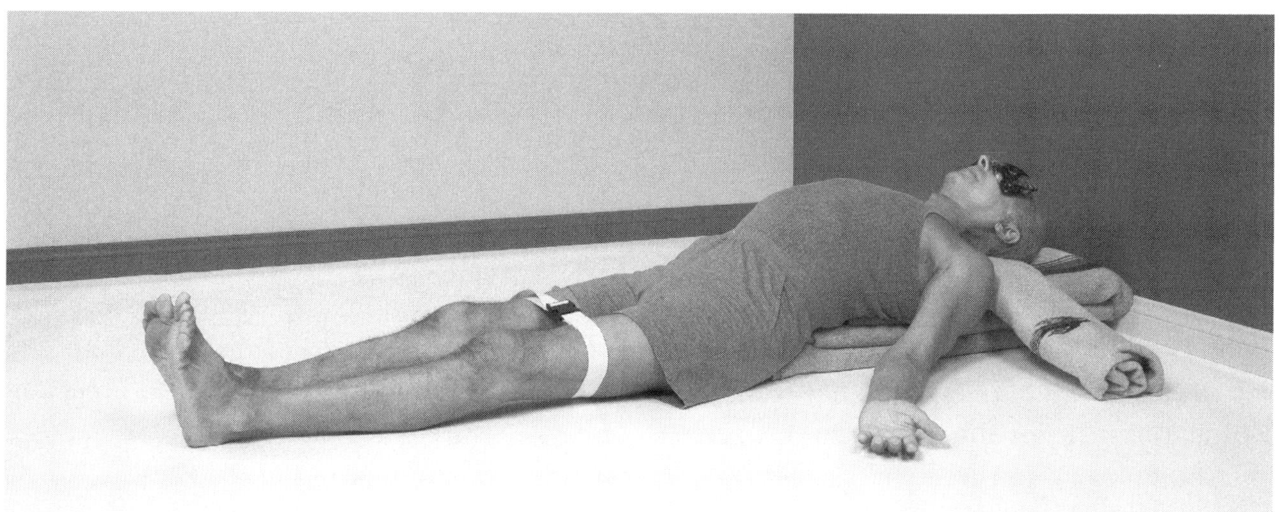

Blankets reaching only to upper iliac crest.

4. At this point you have nice relaxed legs and a very relaxed pelvis. The sacrum, the bottom of spinal column, is well supported. The shoulders are moving back and away from the front of the chest. With just this very small adjustment, this whole area of the thorax, the place where you breathe, has been opened.

5. Place the hands (palms up) and the arms 30 degrees away from the hips. Allow

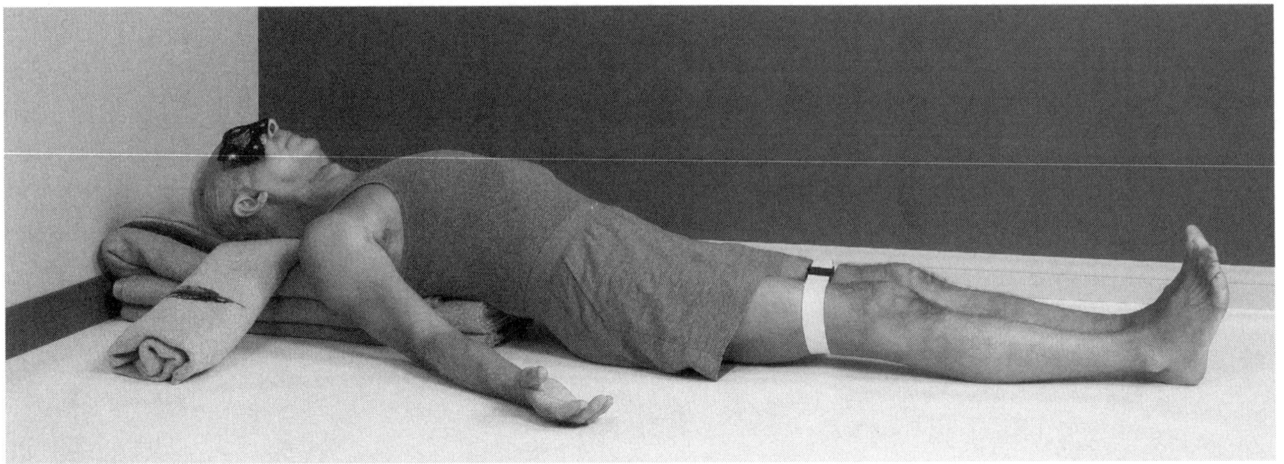

With the leg tie.

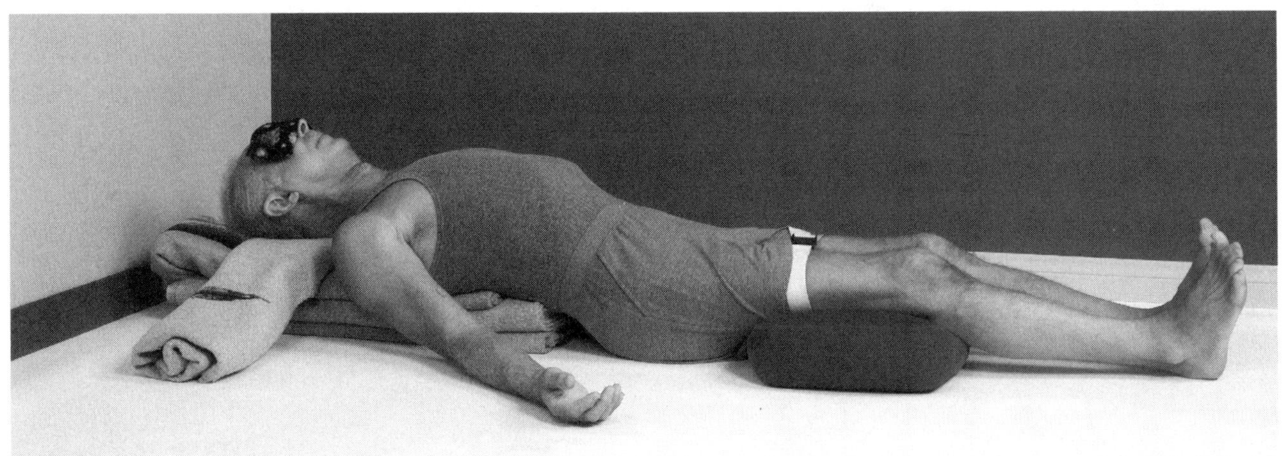

With bolster / With eyebag.

the weight of the thumb to move toward the floor, externally rotating the arms and rotating the shoulders even farther away from the ribs at the front of the torso. Do not force the thumb to go to the floor. Allow it to do so at its own pace. As the thumbs and palms open, so the upper part of the lungs is less constrained and breathing capacity increases accordingly.

6. The breath in this posture begins from behind the navel as it moves toward the spine, allowing the diaphragm to pull downward in the lumbar region and opening the chest. This helps the ribs to catch the breath and bring it toward the sternum. The breath in the restorative posture should always come in through the nose in a particular way. Inhale through the bottom of the nose near the upper lip, and as you exhale, the breath comes out at the tip of the nose. This creates a particular rhythm. Within just a few moments, you will notice that the breath changes its rhythm from a short inhalation-exhalation to a fuller inhalation and long slow exhalation.

Mr. Iyengar has explained that inhalation energizes the body, and exhalation is a matter of surrender. Exhalation permits the physical body to release and relax, especially the central nervous system. In this posture the body is well supported by the blankets, and we attempt to just gently open the breathing apparatus, which is the lungs, the bronchial tubes, and the diaphragm. The pose is also kind to the liver, and in this posture the breathing itself gently increases blood flow to the brain.

7. In addition, an eye bag can be applied at any point during this pose. It is applied from the eyebrow. You gently draw the forehead skin down toward the nose and allow the weight of the eye bag to go toward the temples and ears. The eyes are not looking into the bag or into the lid. The eyes are looking down toward the heart to release any tension from the frontal lobes of the brain. By eliminating stimulation that comes through the eyes and by activating your ears to listen to the breath, you have reduced the outside stress that comes to the body and are now starting to explore the power of the mind.

Smooth Breath

1. After assuming the appropriate posture, as outlined above, allow the body and the mind to relax with normal breathing for at least 5 to 10 minutes. At this point the breath can be directed in the following manner: The inhalation arises from behind the navel into the side chest. The breath enters the nostril at the base of the nose, above the upper lip. There can be a slight dilatation of the nostril if possible. The exhalation exits from the tip of the nose, with the nostrils relaxed. The chest is kept open, and the navel moves back toward the spine.

2. In the Smooth Breath, as in all the pranayamas, start with an exhalation to clear the lungs and release tension. Inhale, allowing the breath to arise from behind the navel into the side chest, dilating the nostrils slightly. Then exhale slowly through the tip of the nose, keeping the chest open, the torso relaxed, and the eyes resting in the cheekbones. Continue the smooth breath as long as it is comfortable to do so. One round, or a cycle, is an exhalation, an inhalation, and an exhalation.

3. Then breathe normally for 1 minute and start the next round. You will soon discover that the exhalation is becoming longer than the inhalation, and that is desired. The number of rounds is entirely a personal choice.

Ujjayi

This pranayama is the process in which the lungs are fully expanded and the chest is puffed out like a pigeon. There is also a sound created by bringing the breath in along the upper palate, which sounds similar to the surf rushing onto the shore. The exhale sounds like the surf pulling away from the shore.

1. Begin with a smooth exhalation. Completely empty the lungs without pressure.

2. Take a slow, steady, deep breath through both nostrils creating an "ah" sound. Bring the breath across the upper palate. The sound should be audible.

3. Fill the lungs to the top or whatever is possible. It is important that the eyes stay down resting near the cheekbones on the inhalation. Then without retaining the breath begin the exhalation.

Please note that it has been suggested that breath retention for those of us with MS is not beneficial in the beginning stages of the practice. It can cause the nervous system to become agitated and overheated. There is the possibility of too many adverse effects.

4. On the exhalation the breath is released in a slow and deliberate manner through both nostrils. The chest should remain as open as possible. The navel moves gently toward the spine. Avoid any tension in the neck and shoulders. The "ah" sound should not have any rasping or catching sounds. At the end of the exhalation, without any forcing or pressure, begin the smooth breath.

There is a variation to the classic approach. For those of us with MS, Mr. Iyengar has indicated that the nervous system has to be protected from overheating and agitation. Therefore 3 smooth breaths are recommended between each of the pranayamas, as follows: 3 smooth breaths; on the 3rd exhalation begin the Ujjayi inhaltion/exhalation; then 3 smooth breaths complete the cycle.

5. Begin the 2nd cycle at the end of the 3rd smooth exhalation.

After a time, this practice becomes very comfortable and the results are very satisfying. Remember that this particular pranayama can be done at any time, conditions permitting.

Viloma One

This pranayama consists of a three-part breath on the inhalation and a smooth ujjyai breath on the exhalation. Its basic purpose is to raise awareness of the breathing apparatus and the control that is possible.

The inhalation is separated into three parts.

1. Begin with 3 smooth breaths

2. On the third exhalation of the smooth breath, begin the inhalation from the navel and bring it to the edge of the rib cage at the diaphragm. Pause. Observe that the diaphragm is soft.

3. Then lift the breath to the middle of the rib cage, encouraging the ribs to move outward. Pause.

4. Lift the breath to the collarbones or sternum, raising the sides of the chest and releasing the eyes down toward the heart.

5. Then release the breath in a long smooth ujjayi descending to the area below the navel.

6. The next inhalation then begins the 3 smooth breath cycle.

Because of the energy used in this pranayama, do only what is appropriate for you. Do not force the number of repetitions.

The classic instruction for this discipline is to retain the breath at each portion of the inhalation. That does not apply here, as breath retention at this stage of the practice is not recommended.

Viloma Two

In this pranayama, the exhalation is separated into three parts.

1. Begin with 3 smooth breaths
2. On the 3rd exhalation, lift the breath up through the rib cage to the top of the sternum, using a soft ujjayi.
3. Release the breath from the collarbones to the middle of the rib cage.
4. Then release the breath to the bottom of the rib cage at the diaphragm.
5. Allow the breath to settle gently at or below the navel.
6. Inhale and start the 3 smooth breath cycle again.

The same rule applies here as it did in Viloma One. Do not force the number of cycles, and do only what is appropriate for you.

Viloma Three

In this pranayama, the previous disciplines are combined. It is important that all three be done as a unit. If at any time fatigue is experienced, stop the practice and go to Savasana (the deep relaxation, or corpse pose).

1. Begin with the 3 smooth breaths.
2. At the end of the 3rd exhalation of the smooth breath, begin with a three part inhalation, as described in Viloma One.
3. At the top of the inhalation, begin the exhalation as described in Viloma Two.
4. At the end of the exhalation, begin the inhalation with the 3 smooth breaths.
5. At the completion of the pranayama practice, go directly to Savasana. Spend as much time as necessary to feel refreshed and invigorated before starting activities.

BENEFITS

The absorption of oxygen into the body is essential for those of us with MS. Our nervous systems demand an effective oxygen delivery system in order for us to complete our days' activities. We also need an effective tool to handle the stress and tension that comes our way from so many different sources. The study of pranayama is vast and complex and requires a lifetime of practice and dedication. Selecting these five segments to begin with will enable us to experiment and develop a practice and reap the benefits of this most amazing practice. This is only the tip of the iceberg. There are many experienced and dedicated certified teachers who have a daily pranayama practice and who are willing to share their experiences with us. Contact with these teachers would be of great benefit.

Those of us who have a pranayama practice teach from that practice and look forward to students who are willing to make a commitment to enhancing their knowledge and improve their health. We must also recognize that life is often filled with good intentions.

We often start off with a great deal of enthusiasm. Then one thing or another prevents us from fulfilling our plans. We give up for just a little while, which then stretches into a long time, and we lose heart and become frustrated. What is reassuring about pranayama is that the breath is always there, waiting to start again and again. Many longtime practitioners have stopped and started numerous times, until the practice has become firmly established, and now they would not give it up under any circumstances. Having seen the benefits it has brought to our lives, its value is beyond measure.

Floor Savasana

1. Depending on the conditions, it is recommended to lie on the floor with a blanket or on the floor itself. A folded blanket is placed under the head, touching the top of the shoulders. If it is difficult to keep the legs straight and relaxed, please note that a rolled sticky mat is placed tightly alongside each leg. In the event that there is tightness or discomfort in the low back, a rolled sticky mat is placed under the knees and a block placed under the feet.

2 A strap around the mid thigh often helps to maintain a relaxed position. Then place the hands behind the hips, open the chest, and lie down on the floor slowly keeping the chest and neck relaxed. Once prone on the floor, draw the flesh of the buttock down toward the thighs. If an eye-bag or folded towel is available, then place it over the eyes. Draw the shoulder blades toward the spine, with the lower point of the blades moving down and in toward the heart. Lift the space between the shoulder blades toward the heart. Then position the arms 30 degrees away from the hips, with the palms up, fingers relaxed, and the mound of the thumb descending to the floor. This will open

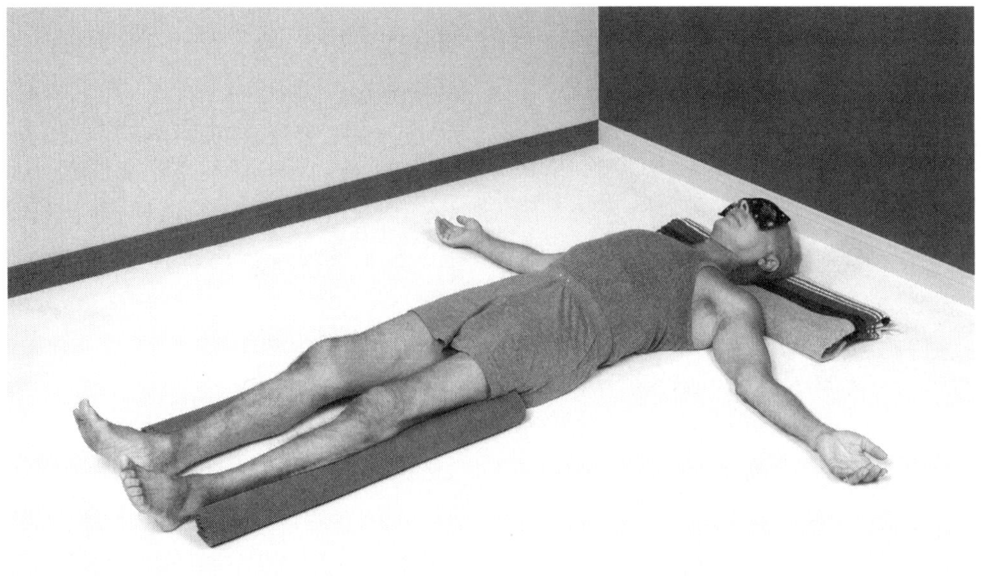

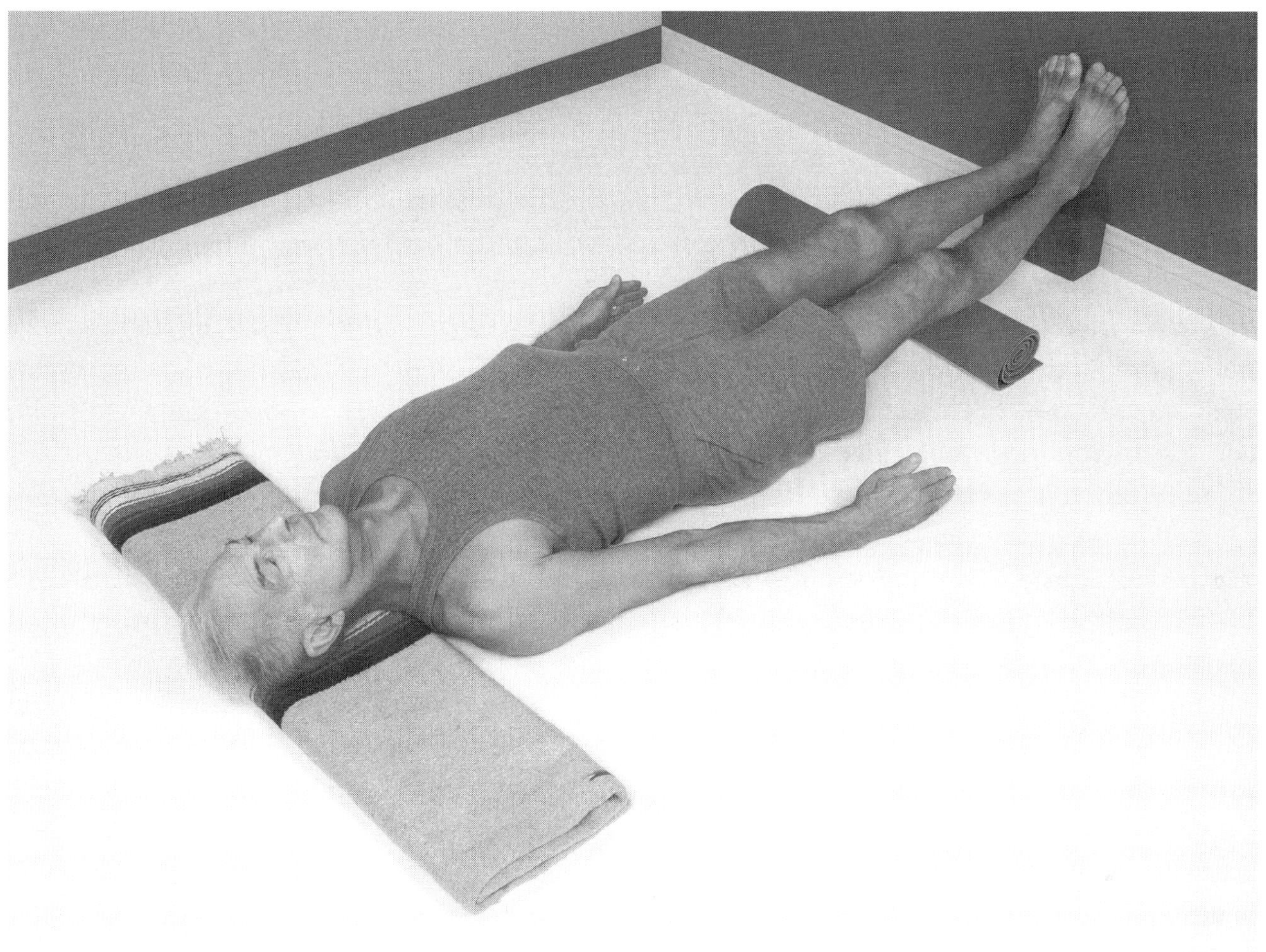

Placement of the sticky mat.

the sides of the chest to allow easy, smooth breath.

3. Be sure that the chin is level with the sternum. If it is not, place an additional blanket or lift under the back of the head. Release the weight of the head into the blanket, balancing the weight of the head between the two points of the occipital bone. Release the weight of the jaw toward the ears. Allow the lips to part so that the upper lip drapes over the teeth. As the face releases tension, bring the eyes down toward the heart from the back of the skull, over the crown, down the forehead, over the eyebrows. The sides of the eye will elongate, easing tension from the temples.

4. A major portion of our nervous energy is used to maintain a pleasant expression. It is important to spend a few moments releasing the facial muscles to achieve a more satisfying Savasana. Allow the weight of the bones of the face to draw down toward the floor. The throat should be soft in the center, with the sides of the neck moving down toward the floor. With that action, the outer edge of the shoulders will descend into the

floor, releasing any tension in the collarbones or upper ribs. The upper arm becomes heavy and the forearm spreads out. The wrist and hands become light together with the palms of the hands.

5. Allow the weight of the torso to rest against the floor. If there is a misalignment of the rib cage due to weakness of the torso muscles or curvature of the spinal column, then place a wedge or rolled sticky mat under the side of the torso that moves toward the floor, from the armpit to the waist.

6. The weight of the pelvis moves downward, causing the lower abdomen to soften away from the rim of the pelvic girdle. This releases any tension in the psoas muscles and the intestinal tract.

7. The heavy muscles of the thighs release toward the femur bones. The hamstrings are supported by the floor, allowing them to relax. The shins descend down without hyperextending the backs of the knees. If there is hyperextension, place a blanket or a sticky mat under the backs of the knees. The feet are at first touching at the insides of the heels, then, as they relax, allow them to separate.

8. The breath is even and soft. Encourage the breath to arise from behind the navel into the side chest. It is important to be focused on the breathing. There is a tendency to allow the events of the day to become prominent or to project ahead to what actions will occur after class or to just drift and dream.

This asana is one of the most important to master. Not only is it an opportunity for the consciousness to absorb the lessons of the class, but also the organic results of the asana practice become part of the healing process that brings vibrant health. Savasana provides an opportunity to become quiet within, to experience the awakening of the inner body, and to learn how to listen to the inner body and address its needs on a daily basis through your hatha yoga practice. There is a sense of security in this pose because you are aware that the instructor is watching and is there to be of assistance. Absorbing the silence around you through the breath is a rare privilege and not often available.

9. When it is no longer possible to remain focused on the breath, then roll to your right. Rest the head in the crook of the right arm. Bring your blanket under the head on top of the arm. Bring the left knee over the right thigh and rest the inside of the knee on a block, blanket or rolled sticky mat. Stretch the right leg out and bring the back of the head into line with the right foot. Lie in a straight line from head to heel, left hand resting on the floor in front of the torso. Remain in this position with the eyes closed for a few minutes.

10. Sit up by pressing down with the left hand into a comfortable sitting position and put the blankets under the buttocks. Keeping the eyes closed, breath easily and softly. Open the eyes on the inhalation and salute the teacher.

11. Be mindful to return all the props to their place so that the yoga space is clean and clear. This applies not only to the commercial space, it is also important for your own practice space in your home.

Namaste.

Part
II

Function-Directed Yoga for Functionally Impaired Individuals

In this section we address how yoga can help with seven different problems that often come along with multiple sclerosis, giving scientific and medical explanations intended for informed patients and the larger medical community. We describe suitable yoga poses for managing each problem. These poses are intended for people with mild or severe multiple sclerosis (MS), those just recently diagnosed who want to retain all possible function, and those "coming back" from more severe MS due to the helpful effects of medications or the vicissitudes of this whimsical disease.

Some of the poses may seem impossible, but most are given in three versions:

- The classical or standard pose is for people with mild MS, pretty good balance, and a lot of guts.
- The entry-level pose is at the other end of the spectrum. It is designed for the earliest attempts at the pose by people with restricted function, and for those who might face yoga with reservations.
- The intermediate pose, as the name suggests, is a transition from the beginning, entry-level pose toward the classical pose.

The poses are grouped according to their benefits. Patients may detect new limitations in vigor, range of motion, spasticity, strength, coordination, or balance. They, their physicians, physical therapists, or other health professionals may begin with the poses that are especially useful for their particular purpose.

The classical poses are immediately suitable for patients with the least MS involvement. They are also valuable for those who cannot perform them at present but who will do the less challenging forms of yoga, at least for a while. For these individuals, getting an idea of what lies ahead—the gestalt of the fully realized forms of the poses they are beginning to work on—can be conceptually important and a source of inspiration.

The classical poses are brilliantly and smoothly put together. Each one is like a Beethoven string quartet, a great piece of art. In this book they are grouped by emphasis, but each has elements of stretch that expand range of motion and oppose spasticity, and each improves strength, coordination, and balance. The poses are like the smooth stones found at the edge of the seas, worn and polished by many years of continual action and thought by the yoga community.

The more difficult classical version of each pose is given first to present the set of bodily relationships that may be preserved more or less in the entry-level pose. The entry-level and intermediate poses offer many degrees of intensity that progress gradually toward the definitive, classical pose.

Remember that each pose is a composition of form and function that has evolved over time by a very large number of yoga participants. Each often incorporates an ingenious and profound interplay of contraction and relaxation, with feedback so well integrated and smooth that they may be difficult to recognize.

Multiple sclerosis (MS) is generally divided into "relapsing-remitting" (which makes up approximately 67% of detected cases) and "progressive." The former manifests exacerbations and remissions, the latter continues to show sporadic but consistent degradation of function over time.

How Yoga Applies

The cause of MS is not known, nor is there any known cure. Therefore it is impossible to say whether yoga directly addresses MS's pathogenetic factors or the process of the illness. Yet there are many examples and some valid studies demonstrating that yoga can be of salutary benefit in each type of MS. It appears that the practice of yoga sets up an antagonistic process that is often more powerful than the degenerative effects of the disease. Being a progressive, self-applied technique for maximal independence, its goals are strikingly appropriate.

Regardless of whether there is loss of energy, reduced range of motion, spasticity, weakness, dyscoordination, imbalance, or numbness or paraesthesias in different parts of the body, yoga can serve to minimize involuntary muscle contraction, maximize flexible range, and improve strength, coordination, and balance. Yoga effectively diminishes the impact of sensory changes by raising functional abilities to a higher level, improving overall concentration, calm, and a realistic sense of well-being. Regardless of other factors, yoga energizes.

Yoga is valuable to people with MS for three reasons. First, the practice of yoga reduces functional deficits. Second, it increases self-reliance since it fosters independence and can be carried out independently. And third, it is one of the principal aims, in fact the principal aim of yoga, to steady and quiet the mind.

Contemporary psychologists Paul Ekman, Joseph Campos, Richard Davidson, and Frans de Waal (9) agree with William James that most forms of emotion are so closely associated with our bodily responses, we hardly know we have them when the body is passive. This applies in dramatically heightened force to people living with MS.

Multicultural studies confirm that if randomly selected individuals are told in completely anatomical terms to open their eyes very widely, part their lips, and protrude their tongues just a little, so they don't quite show (thereby making the facial expression of disgust), then when they are asked what they feel, they will answer "disgust." In other words, we often appear to learn how we feel by observing what we are doing (10). Some folks are mesmerized by a picture of a neuron in the brain lighting up and exciting a chain of neurons that eventually stimulate a muscle to wiggle your finger. Mind over matter: the brain moves the body. Yoga focuses on just the opposite. Touching your toes elongates the hamstrings. They stretch and soon relax. Your brain and central nervous system become calm as you perceive the sustained relaxation of the stretched muscle. Yes, the brain moves the body, but it is the mind making the body act, and the body's fed-back effect on the mind, that is yoga.

A person develops competence in yoga by learning from a teacher and practicing on his or her own. Along the way, not necessarily a very long way (a few months on average), the individual acquires a basic knowledge of the body. This entails particulars of his or her body, initially, and soon, the placement and functions of the common muscle groups. At that point the individual is ready to recognize signs such as the propensity of his or her adductors to cause scissoring, or the gluteus medius to go into spasm when descending more than four or five stairs.

It helps to just be aware of either liability and the circumstances under which it occurs. It serves to focus the efforts of the individual toward the problem and limits the general anxiety associated with it. Once aware of the problem, the individual will either avoid long flights of stairs altogether, or be ready to use appropriate stretch techniques to reduce the incidence of spasticity and limit its effects when it does occur. The same stretching techniques that reduce the muscles' tendency toward spasticity also strengthen them, increase the range of motion at the hips and ankles, and relax the distress that walking and stairs would otherwise entail. This anxiety would, naturally, disadvantageously heighten reflexes all the more.

Knowing that one can avoid certain physiological situations, witnessing oneself "train" for them and handle them, means watching oneself go through them to the end. The fact that people with MS acquire the ability to locate, recognize, and remediate or avoid these situations further adds to their comfort throughout life. This is a good in itself, but it also augments a sense of well-being and confidence that bring forth the adage "nothing succeeds like success."

Promotion and Prevention

Professor E. Tory Higgins of Columbia University, a seminal thinker in modern motivational psychology, distinguishes between two types of "referential focus" (11). Two background attitudes are present in all of us to varying degrees at different times. *Promotion* is oriented toward success, interest in accomplishing whatever one can, brushing mistakes aside as the price of taking the risk to try. *Prevention* minimizes error, giving up opportunities to possibly accomplish more in order to avoid embarrassing missteps. One strains to succeed, the other takes care not to fail.

Both promotion and prevention have their place in the surgical suite, the contractors' office and the artist's studio. Unfortunately, disabilities and deficits incline one to focus on prevention, even in situations where a more positive and even slightly risk-taking attitude might be more advantageous. By affording people a measure of self-initiated promotion and prevention, yoga helps even the scales, a little at first, and more and more thereafter. Increased calm comes with, and also brings, feelings of mastery and control.

Contrary to the romantic view of the unbalanced and erratic genius, in patients with MS emotional stability promotes cognitive capacity and a creative approach to life.

Different Uses of Yoga in Relapsing and Progressive MS

Between its onslaughts, relapsing MS, like a retreating army, leaves a vacuum in its wake. Unless immediate work is done, the functional damage will outlive the neurological (since by definition the neurological damage often remits, at least in part). At that point, what is called for is exactly the job of work at which yoga excels: regaining energy and focus, stretching to expand range of motion, counter residual spasticity, and improve strength, coordination, and balance. These goals can be reached through sustained and variably complex postures.

The same applies to any neurological compromise with functional sequelae, such as cerebral palsy, stroke, Parkinson's disease, head trauma or spinal cord injury.

Progressive MS is a slightly different story, but there may be significant regaining of lost ground even though there are no remissions. In these situations, all the experience and technical competence of the teacher or therapist, and all the resourcefulness of the student or patient are called forth to resist and flexibly adapt to diminished capacity. This may involve unconventional uses of faculties. Extreme examples of this are the many individuals who have learned to paint by holding a brush between their toes. Some people simply use their normal abilities in the same ways, but more so, such as the wheelchair victors of marathon races who finish long before the fleetest of foot. Still others will use sufficient focus and care that neurological phenomena simply don't get a chance to interrupt things, at least for a set period of time, until the job gets done. In Gilles de la Tourette syndrome, for example, tics can be voluntarily suppressed during a public presentation. The same suppression is often possible with tremor.

In rehabilitation medicine people often distinguish *impairment*, the loss of or injury to living tissue through amputation, stroke or illness, from *disability*, being incapable of performing basic tasks such as dressing, bathing, walking, and both of these from *handicap*, losing the capacity to fulfill common roles in society such as parent, student, employee.

Yoga's major role in both forms of MS, where impairment is not much under control, is to limit disability and thereby reduce handicap: to enable people with less control of their right leg still to walk safely and reliably (reduce disability), and therefore to be able to work (avoid handicap). Whether yoga affects the underlying impairment – plaque that impedes neural transmission to the quadriceps, let us say – is less certain. However, while speculative, there is another way in which yoga may prove beneficial. It *may* reduce impairment.

Motivation, Feedback, and Miracles

The work of D.V. Buonomano andl M.M. Merzenich has shown that monkeys who are deprived of sensation in their middle fingers have changes in the parts of the cerebral cortex that register sensations (12). The neurological tissue that was devoted to registering sensations coming from that finger

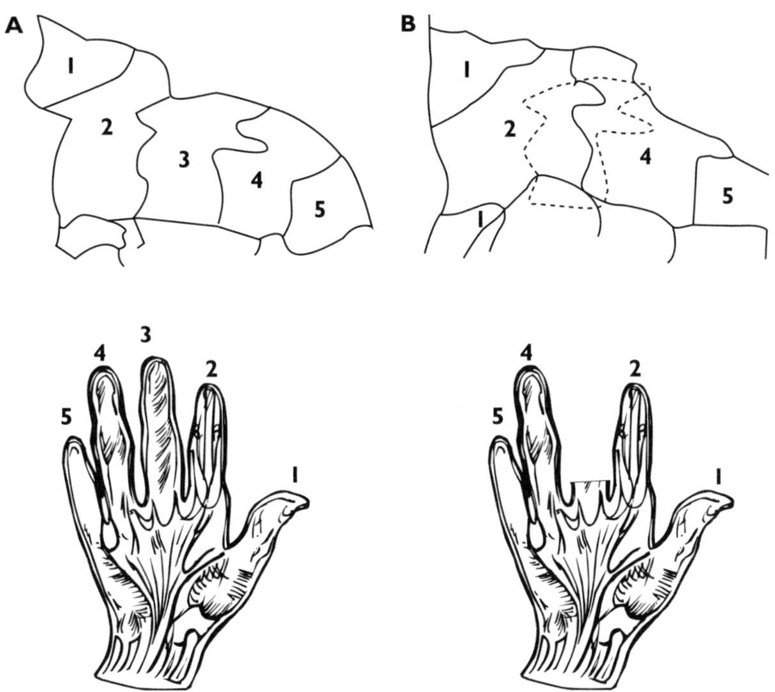

becomes aroused with stimulation of the index finger, or the ring finger, or the thumb. Fascinatingly, when sensation was restored to the middle finger, that same brain region began again responding only to sensory stimulation of the middle finger. The brain adapts to loss of input, then will re-adapt to subsequent gains, remodeling its sensitivities to take advantage of the information available to it. "It is no individual neuron or group of neurons. It is the total integration of the network of the brain that makes a difference" (12).

More recently, Christopher Reeves and laboratory scientists showed that hard, conscious work with attention to muscular anatomy and kinesiology can accomplish seemingly impossible tasks (13, 20).

By a mechanism that awaits even preliminary elucidation, frequent, highly motivated attempts to move a heretofore paralyzed limb are meeting with success after stroke and spinal cord injury. Such changes within the brain and spinal cord were thought impossible. Work by great neuropathologists such as Ramon Y Cajal and Camillo Golgi once appeared to confirm that "By age 4 or 5, the fountain of neurological development is dry, never to flow again" (14, 15). However, numerous counterexamples now exist, including the work at the University of Alabama in Birmingham with patients suffering stroke. A fair-sized sample of people have consented to have their unaffected limbs bound down, requiring them to use their hemiparetic or hemiplegic side. The things they want to do, they must do with the impaired limbs. And this often rehabilitates the affected, even paralyzed, limb(s) (16).

Motivation is critical. To Dr. Merzenich and, it appears, to Christopher Reeves, the activity must matter to the individual. If it is boring and mindless, the mechanisms underlying the brain's plasticity will not kick in. When a person focuses and pays attention, brain molecules turn on the reward circuitry that promotes plasticity (the ability of the neurological tissue to actually change in function, and possibly structure) (17,20). Outcomes measured weeks and months later show that these individuals have strikingly (and statistically, significantly) greater function than matched controls.

In each of these cases, at least some of the plasticity of the central nervous system is seen to continue into adulthood. Most experts agree that before ages 3 to 5, the brain tissue is busy organizing itself according to what is effective signal processing of the external and internal environments. Nobelist Gerald Edelman and others have theoretically modeled some of the processes (18). But it is the recruitment of working tissue to new function, the formation of new centers to perform impaired functions, and the creation of new pathways that has now been convincingly documented to extend quite a bit later in life. This may apply to some of the increased mental and physical activity seen in multiple sclerosis patients doing yoga (20).

The Invisible Treatment

In the laboratory, meditation has been shown to increase cortical thickness. In controlled studies with children, yoga is associated with improved plasticity and motor control per se, and yoga practice is experimentally found to alter signaling molecules having to do with pain relief, such as endocannabinoids, and such basic neurotransmitters as nitric oxide (21-23).

Another critical aspect of recovering function, long known to occupational and physical therapists, is deconstruction of tasks. One does not teach a child the alphabet from A to Z in one sitting. Similarly, a person who has lost right-handed function regains the ability to eat by practicing placing the fork in a tomato, then practicing transferring the fork from the right to the left hand, then using a knife to cut the tomato, then raising the fork carefully and accurately. This breakdown into simple parts is another method of successfully inducing plasticity. For this reason we have numbered each part of each pose that follows. Students and teachers can focus on single directions whenever that is desirable.

Yoga and eating tomatoes involve the same self-conscious and highly motivated obligatory movement of specific body parts. In yoga no body part or movement is omitted or underserved. Intensive yoga practice meets the criteria for the inhibition work in Alabama, New York, and elsewhere, and the consistent repetitive patterns that were linked with Christopher Reeves' success (20).

But isn't this process backwards? Isn't it something like sending out the invitations, buying a dress, renting the hall, and hoping that a bride and a groom show up? Here we are trying to move a foot or finger, hoping that there will be some intelligent reason to do so, that function will return? Yoga is stretching and moving for its own sake. Isn't teaching yoga to improve reaching for the cookie jar practicing the act before there is any motivation to perform it? Haven't we put the cart before the horse?

No. It is different. The yogi is more like the farmer, who cannot create life, but can cultivate the field in even rows, remove weeds and irrigate, distributing sunlight and rainfall evenly so that the crop, when it does come in, will be properly protected, cared for and utilized. Only in the case of yoga there is vigorous, internal human effort as well. It is more like promising to be a faithful partner "for better or for worse, in sickness and in health....," and the fact that one promises goes a long way toward people behaving that way!

The most familiar yoga practice is Hatha Yoga, or, literally "Manual Yoga" in the Sanskrit. This includes the familiar lotus position, the headstand, and extends to the extreme poses that fill the current flood of books on yoga. Many yoga poses or asana are recorded and pictured in a tremendous and elaborate literature spanning six millennia. It has been a focus of attention in many centers of learning and many sites of cave-drawings, from Sri Lanka to Iowa to Beijing. Though each posture is aimed at improving health and increasing personal calm, different poses are noted to have specific effects, and therefore are thought more appropriate for particular conditions.

Three poses are the starting-off point for a number of the asana that follow. One is standing, one sitting, one lying down. It may be wise to go over them first.

TADASANA

The Mountain

For balance, endurance, strength and to oppose spasticity, hip flexion contractures and hammer toes:

This pose requires effort each time it is done. As the yogi strives to quiet the mind, inhibiting all the ways we have of occupying it, the practitioner of this posture inhibits all movement of any kind. How does one inhibit those un-

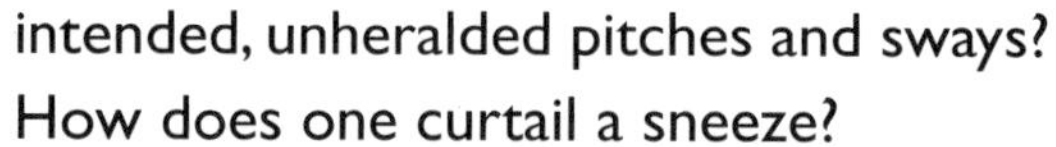
intended, unheralded pitches and sways?

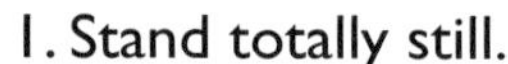
How does one curtail a sneeze?

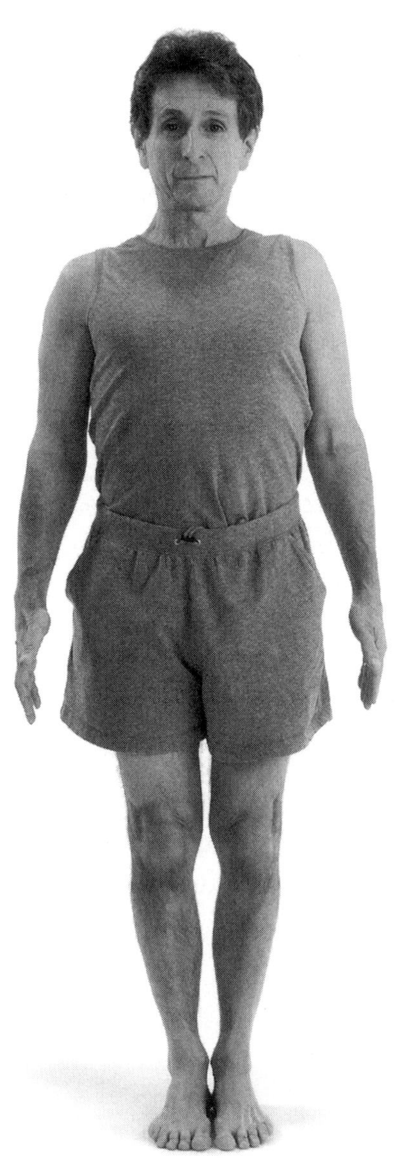

1. Stand totally still.
2. Look straight ahead, balancing right to left and front to back.
3. Let your arms rest at your sides, palms facing each other.
4. Both ankles, hips, shoulders and ears should be in one plane.
5. Balance each foot's weight, half on the heel, half on the ball of the foot and big toe.

Dr. Renee Caillet suggests that if gravity's downward force on the foot is divided into twelve equal parts, then six will be on the heel, two at the big toe and its metatarsal, and one for each of the remaining toes and their metatarsals (24).

Practicing this pose will help you maintain a quieter posture for longer, but no amount of practice will eliminate the need for genuine effort to accomplish it.

Breathe quietly in the pose for 30 seconds to one minute.

Dandasana

The Staff

1. Sit on the "sit bones," inner legs especially stretched out with right and left ankles and big toes and first metatarsal heads in contact with each other.

2. Palms flush with the floor, fingers pointing to the front, straighten your elbows and lower your shoulders, pulling the shoulder blades together, back and down.

3. Keep the spine vertical. Look straight ahead.

Stay in the pose breathing carefully and symmetrically for 30 seconds to one minute. Versions of Dandasana for less mobile people are also described in Section 1 of the book.

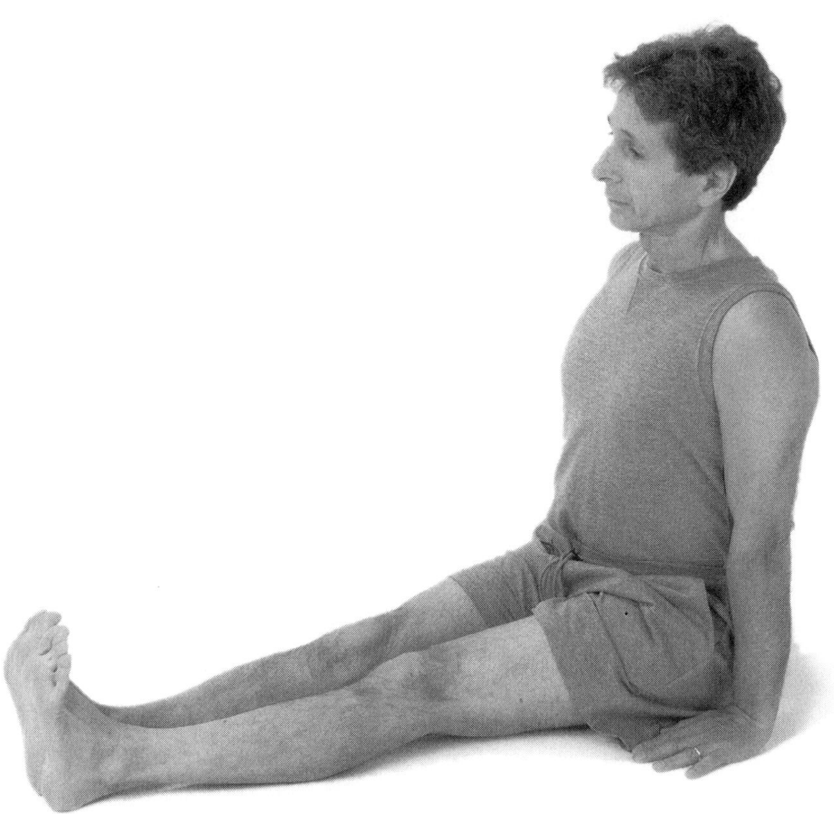

SAVASANA

Corpse Pose

1. Lie on your back, palms up, knuckles down.

2. Elongate the back of your neck and the backs of your legs, advancing your heels and the back of your head as far as possible from your hips and shoulders. Keep the heels together but the forefeet and toes will drift apart.

3. Close your eyes. Let your facial expression dissolve.

4. Relax the jaw muscles, soft and hard palates, and cheek muscles.

5. Empty the mind: no memories, ideas, no dreaming.

Mr. Iyengar allows that at first, this relaxation will lead to sleep. After a while, an alert and calm individual breathing slowly and dispassionately for 10-20 minutes experiences a fine and thorough rejuvenation.

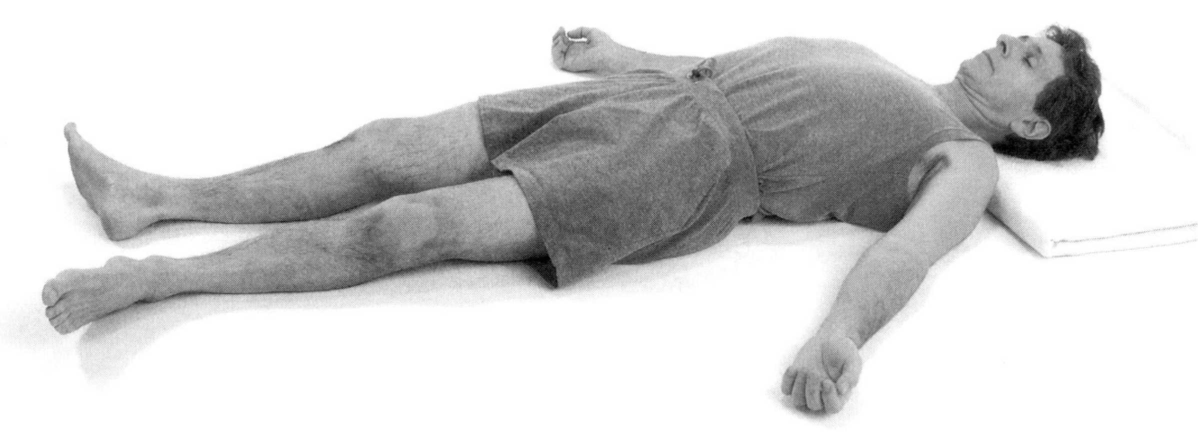

Specifically Directed Poses

There is a flexibility to each pose at each level, especially the entry level and the intermediate ones, which might incline the practitioner to believe that each is representative of an entire spectrum or family of poses. This is true, but one must also bear in mind that the pose itself is the result of many years of refinement and, having been formed by centuries of thoughtful experience, is a kind of ideal to be asymptotically approached by most of us.

A little anatomy may be useful throughout what follows.

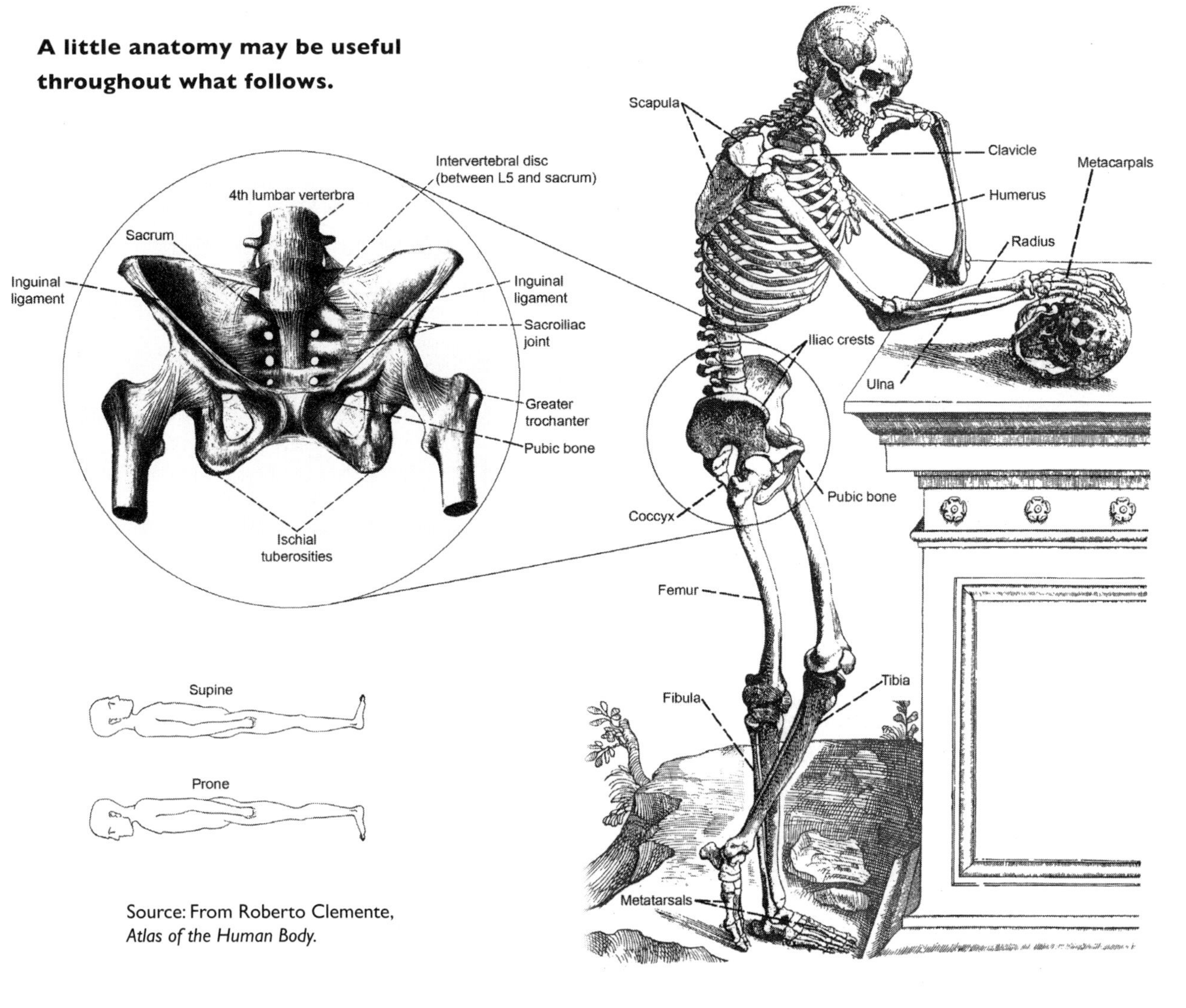

Source: From Roberto Clemente, *Atlas of the Human Body.*

"Props" are listed at the beginning of each pose. Bear in mind that other or additional props may be needed according to the nature of the practitioner and the practice.

Optimally, practitioners should work up gradually to a full minute in each pose on each side, unless otherwise indicated.

The rest of this book focuses on improvement in seven areas central to people suffering from MS and similarly disabling conditions. They are (i) fatigue, (ii) spasticity, (iii) range of motion, (iv) strength, (v) coordination, (vi) balance, and (vii) confidence and calm. In each of these areas, approximately a half-dozen poses will be approached. In each case, the "standard" pose will be described first, then an "entry level" version recommended for wheelchair-bound and bed-bound individuals, and a third, intermediate version for people who are at the border-lines of ambulation and transferring. Naturally, the idea is to master the material at whatever point seems right. For safety's sake, always read through all the versions of the pose, then start out with the entry-level pose and move through the intermediate to the classical. The patience this engenders is part of the process! We have observed people go from a given pose to a more challenging level with encouraging consistency.

Seven benefits of yoga are equally valuable to patients with either type of MS, as well as other patients with similar problems.

1. Reduce fatigue
2. Improve range of motion
3. Reduce spasticity
4. Strengthen
5. Coordinate
6. Improve balance
7. Raise confidence and generate calm.

Yoga raises confidence (#7) through a combination of the first six benefits and because all six can be pursued independently. The practitioner realizes that he or she has much greater control over inner and outer states. Each benefit contributes to one's calm. Each benefit requires possession of at least some measure of the qualities that lie above it.

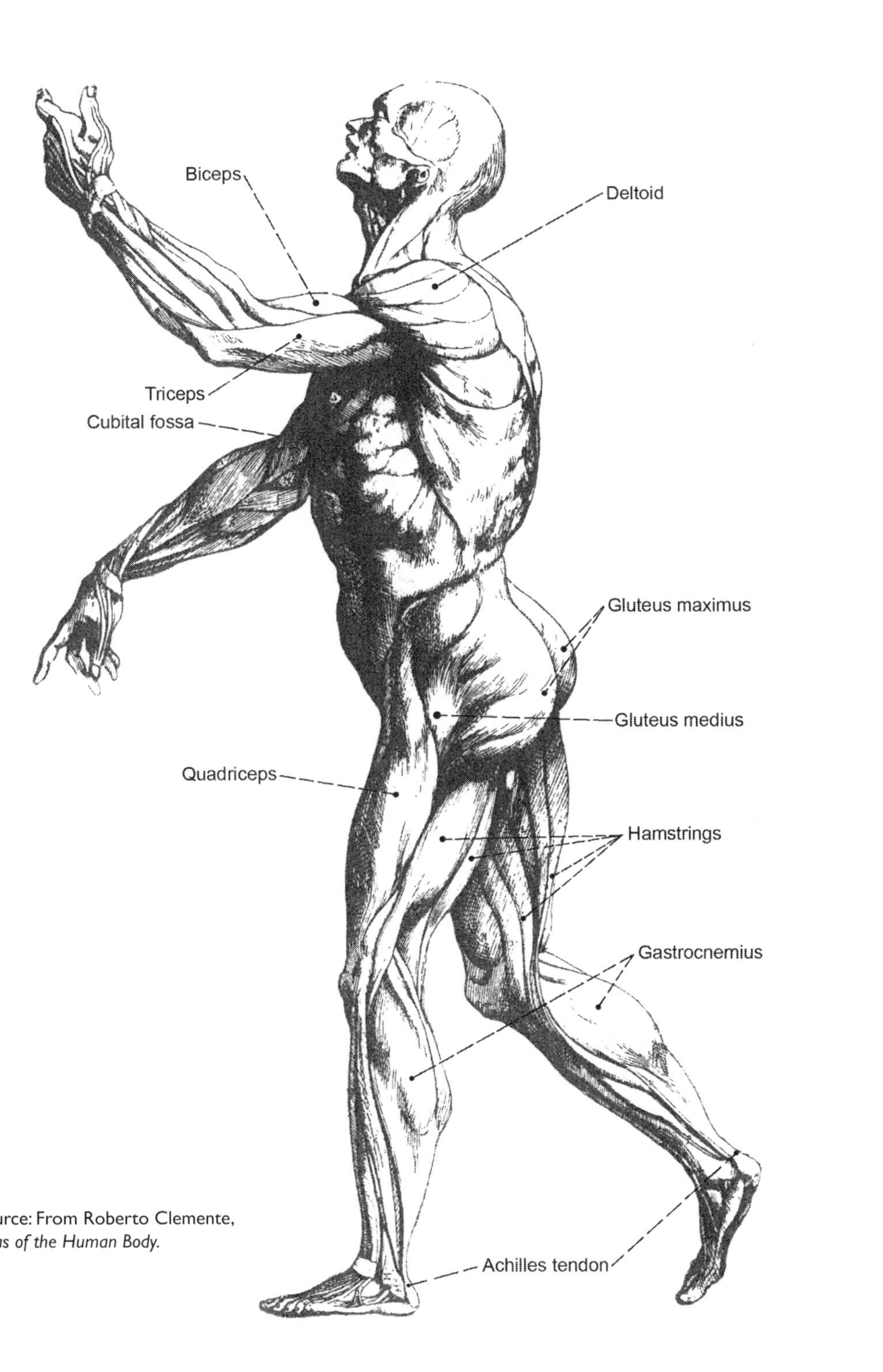

Source: From Roberto Clemente, *Atlas of the Human Body.*

7 Reduce Fatigue

Energy is to the individual what capital is to a company: without it, nothing can be done. Recent research has found that if there is any one thing that can be proven about yoga and MS, it is that fatigue is significantly reduced. (19).

Yoga training is uniquely suited to this endeavor, be it after stroke, cerebral palsy, traumatic injury, in ALS, MS, or other central nervous system damage.

One of the principal handicaps in MS and practically all neurological illness is loss of energy. A person may appreciate the desirability or need to do certain things, with an understanding that is undiminished, but with energy levels that make it much more difficult to embark on and accomplish the tasks. But achieving goals is the essence of success, here in learning Yoga just as well as in every other aspect of life. Combating fatigue is critical, then, to going forward in this book.

Controlled, blinded studies at the University of Oregon confirm that Yoga practitioners with MS have higher energy levels and greater vitality than they did before beginning Yoga, and than other volunteers that did other forms of exercise.(19) Yoga literally lifts one up by the bootstraps, enabling one to go on simply by doing it. It gives more energy than it takes.

First Things First (But Not Necessarily in That Order)

The following five poses are directed toward reducing fatigue. This function logically precedes any further accomplishments or practice. Nevertheless, some of these positions may not be attainable at the get-go, and it may reasonably be returned to after working on range of motion, strengthening, spasticity, or any of the later sections.

VITARI KARANI

The first example is perhaps the best: a pose of universal scope, providing relief and simultaneously boosting energy in a manner that seems to improve on sleep itself. It is invaluable to beginners and past-masters alike, and is an excellent remedy for headaches of cervical origin. Vitari Karani has already been described in the first part of the book, and is repeated here with some differences.

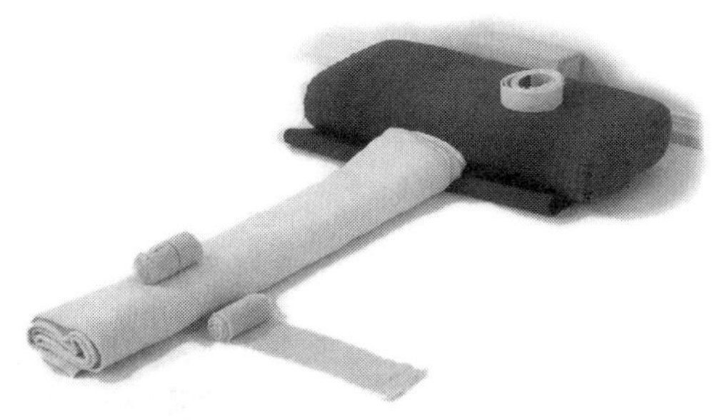

Use a bolster and a blanket folded into thirds so that it is narrower and only supports the spine, and a wall or bed or whatever vertical surface you have.

You may use an eye bag and a sandbag to weigh the shoulders down to the floor. In place of a sand bag one can use a five pound bag of flour or sugar. The weight is the same.

Inverting the body with students who have MS seems to allow them to completely and totally refresh and restore their bodies and their nervous systems.

1. Lie down.
2. Lower your elbows to the floor and move your body as close to the wall as possible.

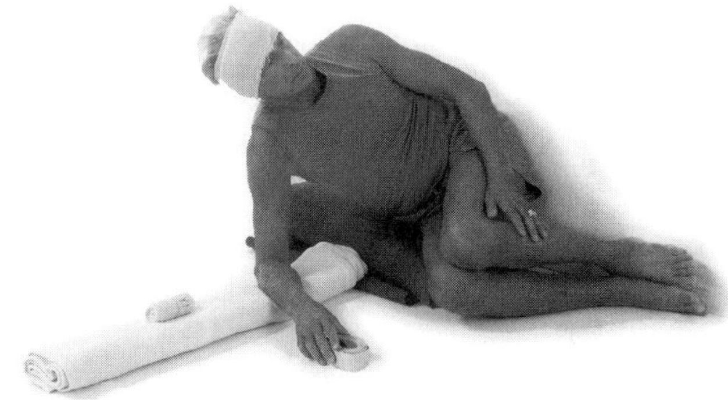

3. Just roll over to the left, keeping your head on the blanket.
4. Now shift your hips into a supine position and then gently bring your legs up on to the wall. The shoulders and chest are supported on the blanket.
5. Arch your back in order to open the chest. Use the sandbags to avoid pitching

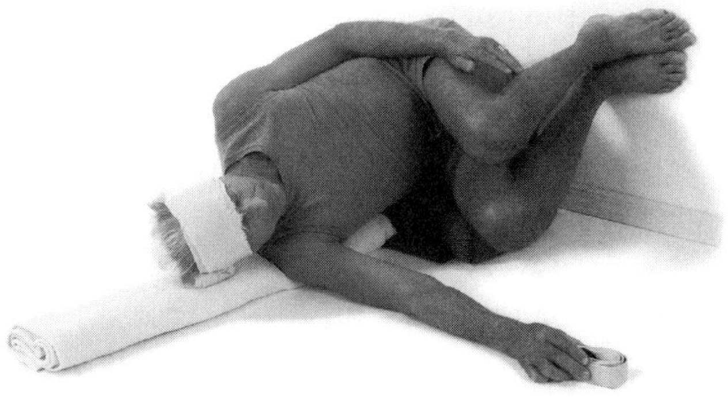

your shoulders forward. Press the shoulders down with the weight. This stretches muscles located in the front part of the chest and allows it to relax.

6. Put an eye bag under your eyes, by simply placing it above the eyebrows, pulling the skin gently down toward the nose and then distributing the sand across the eyebrow lines so that the pressure feels comfortable and the weight is not strictly on the eyeball, but is on the tissue surrounding the eye.

7. Place your hands onto the floor again about 30 degrees away from the hips with the thumb dropping more toward the floor in order to facilitate opening the chest and calming the tension in your shoulders.

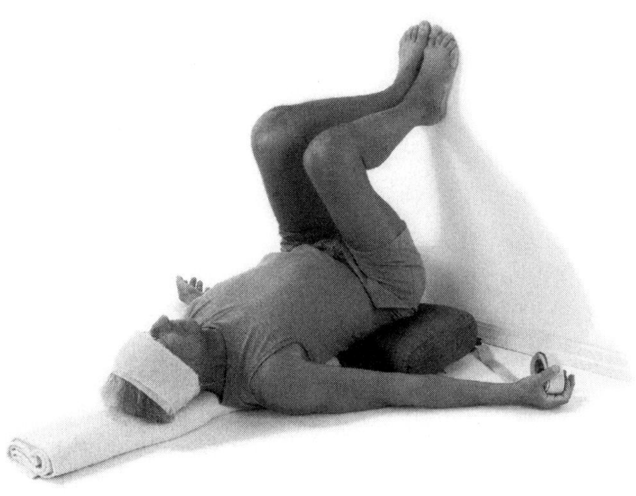

8. Now let us look at the legs. If there is a problem maintaining the legs in this posture and the legs seem to turn out, then you might want to put a strap around the mid thigh region. You or an instructor or assistant can pull the strap gently in order to raise the legs up away from the pelvis and settle the back of the heels on to the wall. This is essentially the same process we will use

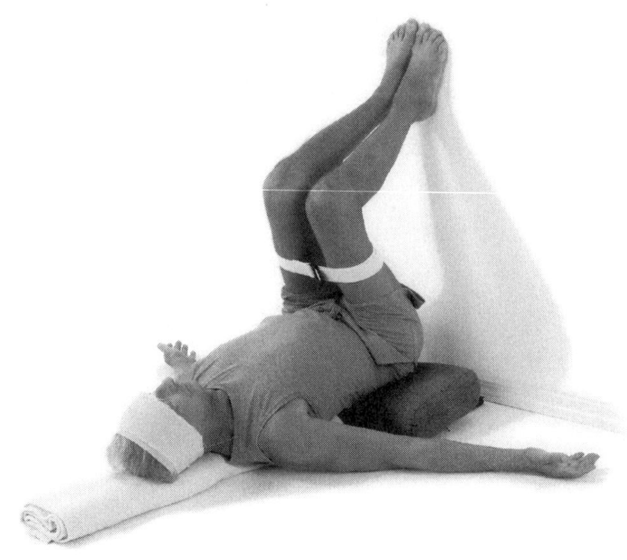

in the back bends which come later in this same sequence.

In this posture the effects of gravity on blood flow are gently reversed. Blood flows "northward" back through the pelvis with some possible additional cleansing due to the fact that the liver's vessels may open more under the increased pressure, All the blood vessels coming up from the intestine, through the hepatic portal system, and venous blood

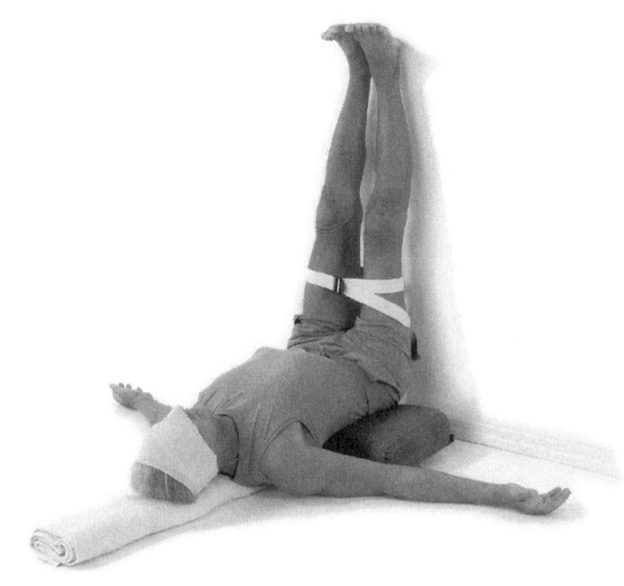

flow from the legs are drained more effectively through inversion. Breathing in this position, changing the pressures in the thoracic cavity with every inhalation and exhalation, will massage the heart and brain gently through "waves" in the blood flow through these organs.

Inhalation is through the base of the nostrils; the exhalation is through the tip of the nose. The practitioner feels rather complete and total release. If you follow the practitioner through this series of pictures, you may be able to notice that he becomes even quieter in successive pictures. You can see that his face is very relaxed and very gentle. Five minutes of this a day and if possible twice a day will offer you considerable calm. It is hard to describe how beneficial this is to people with MS.

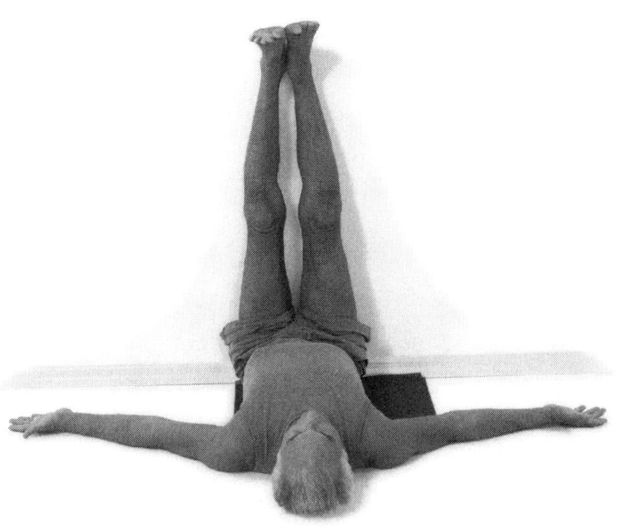

This posture should never be done after eating; it can be done before going to bed provided that the stomach is empty. Still, to do it early in the morning after the bowel and bladder are empty is perhaps the best. Three to five minutes in this pose is more than enough when you first start out. Remember, you are introducing a very effective tool to your system and it must be taken in very small doses even though you would like to take it more often and for longer. It is better at this stage, the introductory level, to stay only 3 to 5 minutes in this pose, the breath remaining smooth and calm.

After that period of time, once you come out of the pose and remove the eye bag and remove the strap, it is best to roll over onto your right thigh to swing your hips completely off the blanket or pad. Cushion your head in your right arm. Allow your left arm to drop gently onto the floor.

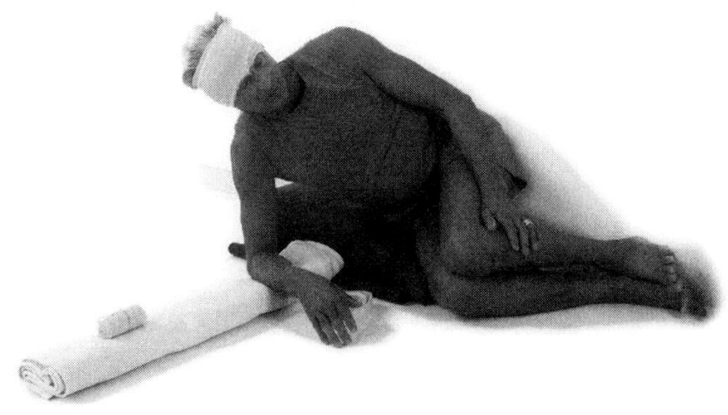

Now remember that your right lung is larger than your left lung, because the heart and stomach are on the left side, taking up a great deal of room. The liver, which is heavy, is now being supported by the floor so the return flow of blood is even and gentle. After you have stayed for at least the same amount of time in the fetal position that you were inverted, then you may sit up, placing your back against the wall. On the bolster or blanket cross your right leg in front your left, put your hands gently on your thigh and allow the total effect of the pose to come to you.

USTRASANA

The Camel

1. Kneel on a flat surface, thighs, calves and ankles together, toes pointed behind you and parallel.

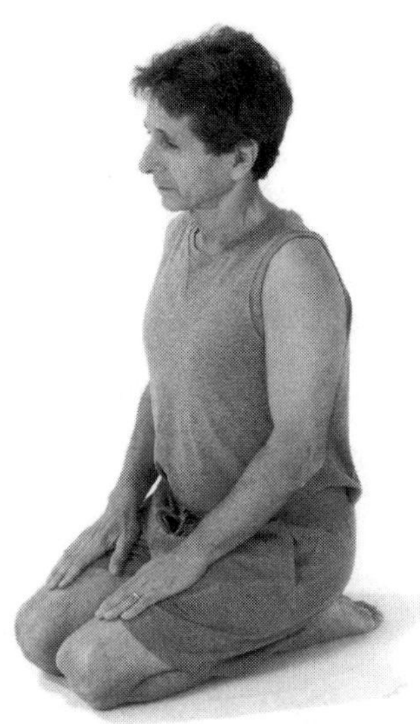

2. Place your hands on your thighs, fingers pointed down.

3. Gradually arch the neck backward to its maximum.

4. Advance the thighs forward to vertical and keep them there.

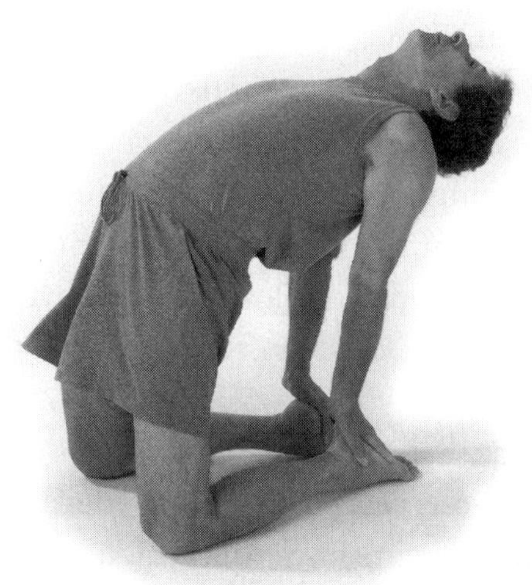

5. Extend the lumbar and thoracic spine, and bring first the right hand, then the left hand backward, resting the heel of the hands on the heels, fingers in line with the toes.

6. Raise the upper lumbar spine and lowest ribs upward as far as you can; tighten the buttocks to improve the arch of the entire spine. Breathe quietly for 30-60 seconds.

7. Exit the pose by sitting back down on your heels and simultaneously bringing your hands in your lap.

Entry-Level *Ustrasana*

1. Place a card chair about 2-3 feet from a wall, and facing away from it. Place another card chair directly in front of the first one, facing toward it.

2. Straddle the chair furthest from the wall as shown.

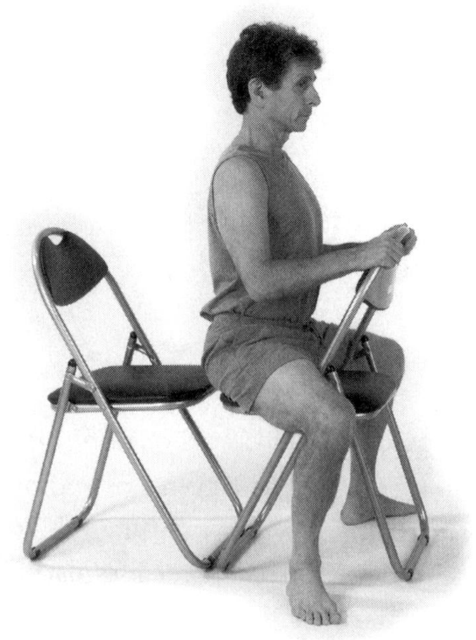

3. Holding onto the arms of the chair, hook your legs one by one under the other chair.

4. Slide backward on the chair until your buttocks are almost at the junction of the seat and back of the chair closest to the wall. Your feet should be flat against the wall.

5. Now raise your hands to grasp the arms or back of the chair that is furthest from the wall. Slowly throw your head back and lift the upper chest still further. Breathe naturally for 20-30 seconds.

6. Lower your legs together or, if necessary, one at a time. You may use pillows under the ribs and upper lumbar spine as needed also.

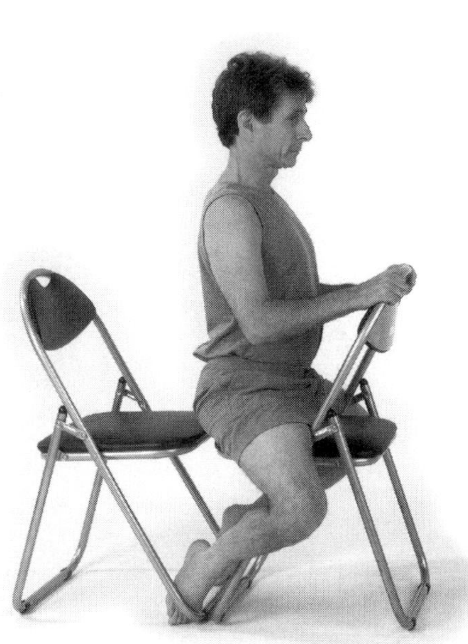

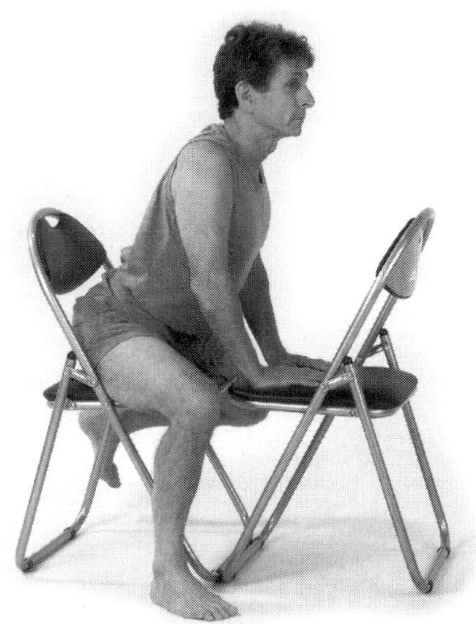

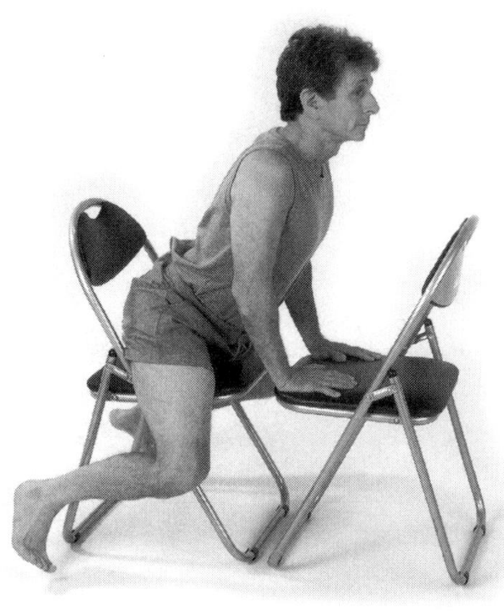

Intermediate *Ustrasana*

1. Slip your legs between the back and seat of a card chair. Be careful not to tip the chair, a common occurrence. If things are unstable or appear to be, place the chair next to a wall and/or use a helper. **[1]**

2. Slide the buttocks forward enough so that when you lie back, only the top halves of the shoulder blades extend off the edge of the seat of the chair. **[2]**

3. Place the feet flat on the floor, toes facing forward, legs parallel and in line with the hips. Hold the chair back when descending. **[3]**

4. Gradually let your head and neck and upper shoulder region descend further and further, puffing out the chest and bending the upper thoracic spine around the front edge of the chair. **[4]**

5. After comfortably remaining in the position at least 10 seconds, and possibly

1

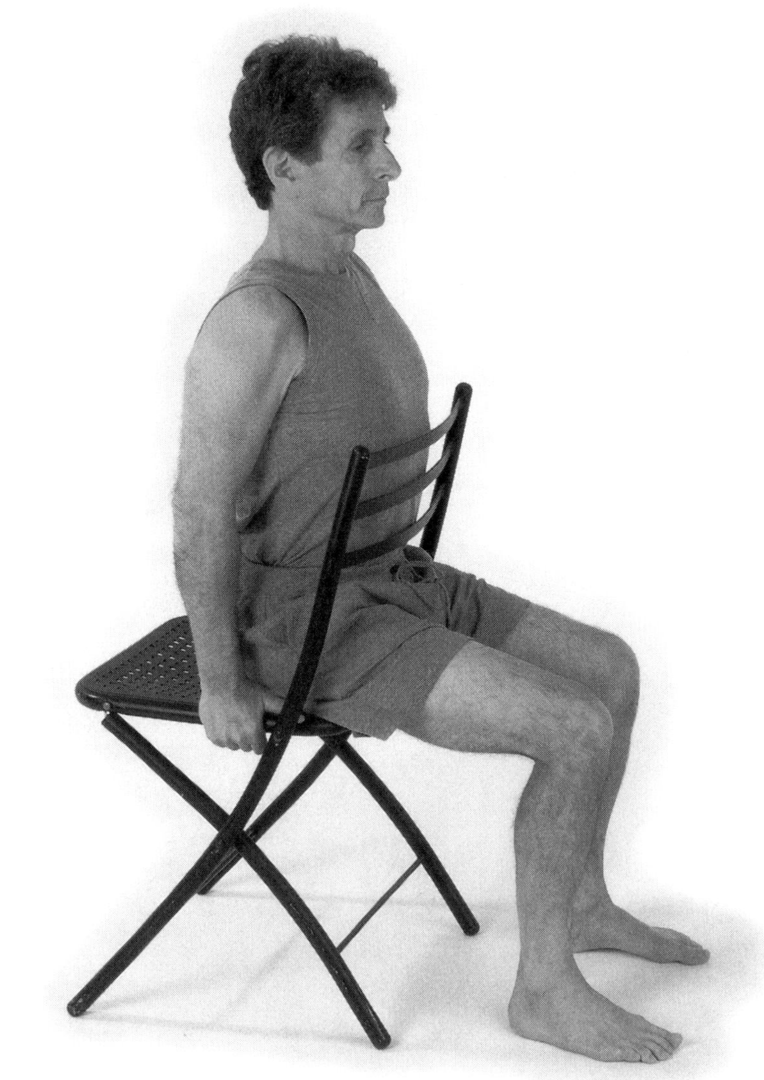

2

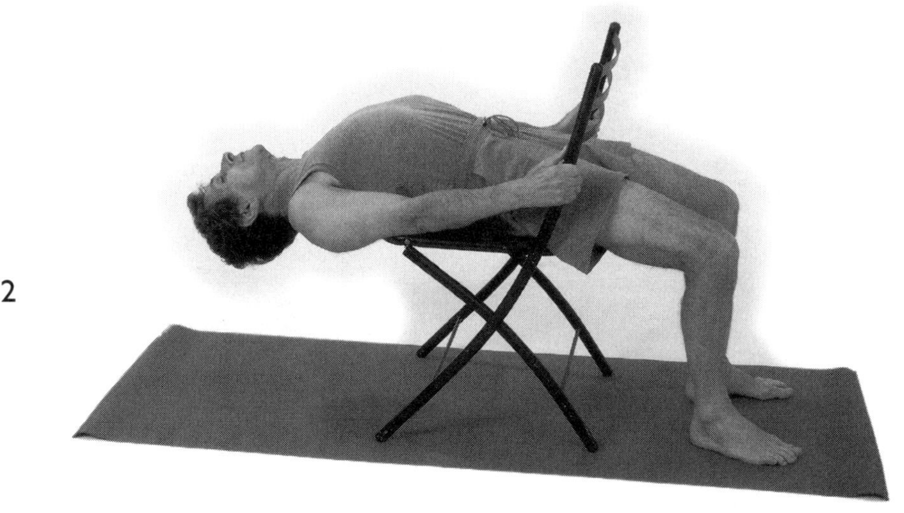

3

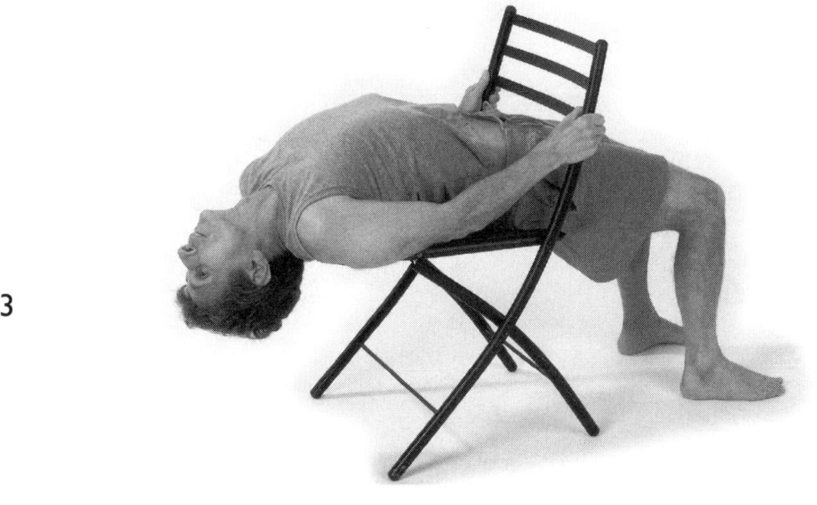

4

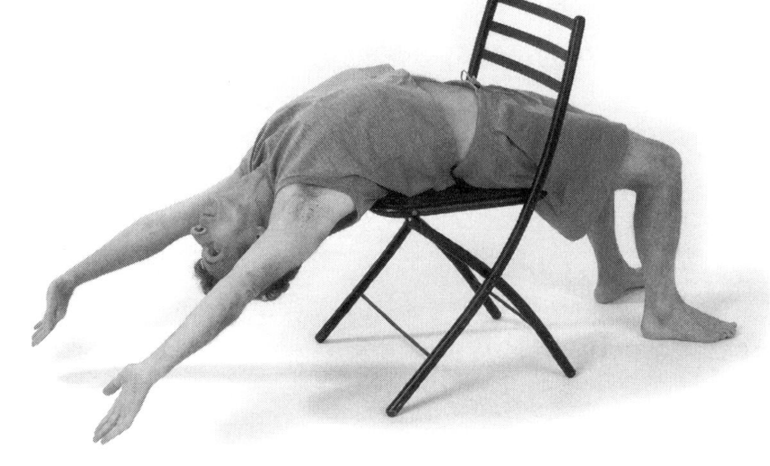

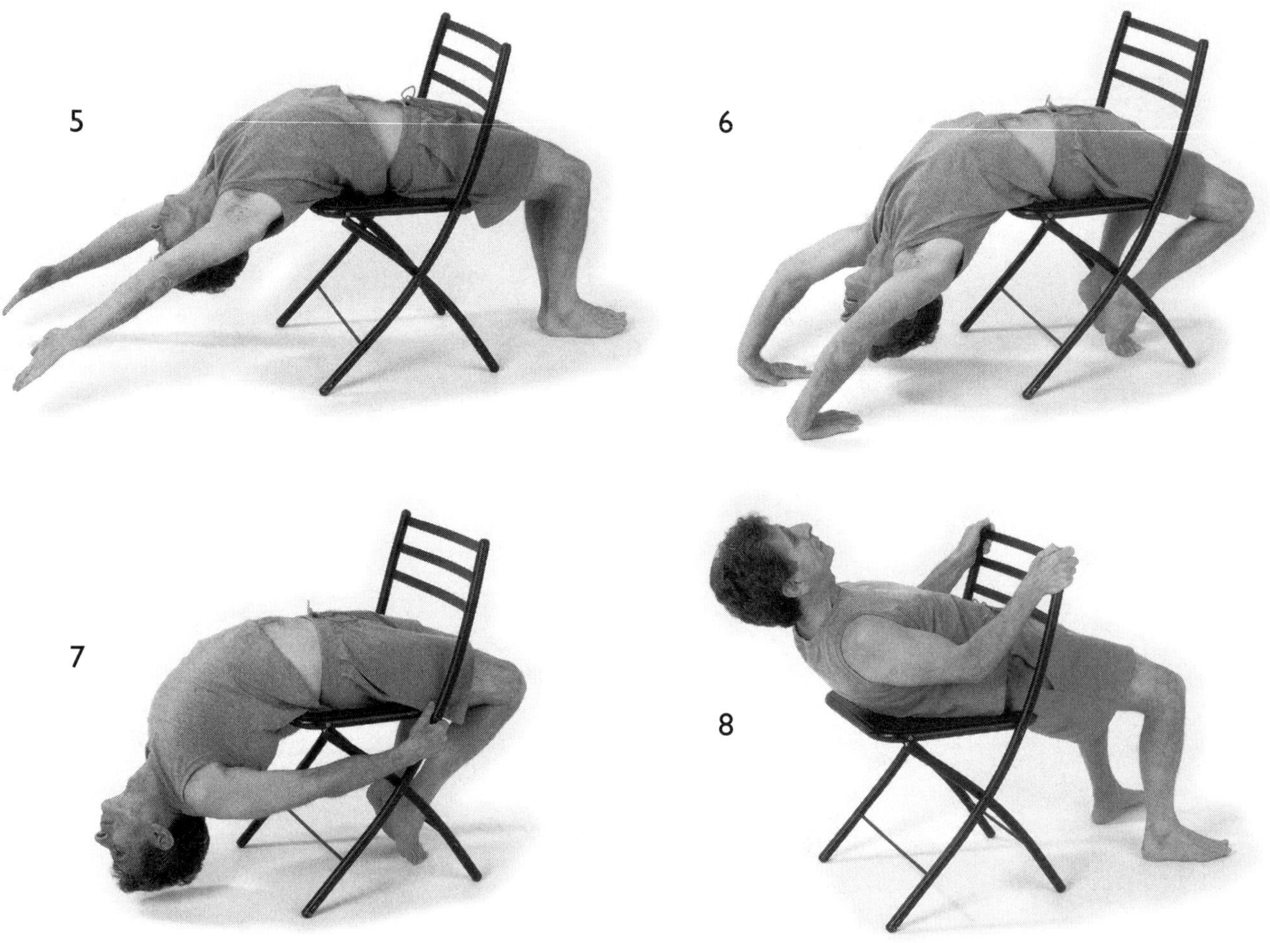

for 20-30 seconds, raise your arms over your head, palms upward, allowing the weight of your arms to further open the chest **[4]**.

6. Remain breathing normally for 20-30 seconds.

7. Grasp the seat or side or back of the chair to return to upright on exiting the pose. Be careful of tipping the chair on entering and leaving.

More Advanced Intermediate *Ustrasana*

Proceed as in the intermediate pose above, but at direction 3, do not slide the buttocks as far between the seat and back of the chair.

1. Allow the entire shoulder blade to hang free beyond the front of the chair seat. **[5]**

2. Raise your arms over your head and behind you, placing palms on the floor. **[6]**

3. Now bring your feet as far beneath the chair as possible.

4. Breathe normally and evenly for 20-30 seconds.

5. To intensify the pose, grasp the chair supports and gently arch still further. **[7]**

6. Then return your feet to flat on the floor, calves and thighs parallel.

7. Reach your hands above and in front of you, grasping the back or seat of the chair to help you ascend back to the straddle position. **[8]**

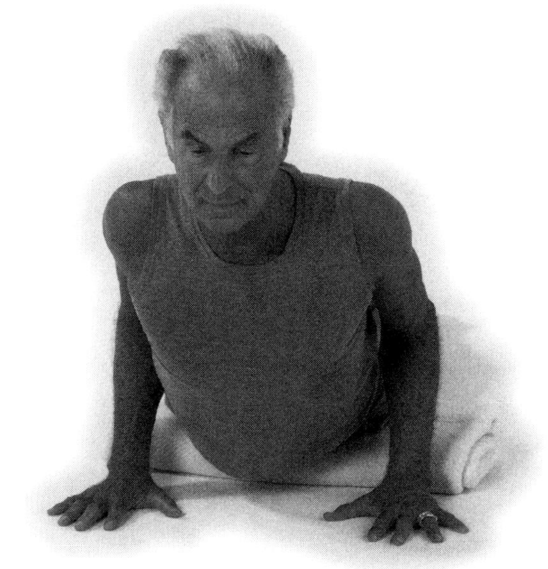

BHUJANGASANA

The Serpent

1. Lie on a surface face down.
2. Place your palms on the surface next to your lower ribs, fingers parallel to your torso.
3. Using your hands for balance and support, raise first your brow, then your eyes, then your nose, then upper lip, then mouth, chin, throat and slowly, the upper ribs from the surface until your head is as far back as possible. The shoulder blades come back, together and down, the pubic bones stay on the surface.
4. Now contract the buttocks and rectal muscles, breathing calmly for 20-30 seconds.

Entry-Level *Bhujangasana*

1. Sit comfortably in a chair with arms, feet flat on the floor, thighs together.
2. Place the heels of your hands on the arms of the chair, as far as possible from the chair back.
3. Press down evenly with both hands, slowly throwing your head back, and your

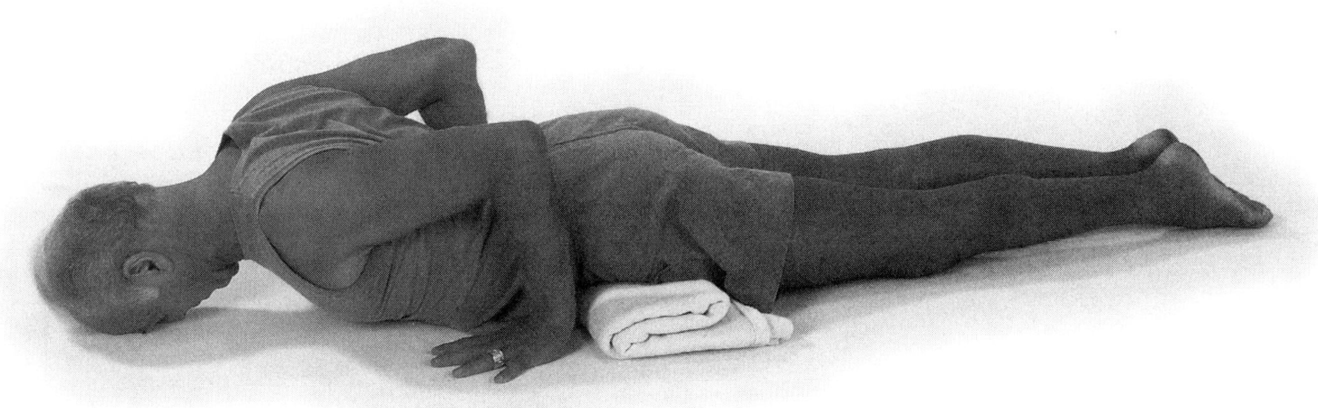

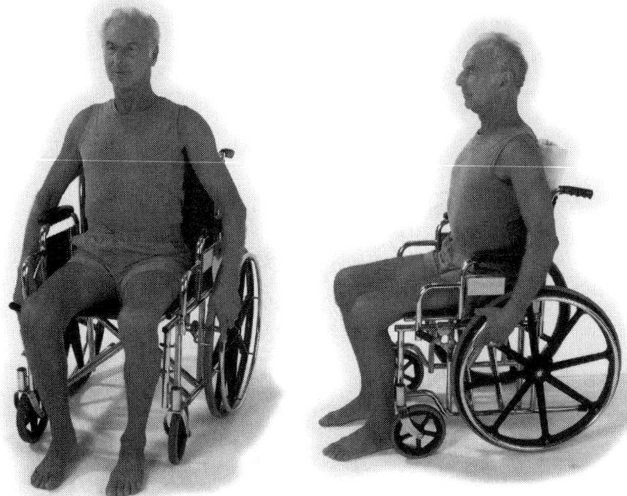

top few ribs forward. Keep your entire lower back in contact with the chair.

4. Hold the shoulders down, the shoulder blades together. Try to press the upper sternum forward and upward. Breathe evenly for 20-30 seconds.

Intermediate-Level *Bhujangasana*

1. Go on all fours over a small pillow and a bolster.

2. Gradually lower yourself into the prone position over the pillows.

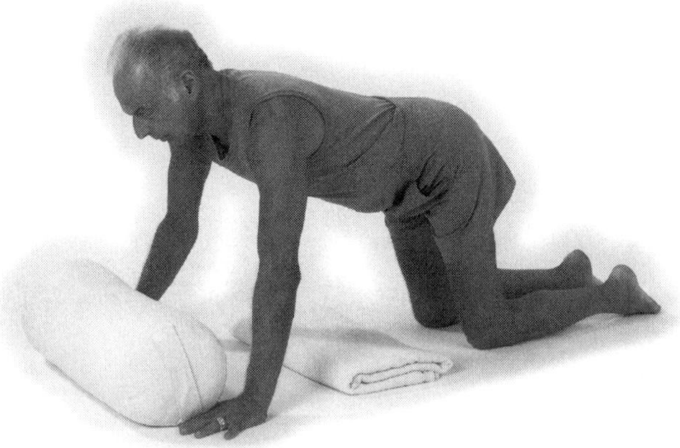

3. Place your palms on the surface next to your lower ribs.

4. Using your hands for balance and support, raise first your brow, then your eyes, then your nose, then upper lip, then mouth, chin, throat and slowly, the upper ribs from the surface until your head is as far back as possible.

5. Keep the shoulder blades back, together and down. The pubic bones stay on the surface. Point your toes.

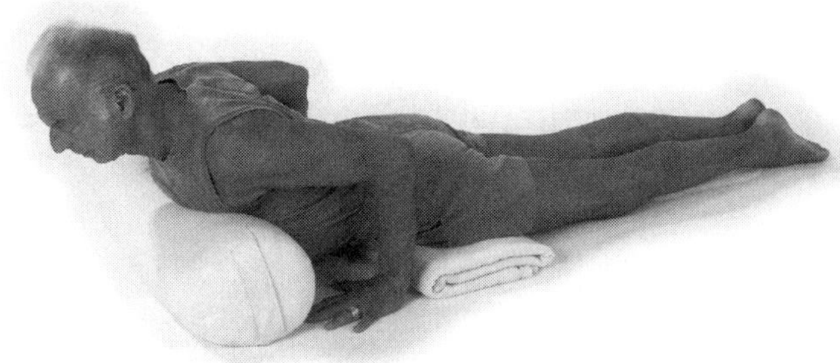

6. Now contract the buttocks and rectal muscles, and remain in the position, breathing calmly for 20-30 seconds.

URDHVA DHANURASANA I

The High Bridge

1. Lie in savasana.

2. Place your palms above your shoulders, fingers parallel and pointing toward them. Keep your forearms and upper arms parallel, and about as far apart as the shoulders.

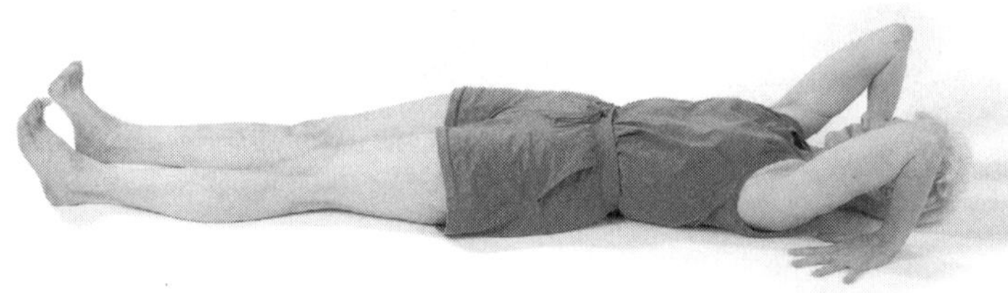

3. Bend your knees until your feet are flat on the floor, and parallel. The feet, shins, thighs, arms and hands on each side should be in the same plane.

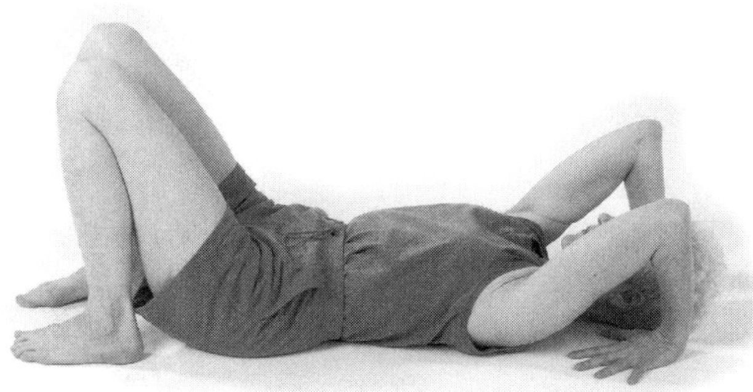

4. Press downward with your hands, lifting your head and shoulders until the apex of your head is on the surface with your hands and feet.

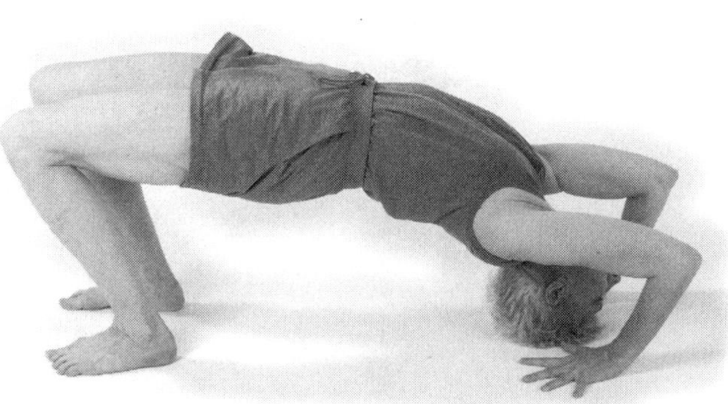

5. As you breathe in, press further with the open hands, balancing weight evenly between them. Raise your head and trunk until your elbows are straight.

6. Straighten the knees somewhat, carefully raising the abdomen and groin regions as high as possible.

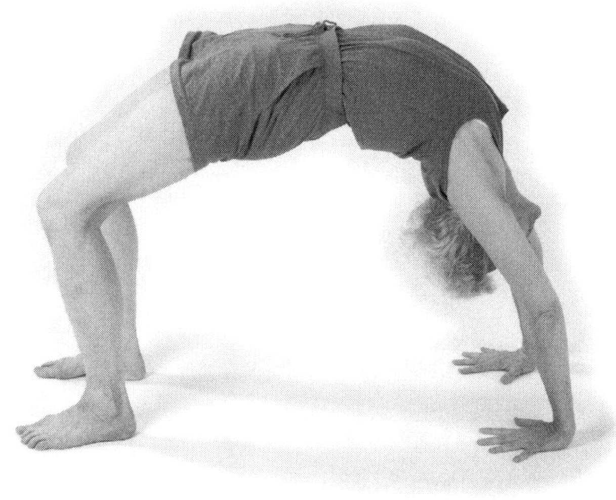

7. Use pressure from your feet and legs to move the shoulders as far forward as is comfortable, opening the armpits wide.

8. Breathe quietly for 30-60 seconds.

9. To leave the posture, first slowly flex the elbows until your head rests on the surface. Then slide your head away from your heels until your shoulder blades rest on the surface.

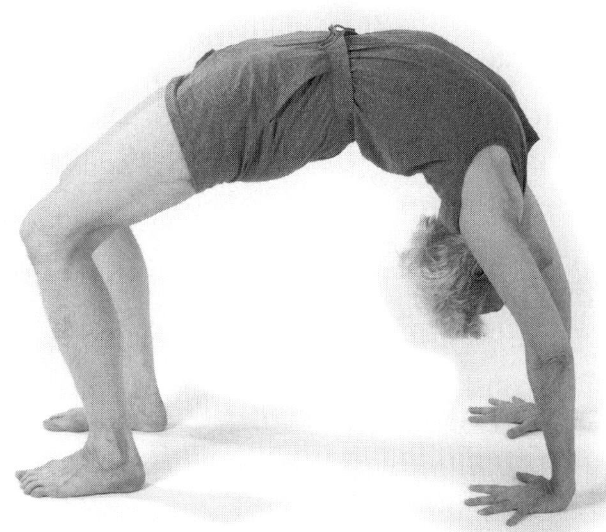

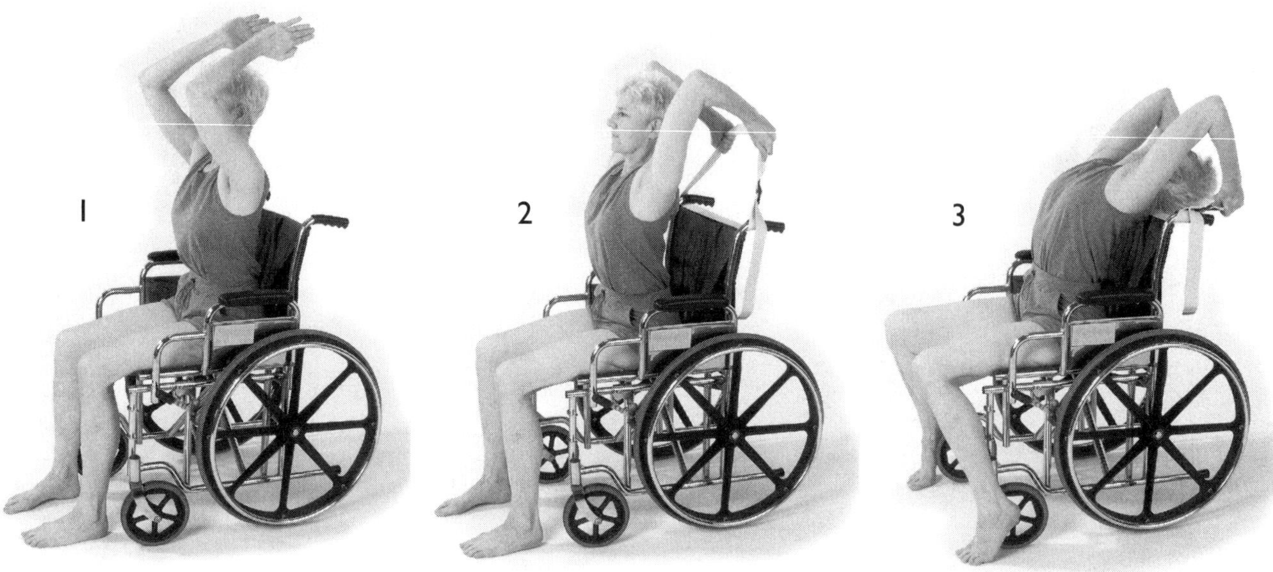

Entry-Level Undhva *Dhanurasana*

1. Sit with feet flat on the floor, knees together, buttocks wedged between the seat and back of a chair or wheelchair.

2. Raise arms in as parallel a fashion as possible, bend elbows 90 degrees, wrists in neutral position, palms facing each other. **[1]**

3. Reach upward and backward, grasping the top of the chair back or a strap that is tied in a sling behind the head. **[2]**

4. "Walk" backwards with your hands, or push backward with your head to maximize the distance backward that the hands, wrists and arms travel. **[3]**

5. Breathe quietly in this position for 30-60 seconds, then release the hands' grip slowly. Return to normal seating position.

Intermediate Urdhva *Dhanurasana*

1. Stand in Tadasana one foot away from a wall, a few inches from the corner of a room.

2. Balance weight evenly over both feet. With an inhalation, bring the hands and

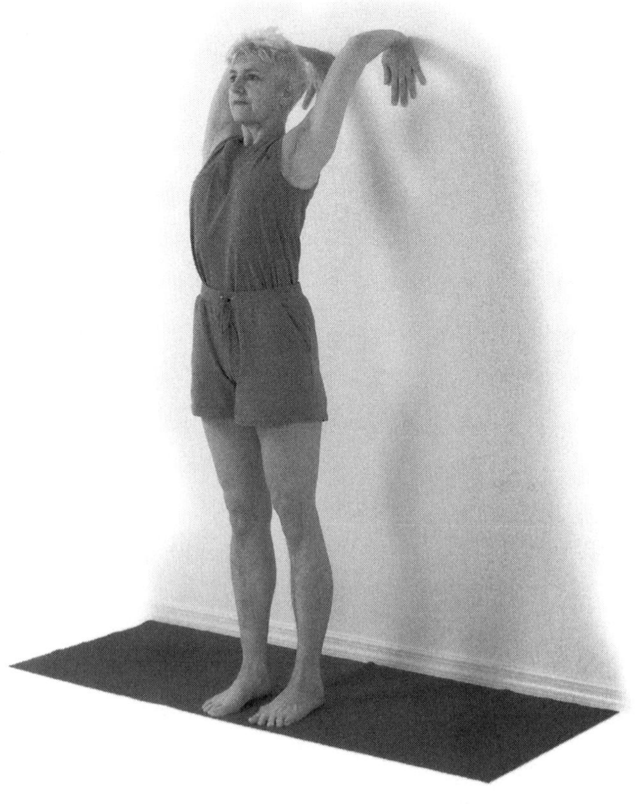

arms over behind your shoulders, fingers and palms touching the wall, right and left forearms and upper arms parallel, and about as far apart as your shoulders.

3. "Walk" down the wall, arching first the neck, then the thoracic spine, then the lumbar spine.

4. Your ankles will dorsiflex slightly, but the weight should still be balanced evenly on each foot. A side wall will help with balance.

As time goes on, you will descend further and further down the wall, and may safely start by standing further and further from the wall. When you have walked down to waist level with your fingers, you are probably ready to attempt Urdhva Dhanurasana. However, if early attempts are unsuccessful, return to the intermediate pose, testing Urdhva again every week or so.

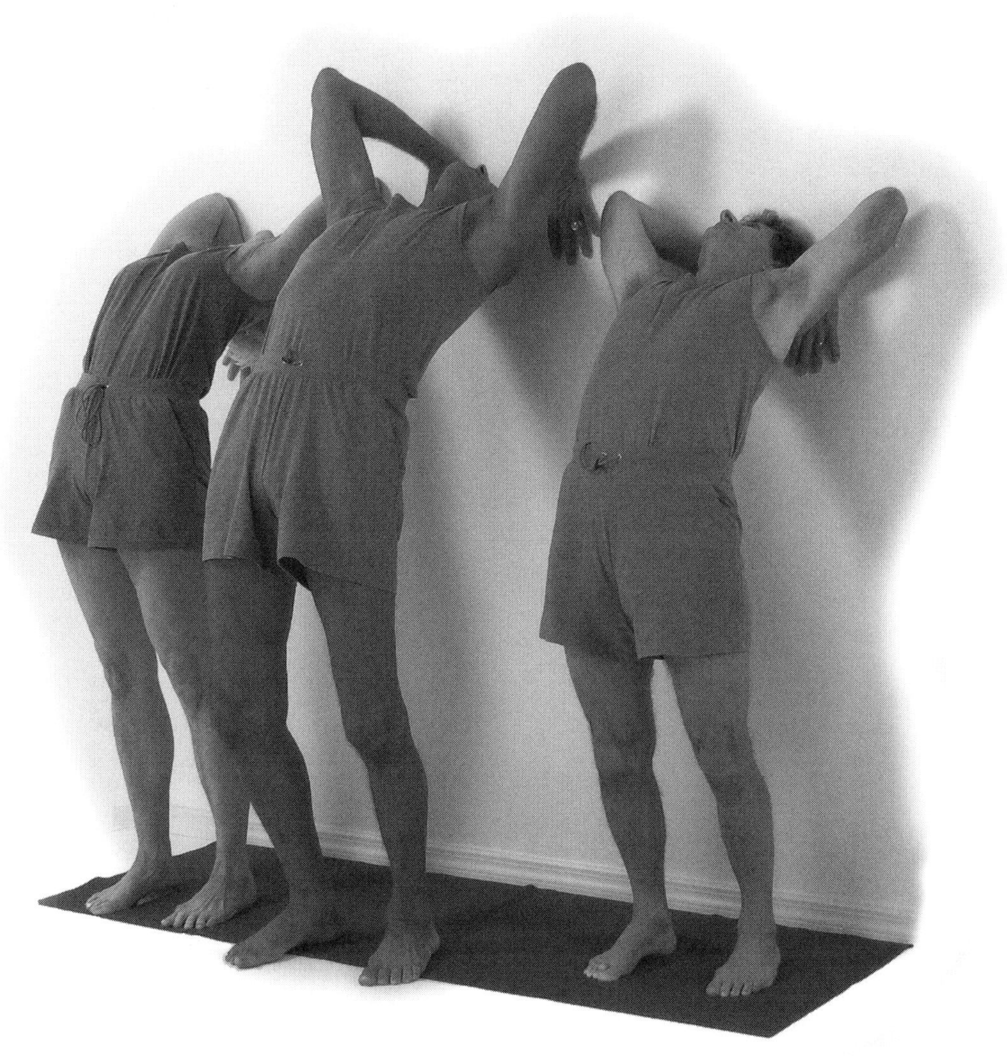

PADMASANA

The Lotus

1. Sit on a moderately sized cushion with legs stretched out before you.

2. Bending the right knee, cradle the foot in both hands and draw it as high as possible onto the left groin.

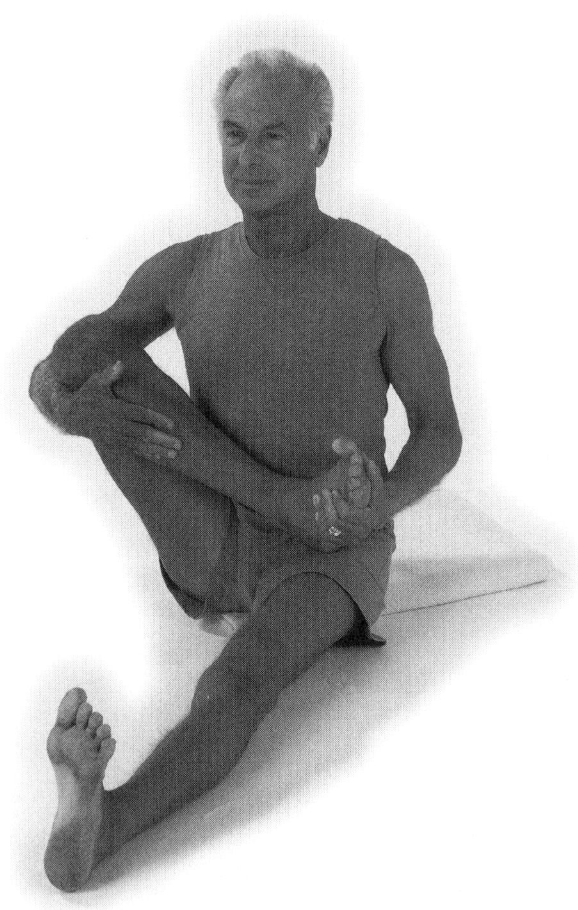

3. Bring the right knee down toward the floor.

4. Now bend the left knee and lift the left foot over the right knee and inward toward the right groin, placing it as close to the abdomen and navel as possible.

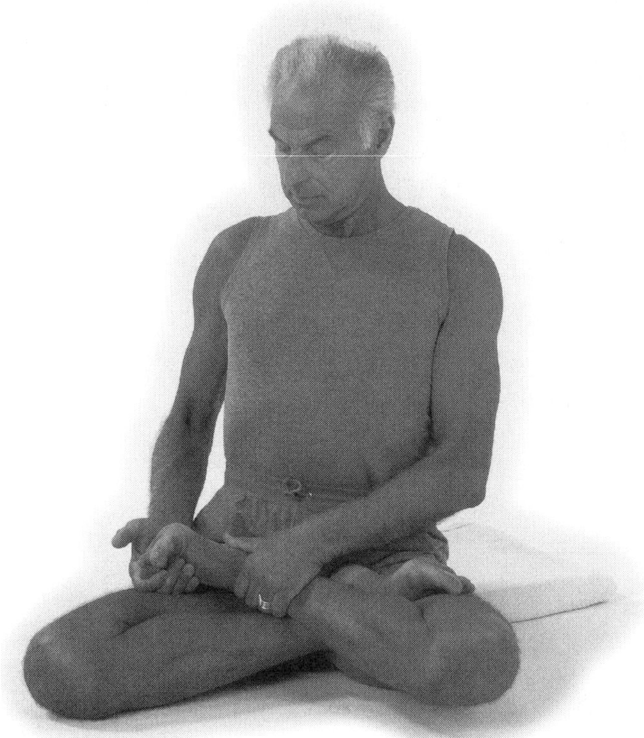

5. Pull in the abdomen, open the chest, straighten the spine from coccyx to the cervical vertebrae.

6. Rest the chin on the chest and the backs of the hands on the knees.

7. Breathe calmly, eyes closed, beginning as tolerated, and gradually extending to 30 minutes.

A certain amount of discomfort is almost inevitable at first, but do not strain too much to attain this pose, nor to stay in it too long. It may require several years to safely and usefully remain in it for 30 minutes. With practice it will become extremely comfortable.

Repeat the pose beginning with the left leg, but consistently practice breathing exercises with legs in one position or the other.

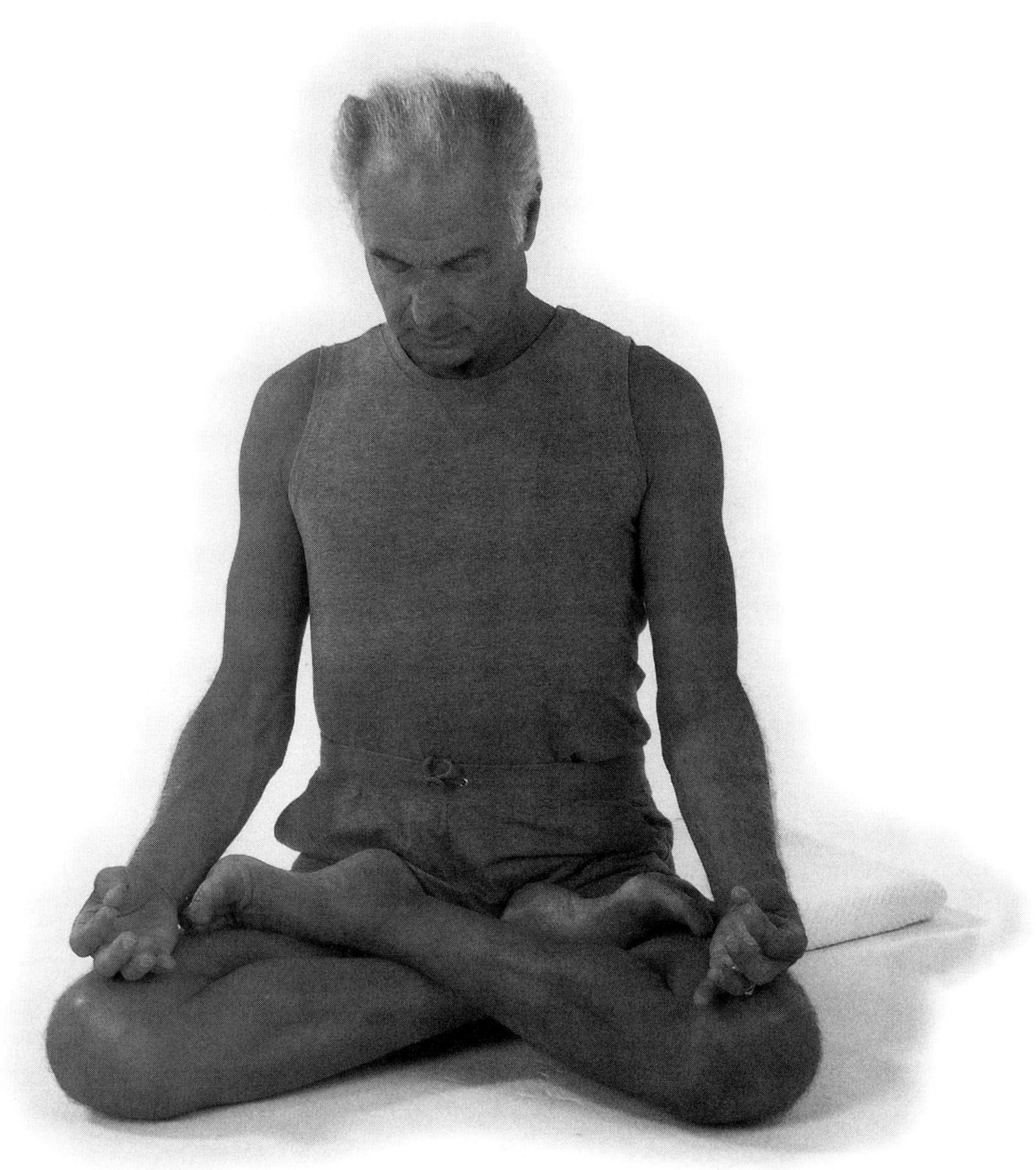

Entry- and Intermediate-Level Padmasana

An excellent means of eventually attaining Padmasana, the lotus, is a smooth continuum of movements. Any division between early and intermediate efforts is, as you will see, entirely arbitrary. Therefore we present it as a single series.

1. Place a blanket next to a wall, and lying sideways in the manner described earlier, raise legs as close to vertical as possible. Spread your arms out, palms up, parallel to the wall.

2. Bend your right knee; slide the heel toward the root of the thigh.

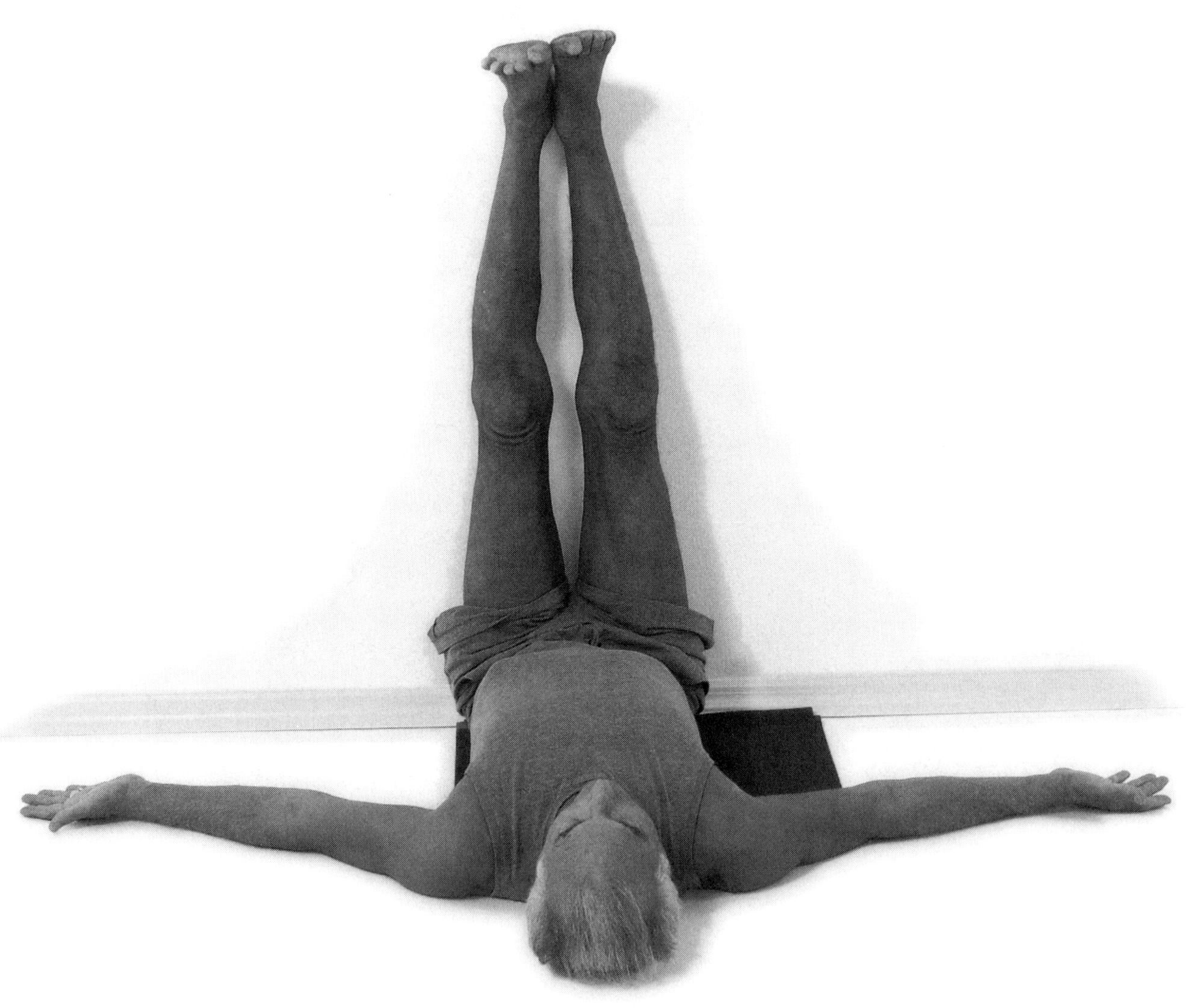

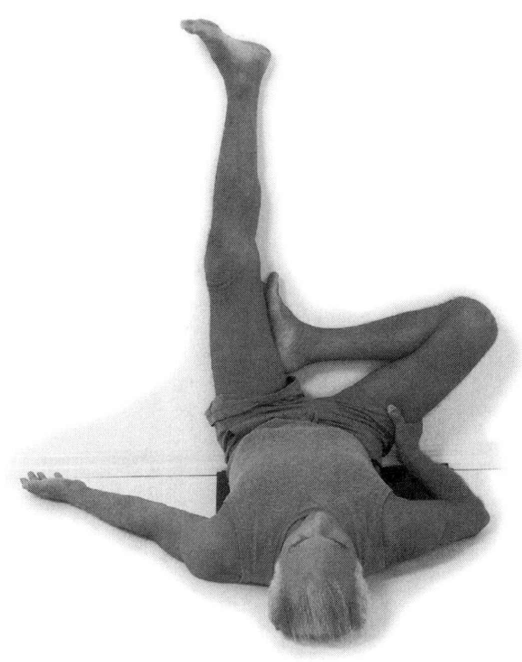

3. Take ahold of your right foot with the left hand and draw it in front of the left thigh as far as is comfortable.

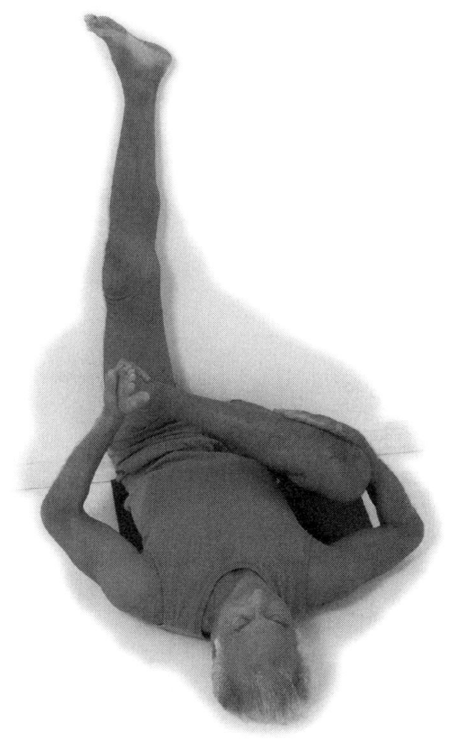

4. Set the right thigh back toward the wall.

5. Gradually bend the left knee. Retain the right thigh's contact with the wall.

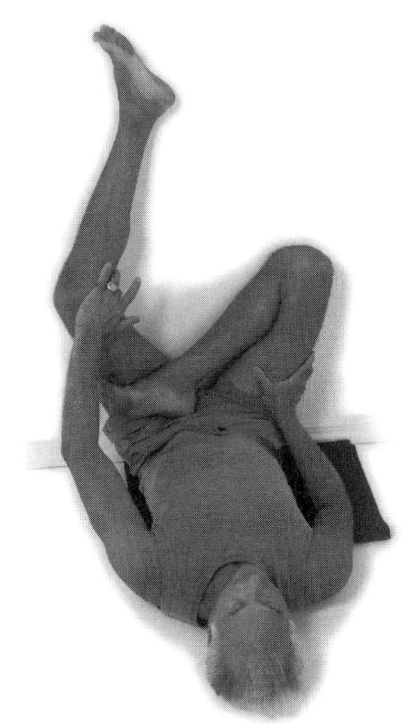

6. After 30 seconds to one minute, reverse the legs and repeat the procedure.

This step is the long one. It may take anywhere from one day to several years to succeed at the next one. Be patient and be careful. Easy does it. There is a proverb: "Be not afraid of going slowly, but of standing still."

7. Try from time to time to place the left ankle over the right thigh. When this occurs, hold it just a short time (5-10 seconds) and then try reversing the legs.

8. Gradually increase the timing to 1-2 minutes. Fit the thighs and shins together symmetrically. Comfort may come slowly, but it comes.

9. When this is reasonably stable, return your arms to the floor.

10. Guide your legs to the floor with your arms.

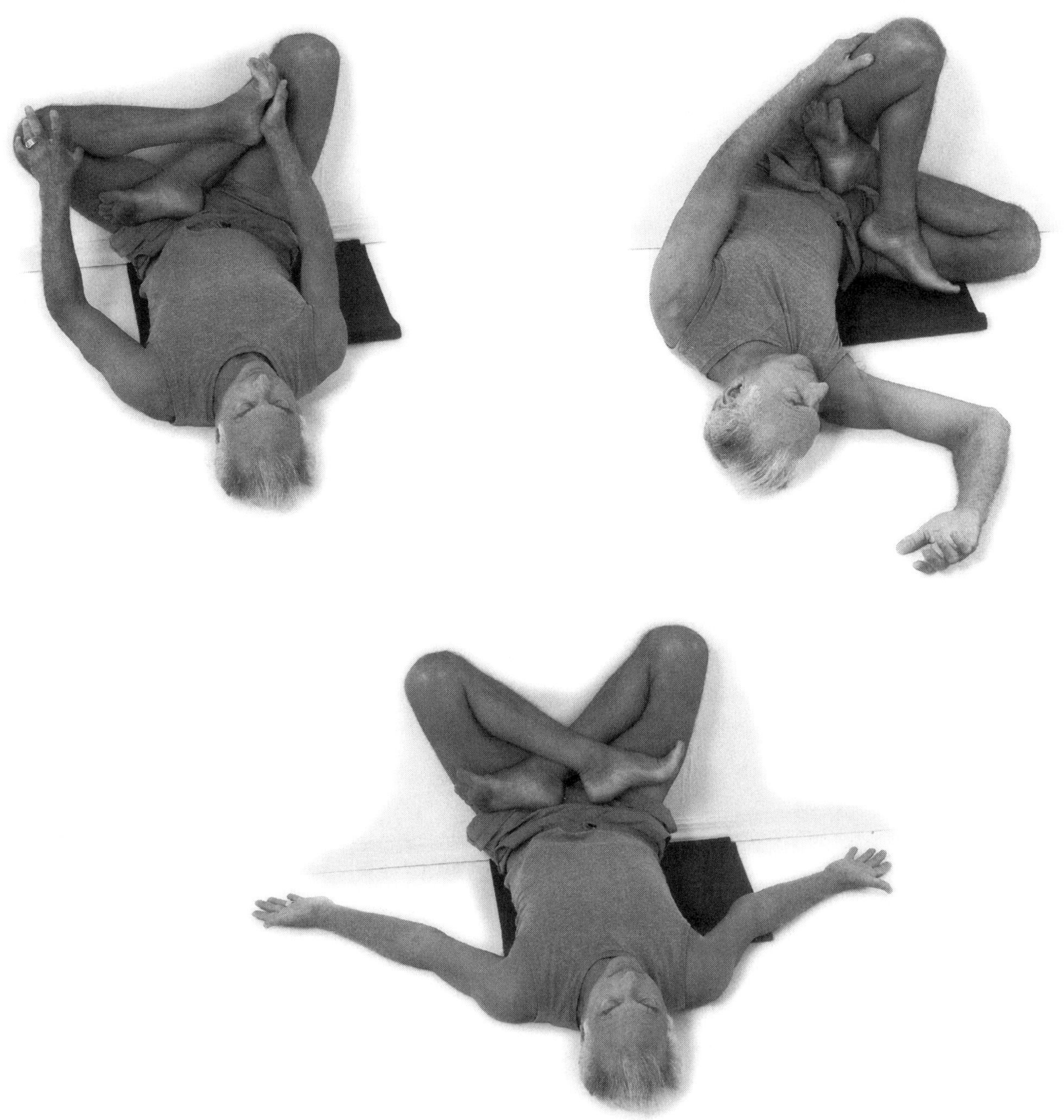

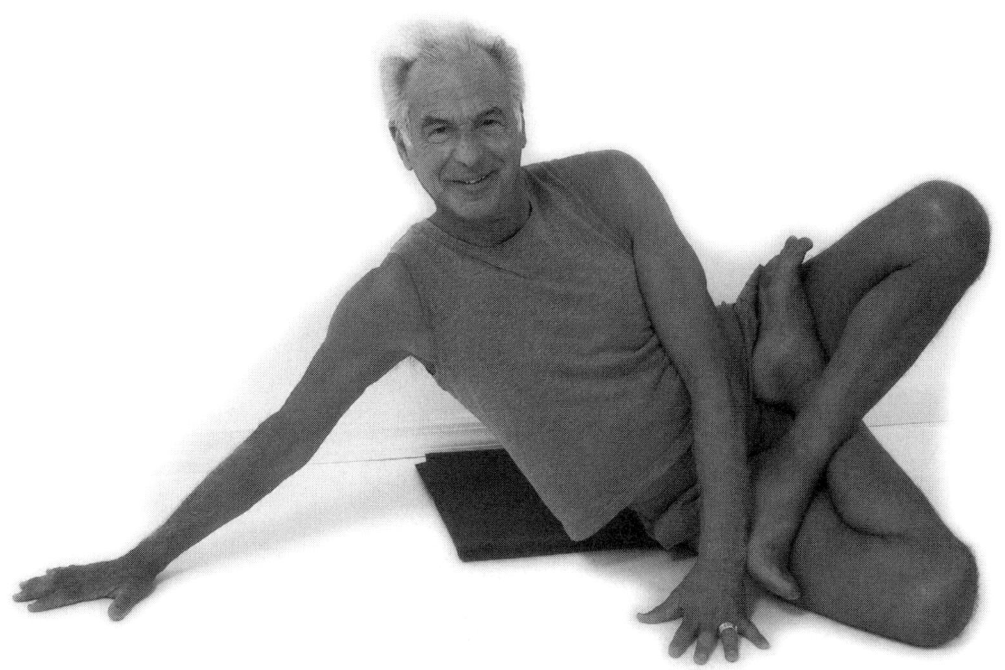

11. Spread your palms widely as you leave the inverted position.

12. Repeat the process, beginning with the left knee bent.

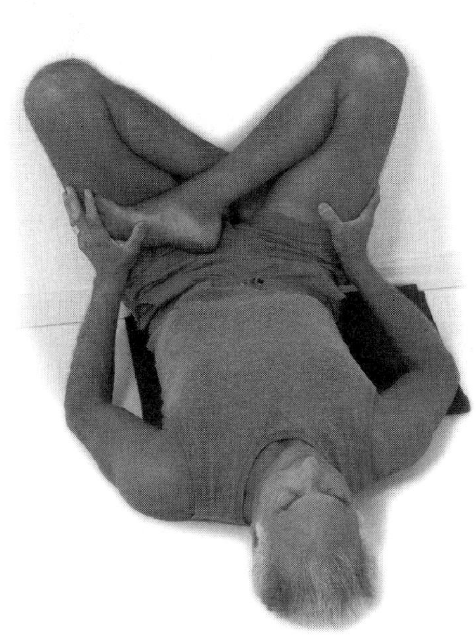

Gradually the pose may provide a stable and quiet sanctuary for you—as it has for individuals over thousands of years.

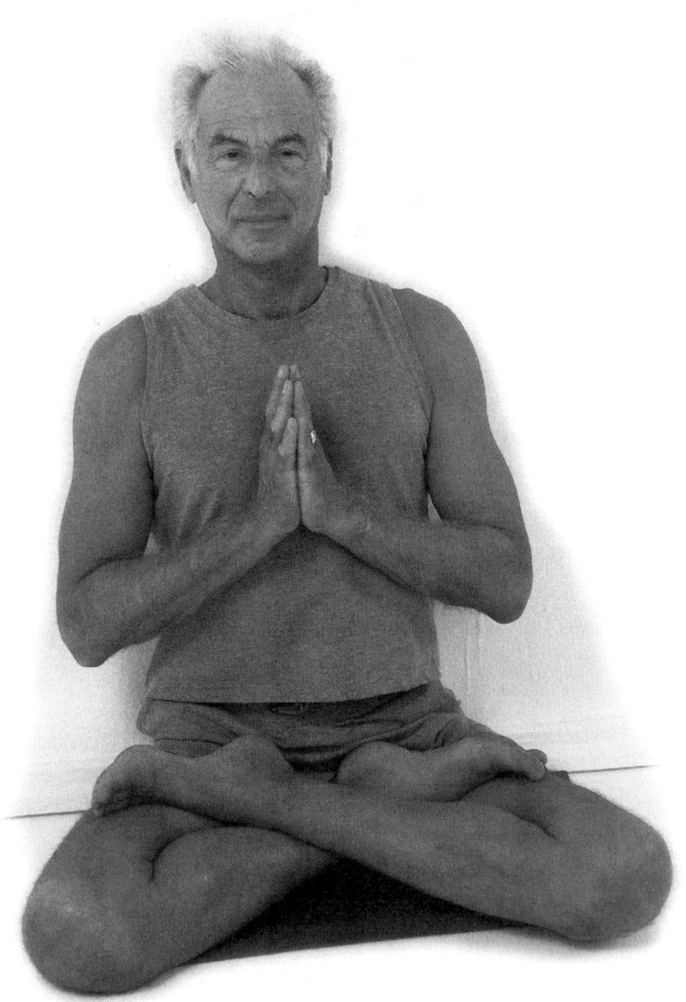

Improve Range of Motion

Whatever else Yoga does, it stretches. Stretching is a natural antidote for two of the most devastating consequences of MS: reduced range of motion and spasticity. First, consider reduced range of motion. There is no better, safer, faster nor more natural way to overcome the restrictions on full movement than lengthening them. This applies to muscles and their tendons, ligaments, joint capsules, and the adventitious scars and adhesions that may develop for a variety of reasons.

Simple as it may sound, range of motion is one of the gravest losses in a host of neurological conditions, for as range of motion decreases, the scope of possible activity diminishes proportionately. A cat with a stiff tail would have impaired balance. A mighty man with restricted range could not bench-press a barbell regardless of his strength. Yet relapsing and remitting MS, with its rising and falling levels of motor and sensory impairment is frequently accompanied by temporarily increased spasticity. But the spasticity, a neurological phenomenon, often subsequently retreats, leaving an unnecessarily long-lived mechanical reduction in range of motion that could be perpetuated by disuse.

As a retreating army of occupation leaves devastation in its wake, the resultant loss of range of motion is often the most serious consequence of an exacerbating episode of MS. Yoga is a safe and sure remedy.

In progressive MS degrees of range of motion may be lost unnecessarily due to failure to challenge the actual limits that impaired function imposes. These add up. Be it the spine, the hips, arms or ankles, unnecessary concessions to the disease work to contract the individual's life-possibilities and opportunities, as well as their joints.

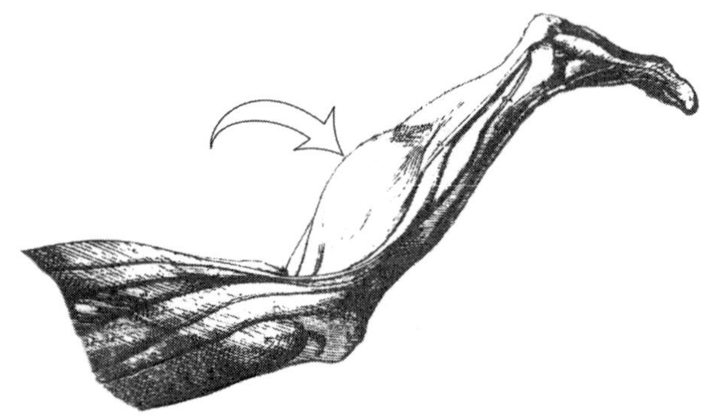

Strategies to Improve Range of Motion

Many important groups of muscles cross more than one joint, and where these muscles are the limiting factors in joint mobility, both joints must be approached simultaneously. The gastrocnemius muscle, for example, crosses the back of both the ankle and the knee. If stretching it at the ankle is attempted without regard for the straightness of the knee, it will be impossible to put it under any tension at all. However, once the muscle is stretched at the ankle, further straightening the knee is often a good method of increasing the range of motion at the ankle joint.

In other circumstances, such as relapsing and remitting MS, it can happen that a given joint is inactive for a period of months due to weakness or spasticity that then remits or vanishes, leaving a competent and properly toned muscle across a joint that is "frozen" by tightened ligaments or constricting joint capsule. Then the critical strategy is to take the muscle out of play, arranging position so that the muscle is slack, enabling one to work directly on the restricting elements. In that case, to disengage the gastrocnemius, one would intentionally stretch the ankle with the knee bent.

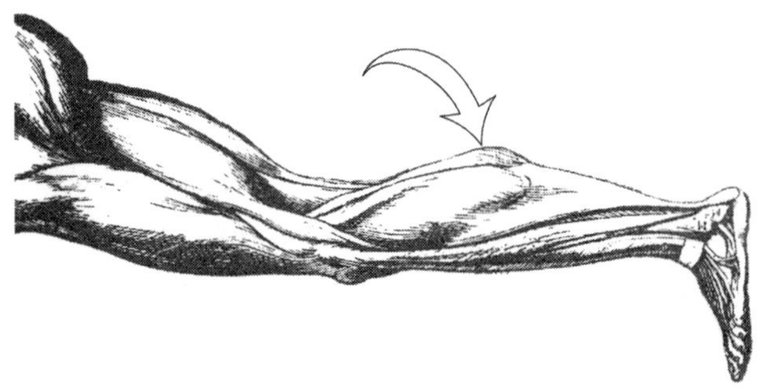

Reduced range of motion and spasticity often work together: tightened muscles serve to decrease range of motion at the joints they cross and decreased range of motion brings on tightened muscles which cannot be stretched, that readily react to everyday stimuli with painful spasticity. In this respect all the asanas given later for spasticity will also serve to extend range of motion. Nevertheless, there are a number of other postures which accomplish this task more directly.

Trikonasana

1. Spend 20-30 seconds in Tadasana, seeking the calm of the mountain pose.

2. Inhaling, spring the legs to 3 1/2 feet apart.

3. Turn the right foot out 90 degrees, and the left foot inward 30 degrees, stretching the arms horizontally as far apart as they will go. Palms down, hands concave upward.

4. Puff out the chest, draw in the abdomen and exhale and descend toward the right

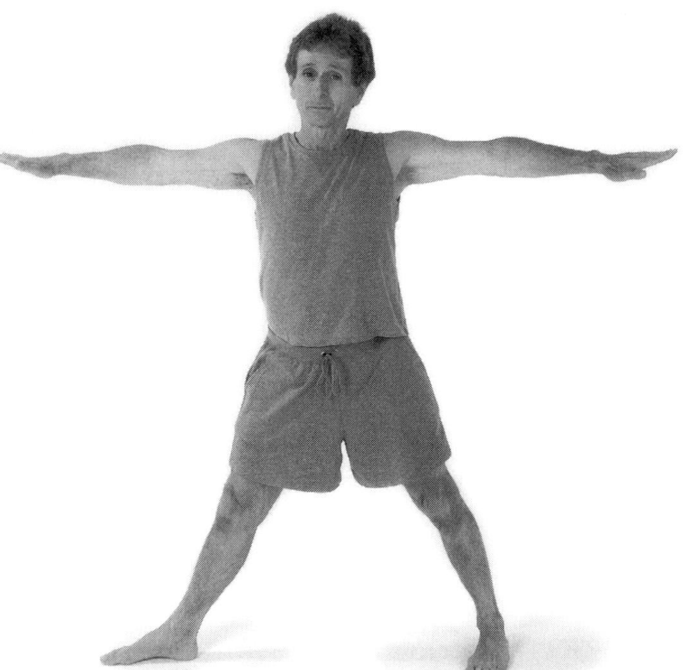

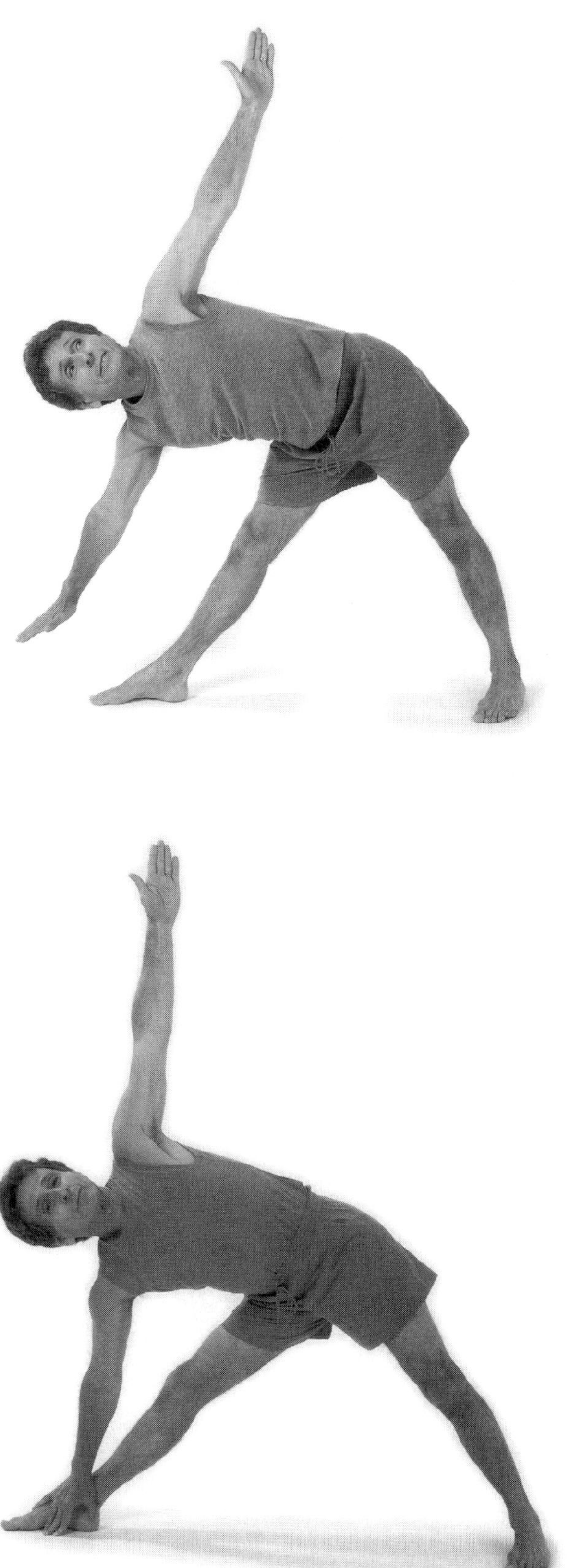

calf, retaining the alignment of the arms, and keeping the torso in the plane defined by the intersection of the two legs.

5. After the right hand reaches the floor, press backward on it to rotate the torso so that a line through the two arms would pass through the center of the earth. Steady the left foot in place as you rotate the left knee outward and curl the left buttock back, so that the lower and upper torso are also brought back, in line with the same plane.

6. The action of the arms and legs will separate the torso away from the root of the right thigh, and raise the left thigh higher, widening the right groin and lengthening the left groin. Breathe calmly and evenly, filling the right and left lungs equally, for 1 minute. Then reverse this for the left side.

Entry-Level Trikonasana

1. Perform the same pose lying supine. Begin with 20-30 seconds in Savasana, quiet and calm.

2. Separate your legs by moving your left leg 2-3 1/2 feet to the left, the right leg still in the savasana position, both feet vertical.

3. Slide the arms out 90 degrees from the torso, keeping shoulder blades down, back and together, and palms horizontal. Elevating the right shoulder slightly will allow the same angling that the vertical standing pose entails.

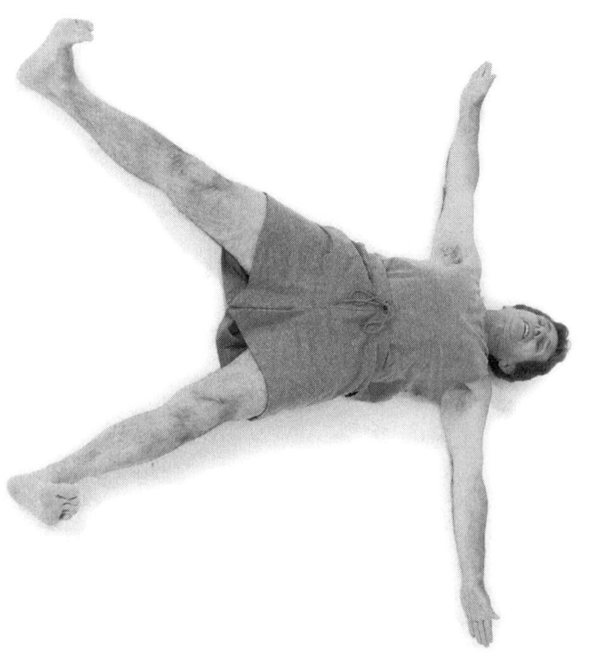

4. Turn your head to the right, attempting to gaze at the left hand with the right eye. Hold the position with regular breathing for 20-30 seconds.

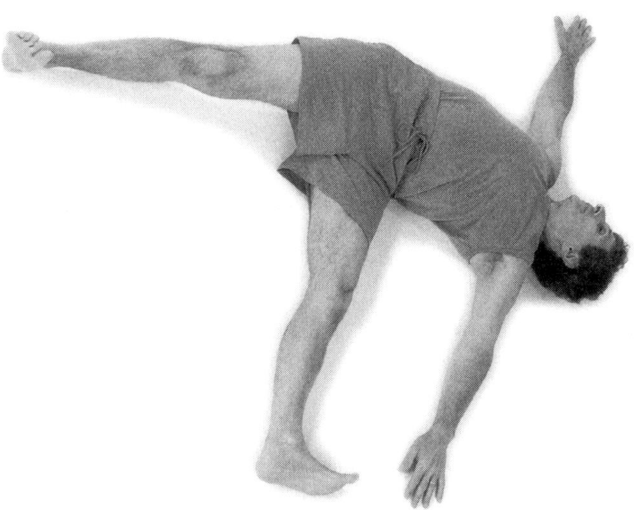

5. Then return the legs to savasana and repeat the pose with the right leg and left shoulder.

Early Intermediate Trikonasana

1. Stand facing a doorway or narrow hall with feet 3-3 1/2 feet apart.

2. Turn the right foot out 90 degrees and the left foot 30 degrees inward, using the right or left arm to keep steady balance. **[A]**

3. Calmly take a few breaths. Keep your weight evenly distributed by turning the left knee outward and tightening the left buttock, while inclining to the right side and slowly sliding the right arm down the side of the doorway or hall. **[B]**

4. Exhale while descending. Remain in the position for up to 1 minute while breathing calmly.

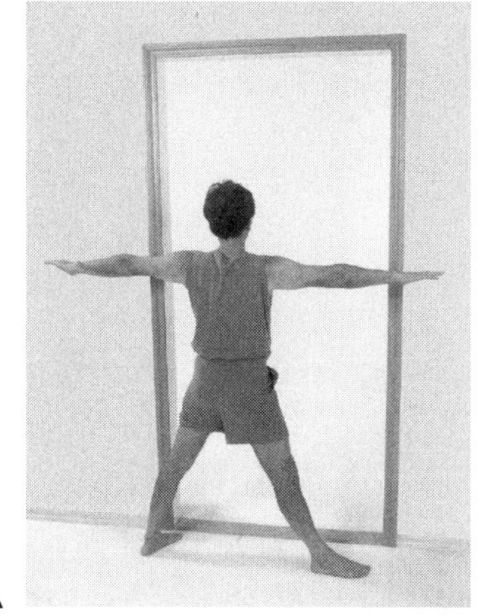
A

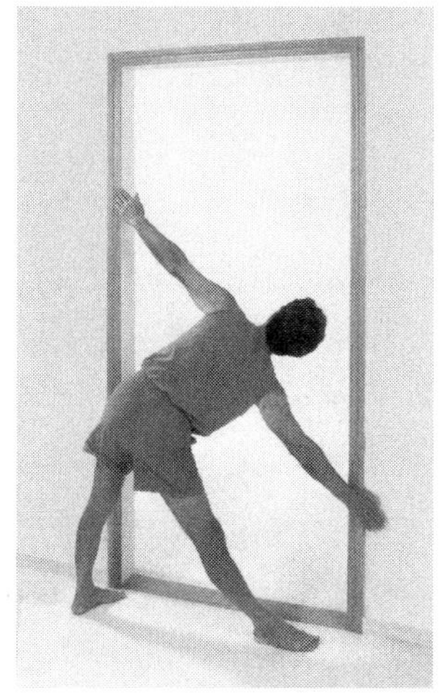
B

Later Intermediate Trikonasana

1. Stand with your buttocks touching a wall, feet 3 ½ feet apart.

2. Turn the right foot out 90 degrees, parallel to the wall. Turn the left foot inward 30 degrees. Stretch the arms out horizontally. **[1]**

3. Briefly turn the palms upward, so that the flexor sides of the elbows, the cubital fossae, turn upward. Then rotate the palms downward. The cubital fossae remain facing up.

4. Take in a good breath, extending the fingertips of each hand as far from the torso as possible. Puff out the chest, draw in the abdomen and descend toward the right calf, keeping the right buttock and the right shoulder in contact with the wall. Retain the alignment of the arms, and keep the torso in the plane defined by the intersection of the two legs. **[2]**

5. After the right hand reaches as far as it can get without disturbing the alignment of the arms, shoulders and trunk, **[3]** press it

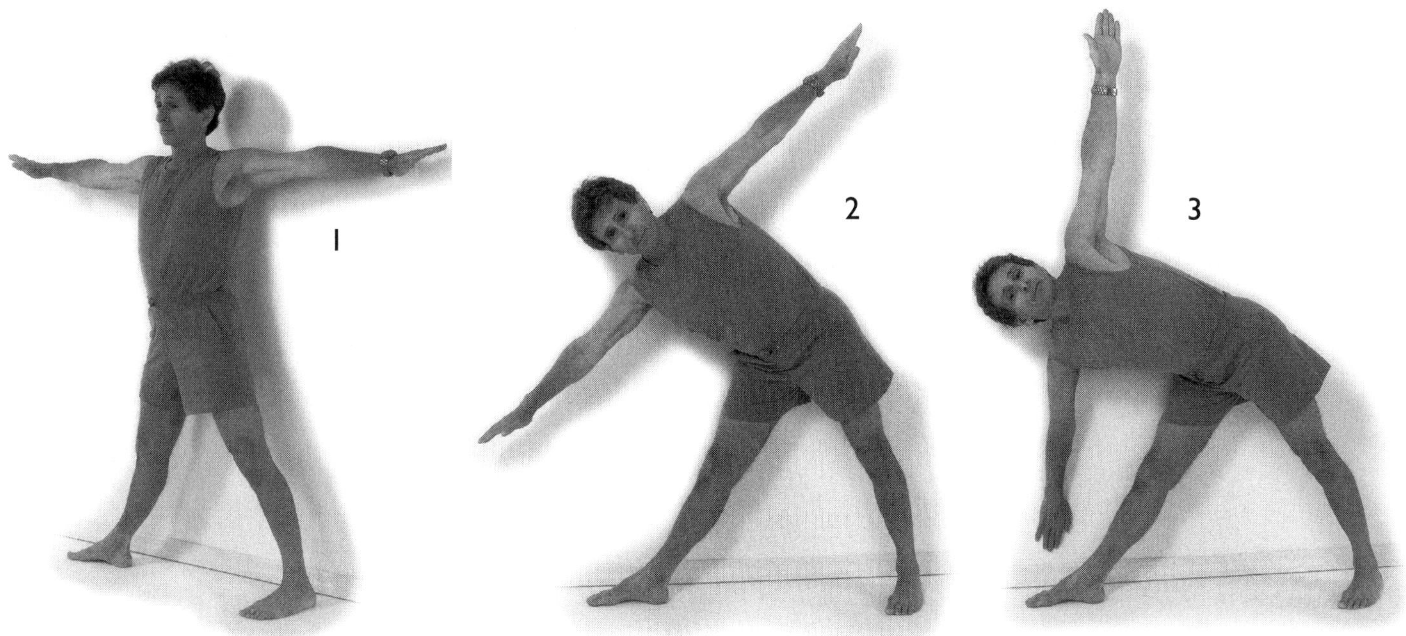

back against the ankle or calf to rotate the torso so that a line through the two arms would pass through the center of the earth, and the torso is still in the plane defined by the two legs. Bending the right elbow will add to the force that can be exerted, but is not the definitive pose. Inhale.

6. Keep the left foot in place, rotate the left knee outward and curl the left buttock back, so that the lower torso is also brought back, in line with the same plane.

7. Attempt to bring the left buttock and the left shoulder blade to the wall behind you, parallel to their right-sided counterparts. Exhale.

The action of the arms and legs will bring the torso higher, away from the thickest part of the right thigh, widening the right groin and lengthening the left groin. Breathe calmly and evenly, filling the right and left lungs equally, for 1 minute. Then do the reverse on the left side.

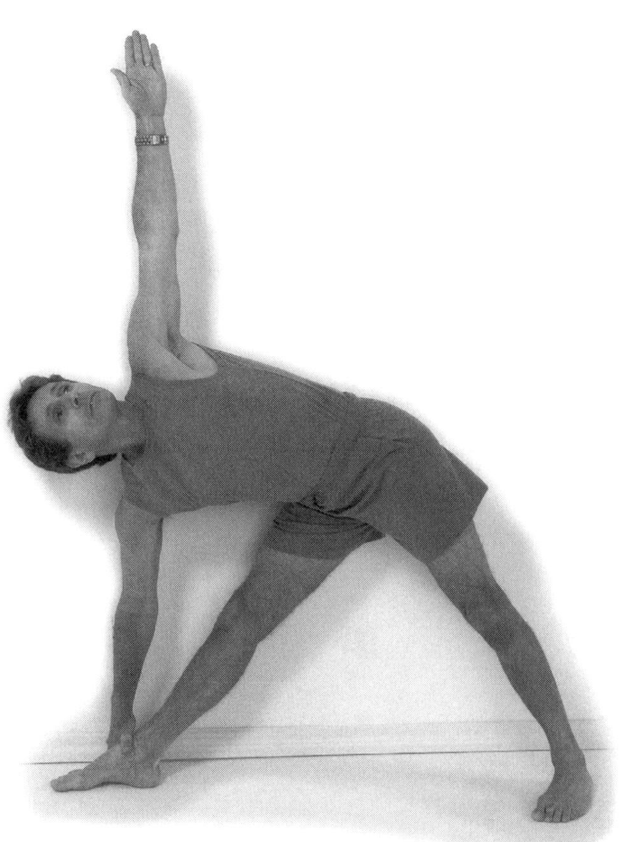

Virasana

This is a powerful and therefore a dangerous way to improve hip, knee and ankle range of motion. Safety first: use a good number of pillows to sit on when beginning this pose. Best to have an experienced person present. After a few trials, the practitioner will be better able to judge what is needed. Stay in the pose for only 10 seconds for the first few weeks, then, over the next 6 months, gradually increase the time to a full minute, increasing by 5 seconds every two weeks. Without an instructor, one should not try performing the first pose described and pictured below for at least six months after taking up virasana.

1. Kneel on a flat surface with knees together but feet barely further apart than the hips.

2. Slowly bend the knees, controlling the descent of your haunches with the fingertips

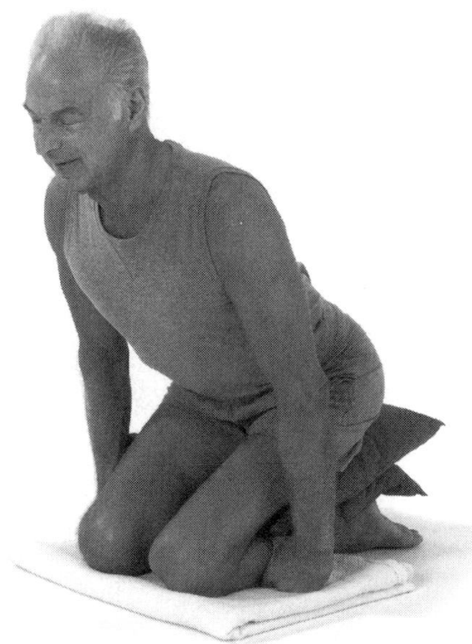

even before knee flexion brings them down to touch the surface or pillows or blocks that have been placed between the arching feet.

3. Gradually settle the buttocks down as far as possible. The inner calves are in contact with the outer thighs.

4. Place the palms of the hands on the thighs, joining the thumb and index fingers.

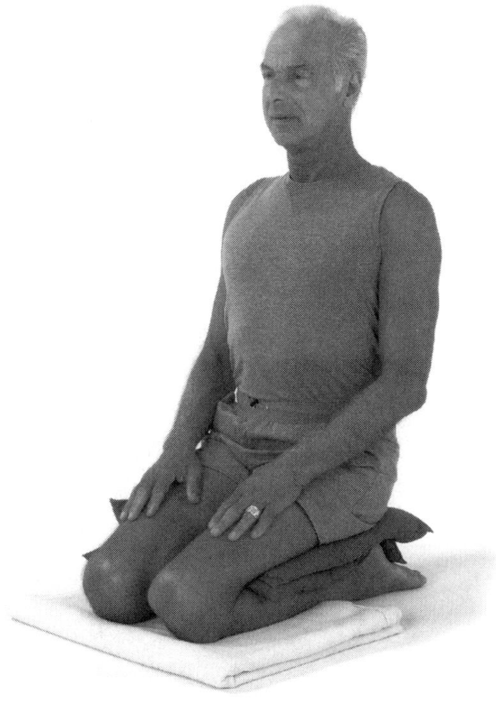

5. Lift the spine from the nape of the neck, pull back the abdomen, and reduce muscular tension in the thighs, abdomen and pelvis. Breathe quietly for 1-2 minutes.

6. Interlock the fingers, palms facing the chest. Bring the hands behind the head.

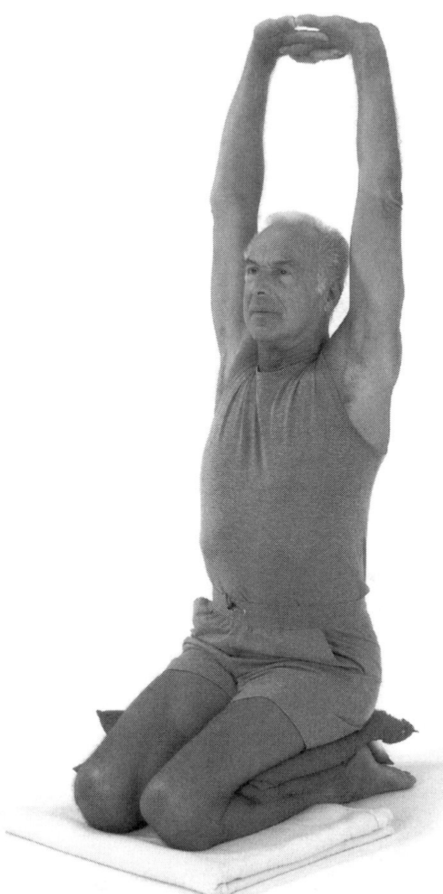

Smoothly flex the shoulders while extending the elbows and wrists, palms facing upwards, biceps behind ears. Keep shoulder blades back, together and down toward the pelvis.

7. Retain the straight back, stretching from the palms to the coccyx. Looking straight ahead, breathe calmly for 1 minute.

1

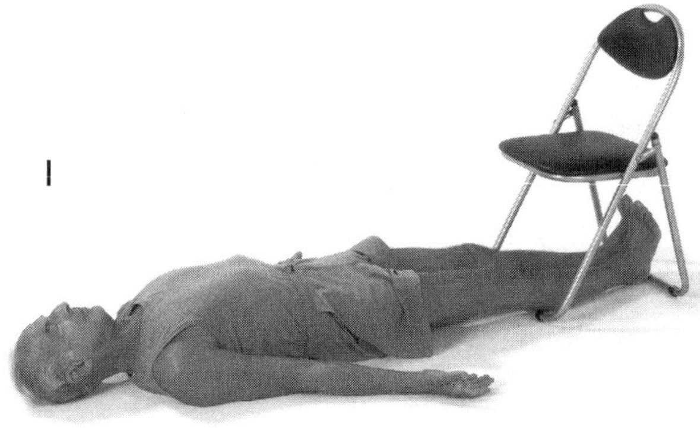

2

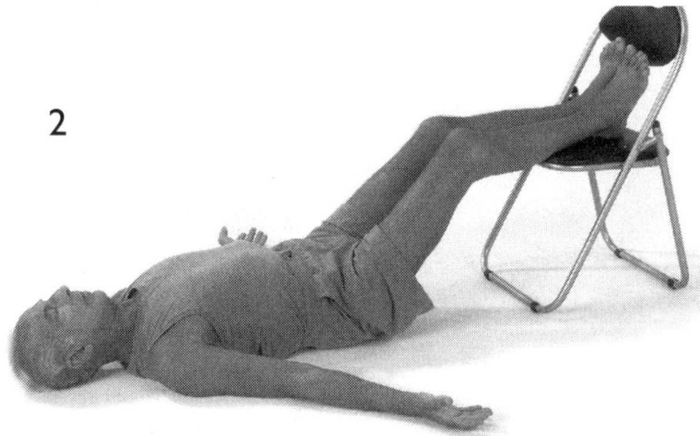

3

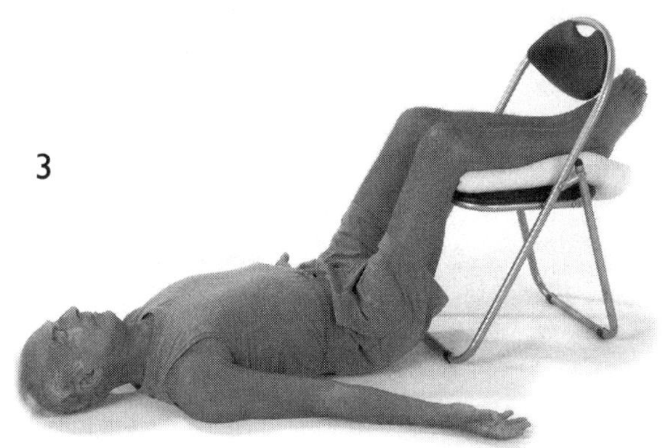

Entry-Level Virasana

1. Lie supine on a flat surface with a chair standing over the legs. [1]

2. Let the backs of the hands rest on the surface, sliding the arms down and letting the shoulders descend to the surface as well. Inhale. [2]

3. Stretch the back of the head far from the shoulders with exhalation.

4. One at a time place the backs of the calves on the chair, moving the practitioner and/or the chair to find the angle at which there is a persistent but safe pull on the knees or the hip joints. Breathe calmly for 1-2 minutes. [3]

Adjusting the chair further away from the body (toward the feet) produces more hip extension but less knee flexion. As the chair stands closer to the hips, the hips and knees are flexed more. Pillows under the sacrum give more knee flexion without increasing hip flexion, and are useful for treating concurrent hip flexion and knee extension contractures.

Intermediate Virasana

An ambulatory person will not have prohibitive hip flexion contractures, but may have knee extension contractures. Therefore this potent and potentially harmful pose still requires great vigilance to improve hip, knee and ankle range of motion.

Safety first. Use four or five pillows or a bolster to sit on when beginning this pose. Scrutiny of an experienced person is better yet. After a few trials, the practitioner will be better able to judge what is safe. Let mild pain and a sense of apprehension be your guide to limitation. Stay in the pose for only 10 seconds for the first few weeks. Then, over the next 6 months, gradually increase the time to a full minute. Without an instructor, one should certainly use more pillows than absolutely needed at first, and place chairs at either elbow to assure adequate balance.

1. Place the pillows or a bolster between two chairs facing each other.

2. With palms and then forearms on the seats of the chairs, kneel in front of the pillows with knees together but feet further apart than the pillows. **[1]**

3. Slowly bend the knees, controlling your descent with hands and forearms. **[2]**

4. Gradually rest the buttocks on the pillows that are between your arching feet. The inner calves are below the outer thighs. **[3]**

5. Turn the palms up, and with the backs of the hands on the chair seats, join the thumb and index fingers if possible.

6. Lift the spine as though from the nape of the neck, pull back the abdomen, and reduce muscular tension in the thighs, abdomen, pelvis, shoulders and arms.

7. Breathe quietly for 1-2 minutes.

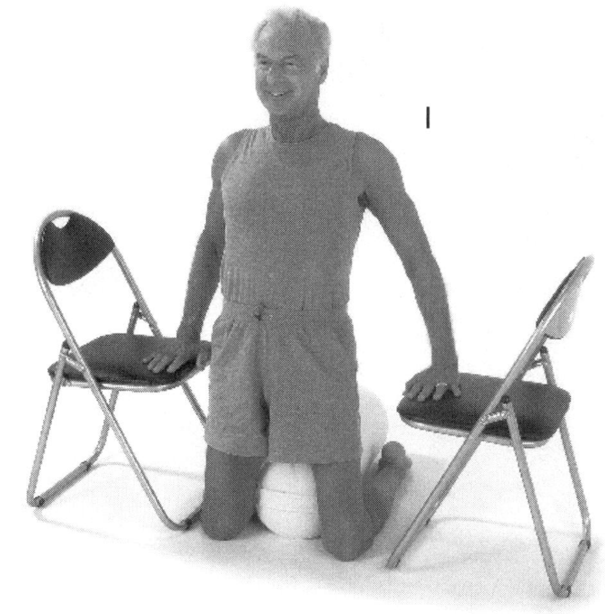

1

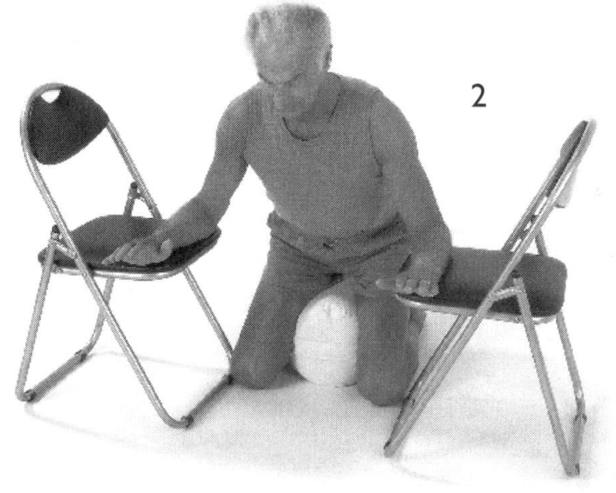

2

If stability is in question, begin the next part with one arm, using the other to improve balance. If possible, lift both arms off the chairs, interlocking the fingers and bringing the arms overhead, flexing the shoulders and extending the elbows and wrists and fingers maximally. Lower and retract the shoulders, opening the chest and pulling in the abdomen. Relax and breathe in this pose for 1 minute.

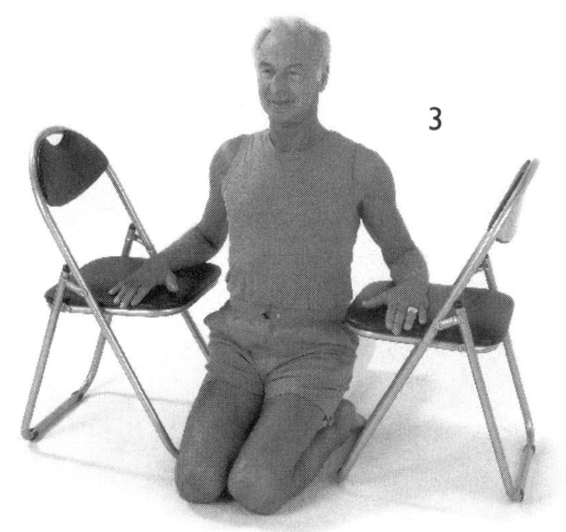

3

SUPTA VIRASANA

Supine Hero's Pose

1. Use the steps on pages 152-153 to enter virasana.

2. Then lower the arms, and carefully lean back, placing the forearms on the surface.

3. Extend the neck, bring the head back, arch the thoracic spine.

4. Slowly slide the arms down toward the waist, palms upward, and straighten the neck, resting the shoulders and the back of the head on the surface.

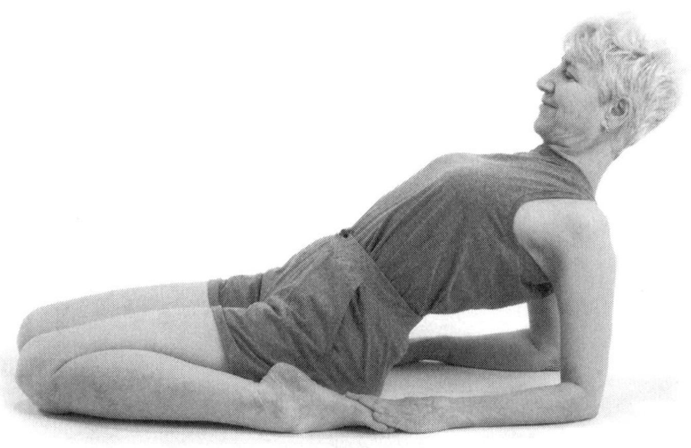

5. Last, slowly rotate the arms as they are stretched out parallel, palms upward, over the head (*see below*).

6. Breathe calmly for 1 minute, putting as much of the back as possible in contact with the surface.

Entry-Level Supta Virasana I

1. Begin with entry-level supta virasana.

2. Raise the arms to vertical and revolve them slowly as they are stretched maximally overhead and placed palm upward on the surface.

3. Breathe calmly for 1 minute.

A bed or couch at the home or a plinth in the clinic are useful for a further stage of beginning virasana.

1. Lie supine on the couch or plinth, using pillows under the thighs if hip flexion contractures prohibit full extension. Take several unhurried breaths. **[1]**

2. Let the shoulders descend into the couch or plinth. Keep the shoulder blades symmetrically placed.

3. Now inch down so that the heels, then the ankles, then the distal calves are off the end of the couch or plinth, causing the knees to bend slightly. **[2]**

4. Keep inching until there is a gentle but persistent tug of tension at the knee and/or hip joint. Then slide the backs of

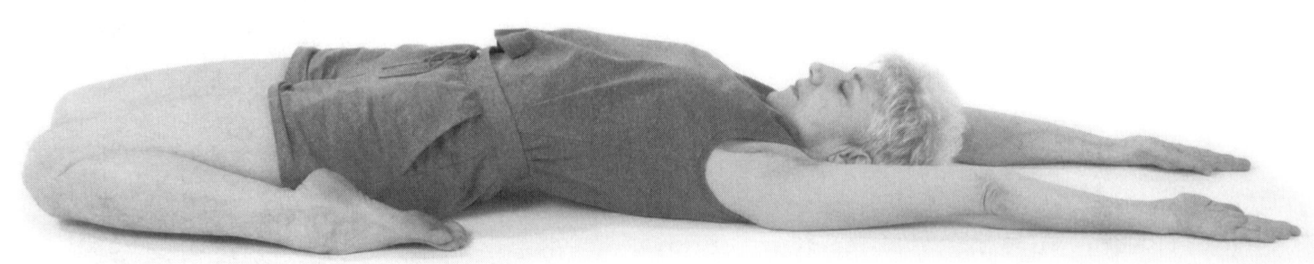

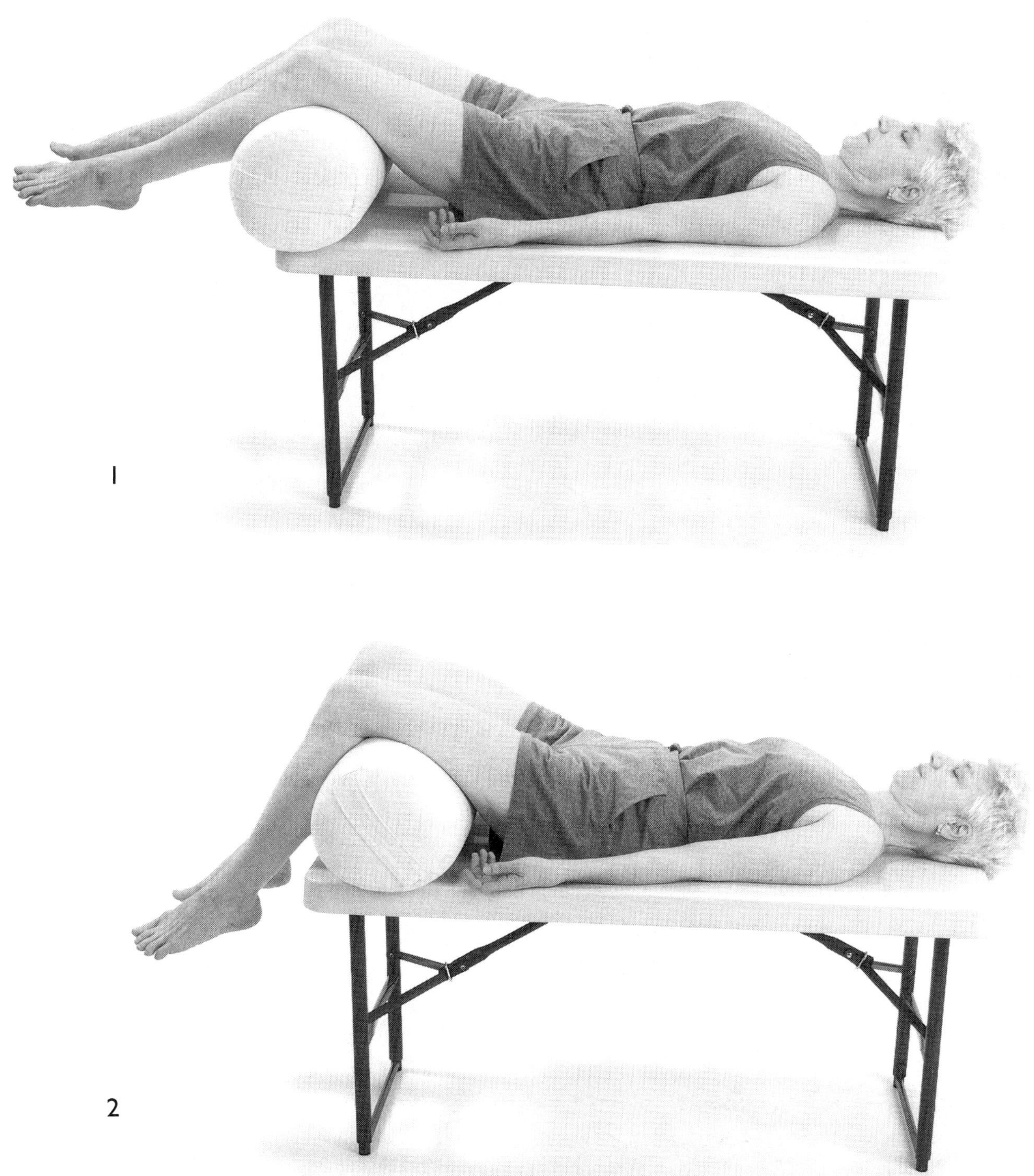
1
2

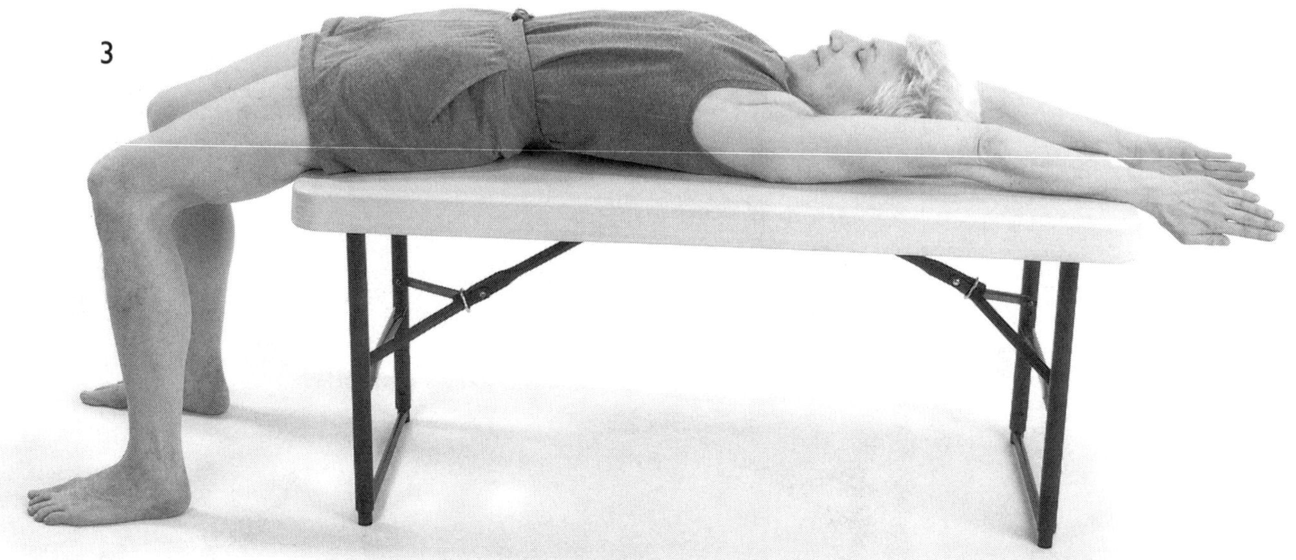

3

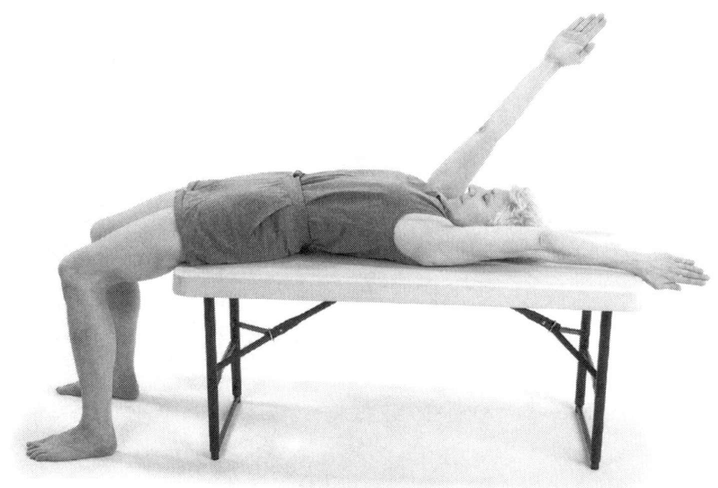

the hands as far away from the hips as possible, let the shoulders fall once again.

5. Straighten the spine and the back of the neck, increasing the distance between the shoulders and the ears.

6. Breathe slowly and symmetrically in this position for 1-2 minutes. [3]

Entry-Level Supta Virasana II

A more demanding variant of these two intermediate poses raises the arms over the head, stretching them in parallel along the couch or plinth, palms stretched open wide.

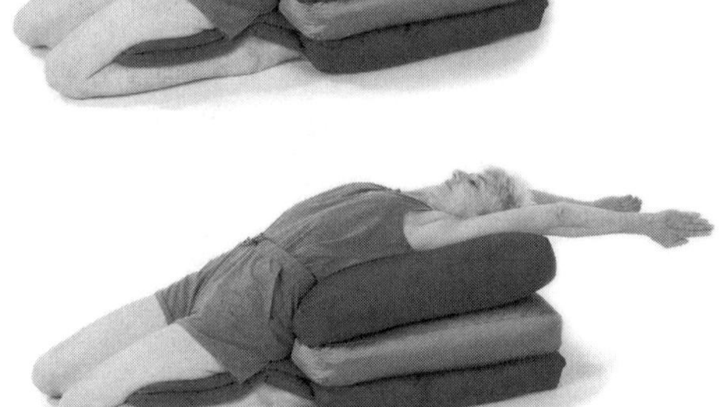

Intermediate Supta Virasana

An intermediate supta virasana requires as many or more pillows under the back as under the buttocks.

Three possible variations are pictured here.

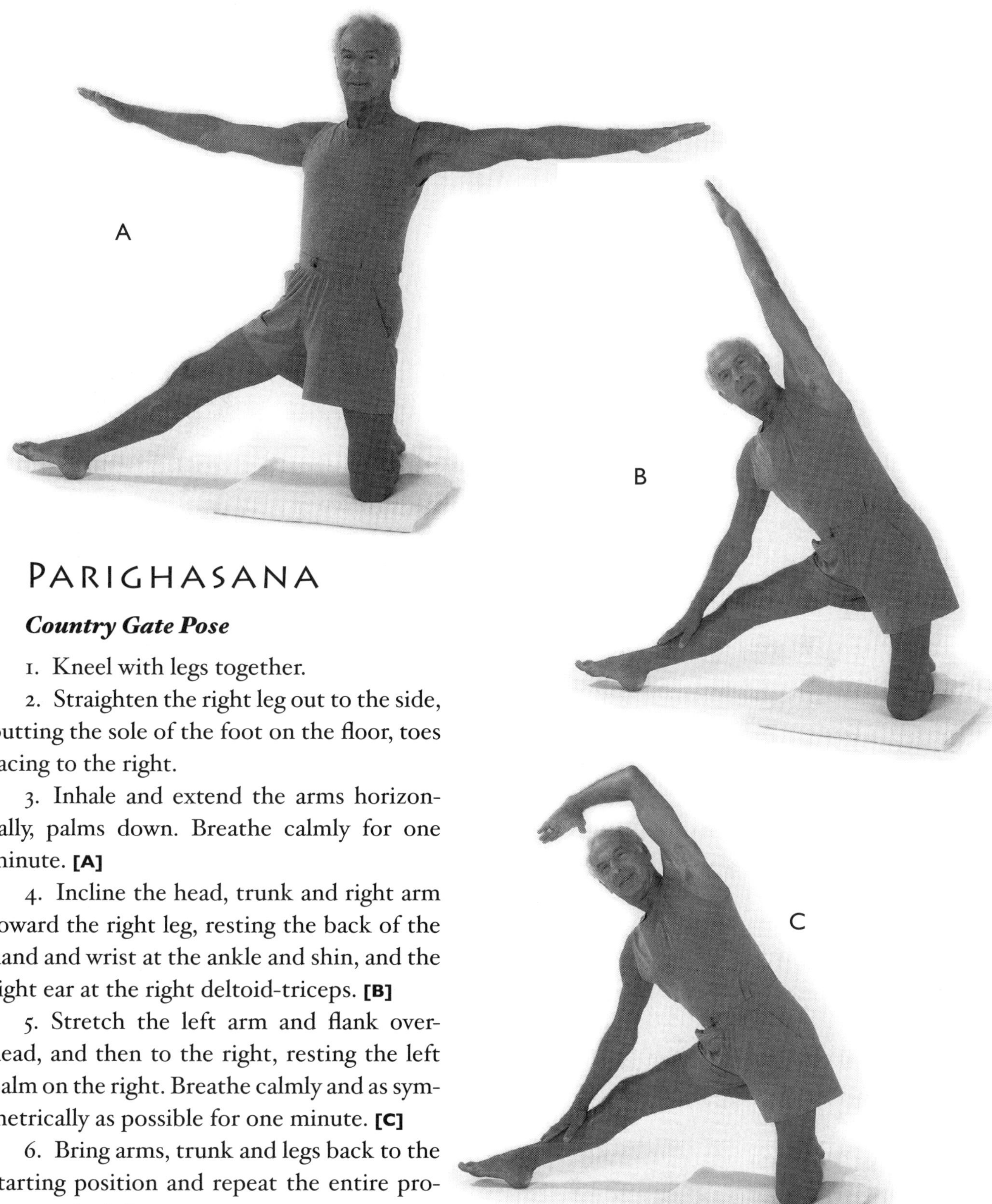

PARIGHASANA

Country Gate Pose

1. Kneel with legs together.
2. Straighten the right leg out to the side, putting the sole of the foot on the floor, toes facing to the right.
3. Inhale and extend the arms horizontally, palms down. Breathe calmly for one minute. **[A]**
4. Incline the head, trunk and right arm toward the right leg, resting the back of the hand and wrist at the ankle and shin, and the right ear at the right deltoid-triceps. **[B]**
5. Stretch the left arm and flank overhead, and then to the right, resting the left palm on the right. Breathe calmly and as symmetrically as possible for one minute. **[C]**
6. Bring arms, trunk and legs back to the starting position and repeat the entire process on the left.

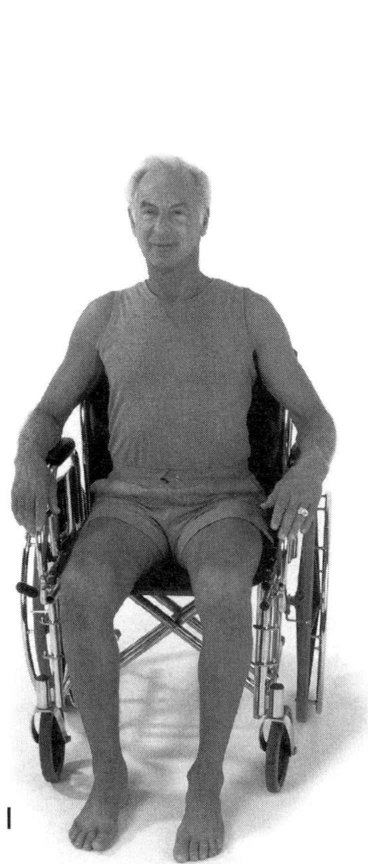
1

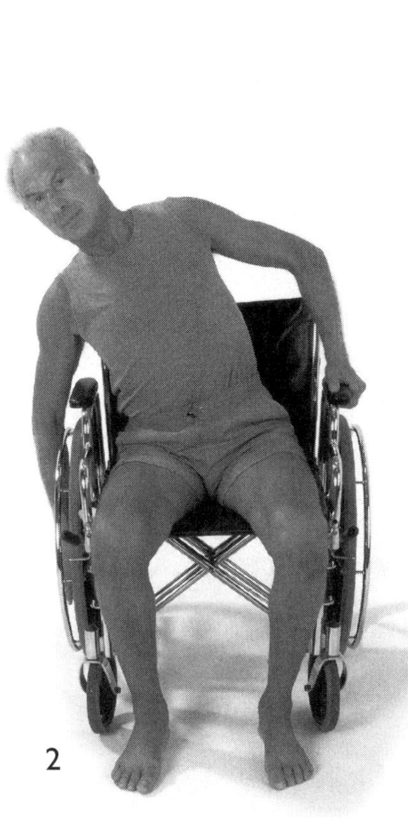
2

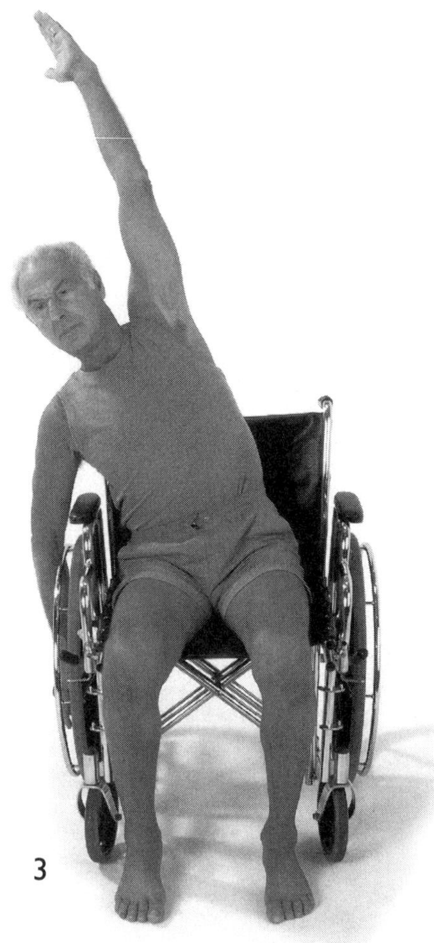
3

Entry-Level Parighasana

1. Sit far back and grasp the arms of the wheelchair or armchair.

2. Balance weight evenly over the two ischial tuberosities. **[1]**

3. Breathe calmly for 1 minute.

4. Use arm pressure to maintain an equal distribution of weight as the head and ribs incline to the right. **[2]**

5. Release the left hand, straightening the arm, then raise it up to vertical, and continue as much to the right side as possible, so that the left bicep is close to the left ear.

6. Still balancing the weight evenly, stretch the left flank from the iliac crest, ribs and scapula to the triceps, forearm extensors and the back of the hand. **[3]**

7. Now breathe evenly and calmly for 1 minute.

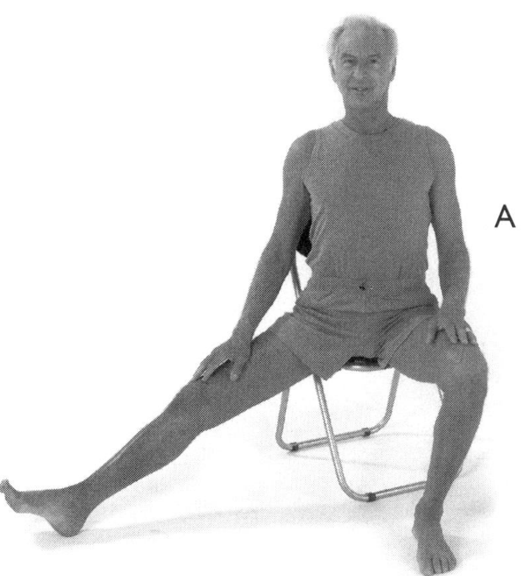

Intermediate Parighasana

1. Sit on the edge of a wheelchair or chair.

2. Swing the right leg out maximally to the right, and straighten the knee to tolerance. Blocks may help to make it straighter. **[A]**

3. Release the right armrest (if there is one) and slide the right palm down the right thigh, while inclining the head and trunk to the right. Use both hands to support, guide and control the lateral descent of the trunk and head. **[B]**

4. When motion to the right has gone to its safe maximum, take a few calm breaths. Then, if balance permits, raise the left arm straight upward, using the right arm and hand for stability. Take a few more calm breaths.

5. When possible, bring the left arm over to the right side, stretching from the pelvic rim and iliac crest along the ribs. Bring the left shoulder as far to the right as possible, and elongate the left lateral arm, the extensors of the forearm and the back of both hands as far as possible to the right. The left wrist and hand stretch straight on from the forearm, neither flexing nor extending. **[C]**

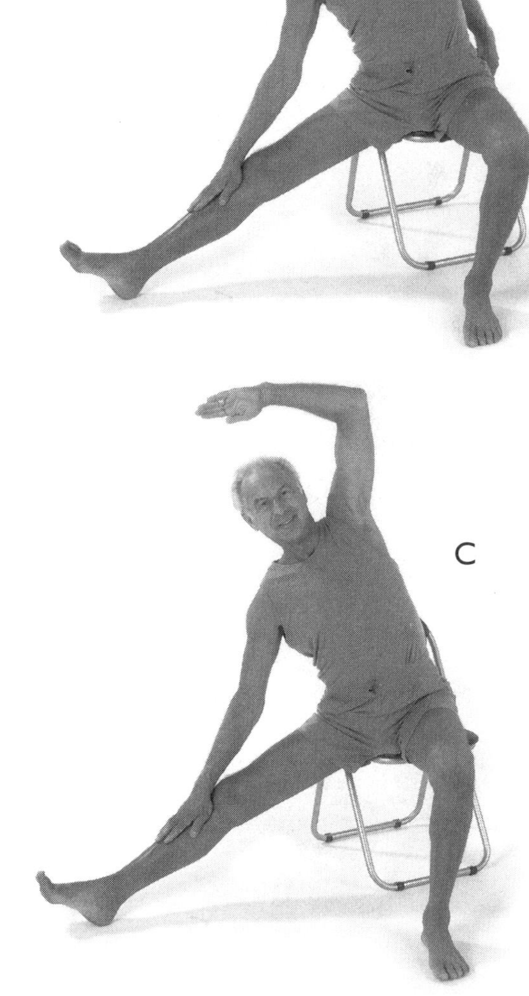

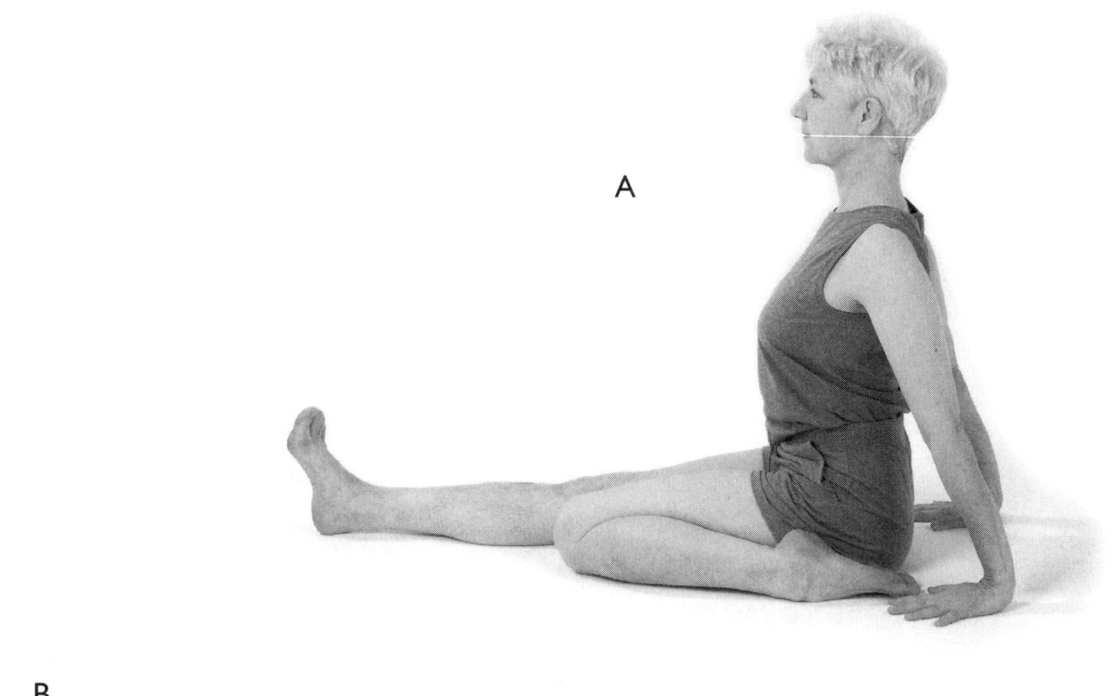
A

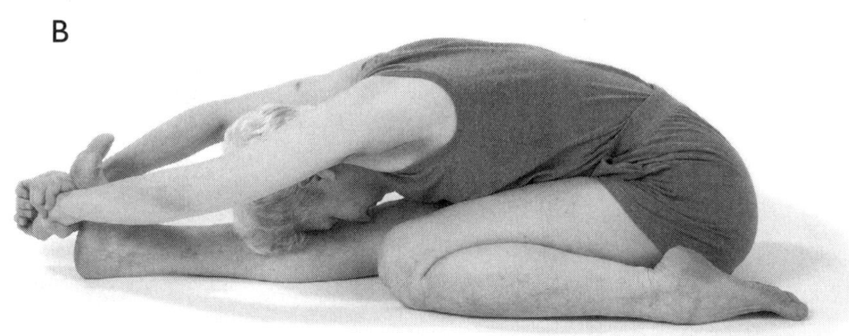
B

Triang Mukhaikapada Paschimottanasana

Three Limbs to the West Pose

1. Sitting on a flat surface, extend the right leg and bend the left underneath, so that the left shin is on the surface, the calf is in contact with the back of the thigh, and the left toes point backward. Rest as evenly as possible on the left buttock and on the right, taking several calm breaths. A pillow under the straight leg's buttock may help. **[A]**

2. Incline the torso forward and slightly to the left, retaining the majority of weight on the left side. Keep the left knee in contact with the inner right thigh.

3. Clasp the left wrist with the right hand, making contact first between the abdomen and the thighs, following with the lower chest against the knees. Let the head and cheekbones rest against the inner right thigh. **[B]**

4. Disengage the muscles at the lateral edges of the back (latissimus dorsi) and the paraspinal muscles, and the muscles that surround the hip joint. Breathe serenely for 1-2 minutes.

5. Then repeat this exchanging left and right.

Entry-Level Triang Mukhaikapada Paschimottanasana

1. At first almost everyone has difficulty sitting firmly on the bent-leg side of this pose. Move close to the edge of a chair, possibly with some small cushion under the right buttock, and extend the right leg maximally. **[1]**

2. Plant the right heel firmly on the floor. If balance is an issue, sit further back in the chair, using pillows and/or blocks to support the straightened right leg.

3. One way to proceed hooks the left ankle under the footrest or supporting strut of the wheelchair or chair. **[2]**

4. Gently and firmly grip the armrests (if there are any) and use them for balance.

5. Extend the spine upward from the coccyx to the nape of the neck. At this point take a few calm breaths, gradually placing more weight on the left buttock.

6. Relax the muscles that normally extend both hips and the left knee, the bilateral hamstrings and the left quadriceps, and flex the left knee still further.

7. Use the chair again, this time to draw the torso forward, while keeping the majority of your weight on the left side. **[3]**

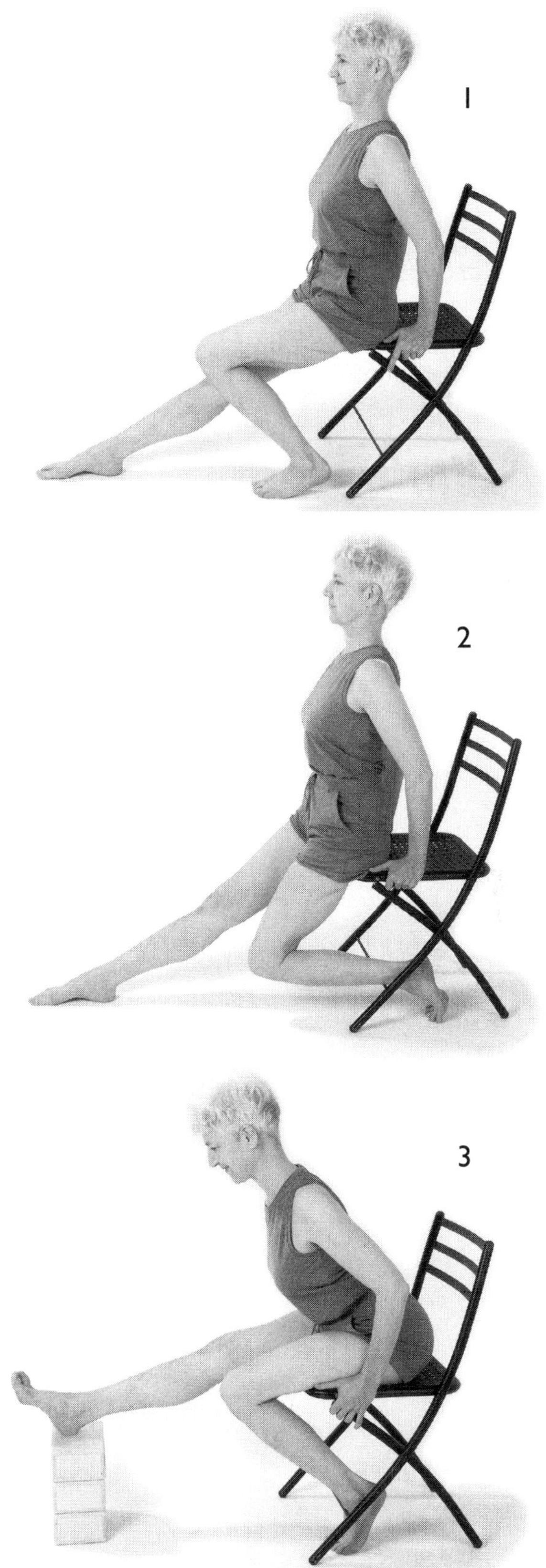

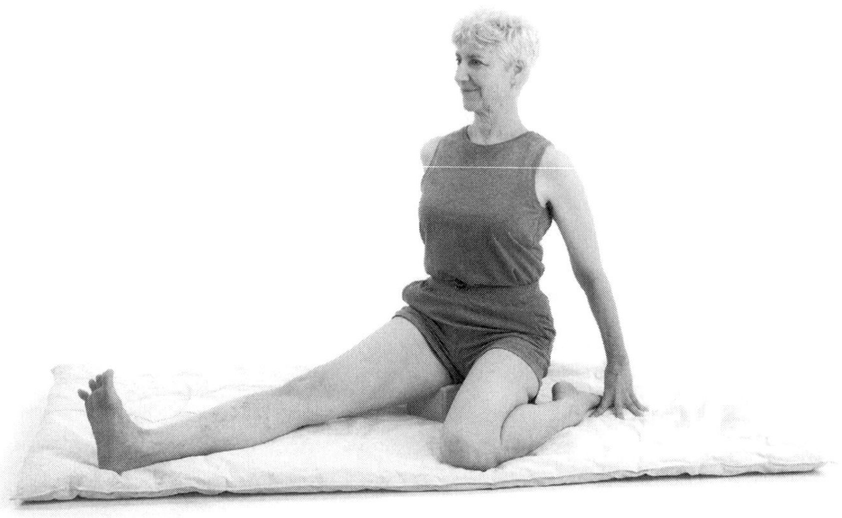

1

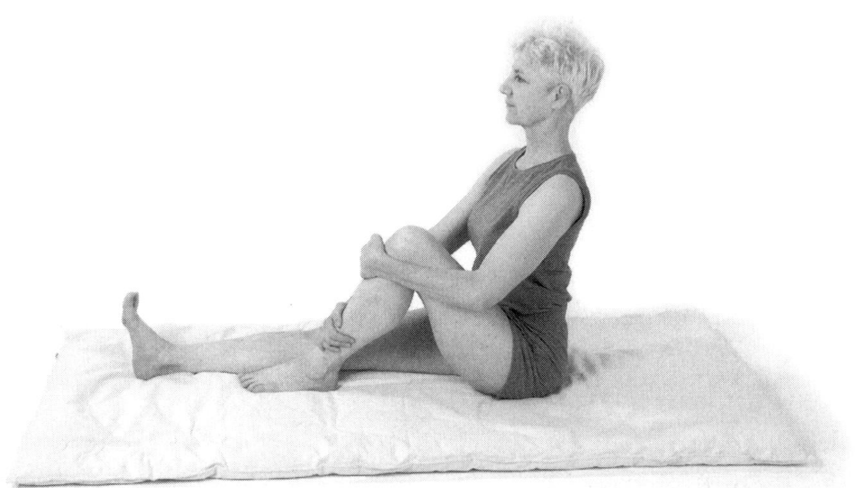

2

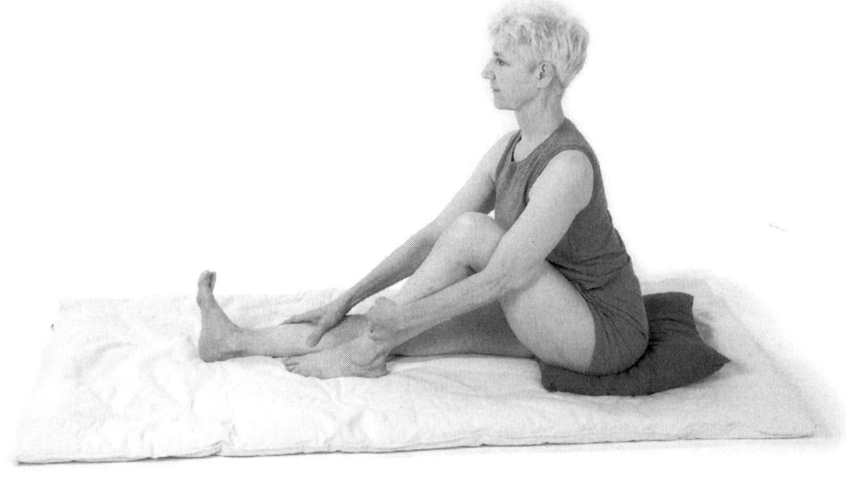

3

counteracts spasticity. It also serves to sharpen balance in all three planes, and strengthen the upper extremities as well as increasing range of motion at all three major joints of the bent leg, and hip flexion and knee extension of the straight leg, e.g., in the presence of flexion contracture. It is a way to approach joint capsule or ligamentous tightening, taking muscular opposition out of the picture while increasing passive range of motion.

Intermediate Triang Mukhaikapada Paschimottanasana

Where range of motion is the greatest issue, this is best done in bed. When balance is also at issue, a firmer surface is preferable, along with supportive props. One has carefully to adjust the amount of pressure that will not injure the joint or throw the practitioner off balance, while making sure it is sufficient to extend the range of the joint. Pain is not always the most accurate barometer: actually testing the leathery resistance at the ends of the joint's range is the best way to tell.

Also, imbalance can cause sudden weight shifts that are best anticipated and managed in advance. This pose is especially helpful in Parkinsonism also.

1. Performed on a bed, begin by folding the left leg off to the left side, shin against the sheets. Use pillows to elevate the buttocks as needed. Even though the left buttock needs elevation, raise the right buttock further still, in order to apportion weight on the bent-leg side. **[1]**

2. If flexibility does not allow sitting on the shin, the thigh and knee may be flexed directly in front of you, parallel to the extended right leg.

3. Although probably not oriented exactly vertically, straighten the spine. **[2]**

4. Then grasp the left shin and rest there, calmly breathing, relaxing the extensors of the left and right hip and left knee.

5. After reaching a comfortably stable and balanced posture, bend the elbows, keeping the upper arms in contact with the torso, bringing the entire torso forward and down as a unit toward the left thigh.

6. If necessary, extend the right arm out to the side, or grasp the side of the mattress with the left hand to exert pressure on the left side while maintaining safe balance. **[3]**

7. Deliberately calm your entire form, head to toe. Breathe symmetrically for a full minute. Then repeat the sequence on the other side.

9 Spasticity

Involuntary, often protracted muscle contraction, or spasticity, is also countered by stretching, but it is a longer story. In the presence of spasticity, it is difficult or impossible to measure true range of motion or strength.

Whether relapsing and remitting or progressive, spasticity plays the part of an impatient and continually painful chaperone of individuals with MS. But Yoga's influence is just as constant in its presence; intelligently and diligently applied, it takes the dominant role!

Science is on our side here. A few common mechanisms appear throughout most of the hundreds of widely practiced poses. One simple mechanism is almost ubiquitous in Yoga. Bear it in mind from the outset.

The Stretch Reflex

It is well-known that when one is dry, there is an increased urge to drink; as blood sugar falls, hunger rises. But the body's check-and-balance systems are not limited to autonomic functions. There are restraining and promoting influences in every voluntary movement. Tiny receptors built into all muscles' anatomy hold back or egg-on each muscular contraction. Every movement involves activating and inhibiting influences that balance its strength and enhance its control. The antagonistic influences of intrafusal (facilitating) and golgi tendon-organ (inhibiting) feed information back to spinal motor centers and pontine coordinative centers in the brain (25, 26). These higher functions regulate the speed, power and contour of each muscle's contraction over time.

Small spindle-like receptors in muscles themselves are activated by the muscle's contraction. They excite or *facilitate* further contraction of that muscle. Yet each muscle has at least one tendon, and in each tendon are golgi tendon organs which are activated whenever they are stretched. Naturally, they are stretched each and every time the muscle contracts. And when stretched, these golgi tendon organs send out signals that *inhibit* the muscle from contracting.

One basic mechanism present in many Yoga postures utilizes the fact that the intrafusal fibres are known to respond to the speed of motion, and generally have their greatest influence early in muscle stretch (27), while golgi tend organs continue to exert their inhibitory influence at their original strength, for a long time (28). (See the figure.)

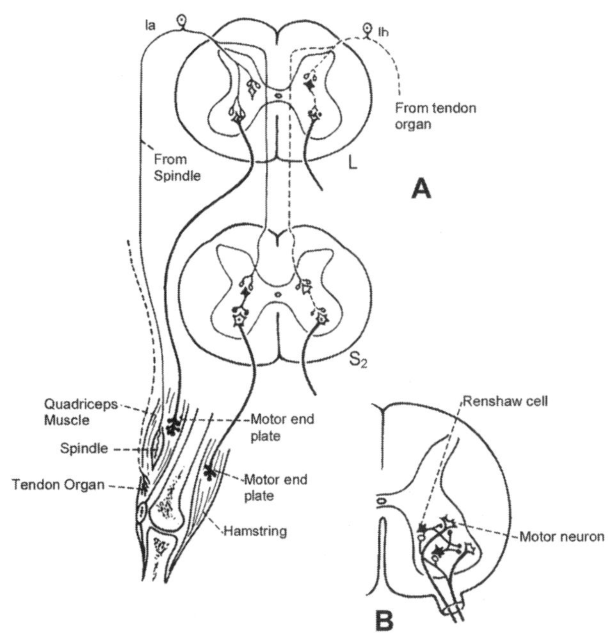

In general, every sustained muscle stretch will, over time, tend toward a relaxation response in that muscle (29). Naturally, any painful stimuli that are activated during that same time period will have a contrary, unsettling and excitatory effect. The Yoga poses that have endured over the centuries succeed in accomplishing sustained stretch and relaxation, without undue antagonistic, painful or arousing side-effects.(29,30)

In multiple sclerosis, any central portion of the intrafusal and/or golgi tendon reflex arcs can be affected. This can lead to spasticity, undue weakness, or a combination of both, depending on which feedback system is affected. For practical purposes, it does not seem to matter whether plaques affect the spindle and tendon organ systems directly, somewhat indirectly through reducing regulating signals sent from higher centers, or very indirectly, by changing the regulation in the higher centers themselves. The point is the same: emphasizing the inhibitory influence while cautiously avoiding undue stimulation of the excitatory systems will reduce spasticity.

Feed Forward from Reducing Spasticity to Improving Range of Motion

There are several advantages to relaxed and extended muscles in a comfortable and calm individual. For the involved patient with multiple sclerosis and others threatened with decreased range of motion, reducing resistance to motion is an obvious, (and painless) means to increase that range. This will not be true when avascular or aseptic necrosis, bacterial arthritis, trauma or neoplastic causes grossly reshape or destroy joints. In the vast majority of joint restrictions of neurological origin, however, where a leathery resistance is felt at the endpoints of movement, the cause is constricted joint capsules, tightened ligaments, or shortened muscle. Yoga is the perfect "minimal medicine" in such situations. We've encountered this simple situation in working with range of motion. But with spasticity there is more to it than that.

The Agonist–Antagonist Reflex

Have you ever noticed that when you contract one muscle, its opposite relaxes? For example, when your biceps (the agonist) contracts to flex your elbow, the triceps (the antagonist), the muscle with the opposite job of extending the elbow, relaxes. Without this automatic response, a great deal more conscious effort would be necessary for even the simplest acts, and movement would be much less smooth, and much, much more hectic. This timing and coordinating mechanism that governs reciprocal muscle contraction and relaxation is "hard wired" into us at the spinal cord level. It has been called the agonist-antagonist reflex. It holds for every pair of agonist and antagonist muscles in the body. Yoga makes use of it to stretch muscles and joints, and also to wage successful campaigns against spasticity. They may be long term and strategic, or conveniently momentary.

To oppose spastic ankle flexion, one contracts the extensors, thereby relaxing the spastic flexor muscle on the spot. If one continues to contract the extensor muscles, and stretches the flexors for any length of time, the golgi tendon organs' influence overcomes the muscle spindles' tendency to stimulate contraction, countering the spasticity in a second way, with a single action.

In this example the inhibitory influence dominates muscle behavior after 90 seconds.

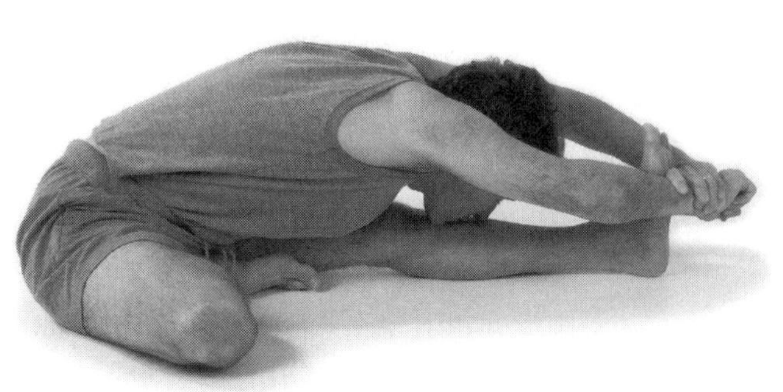

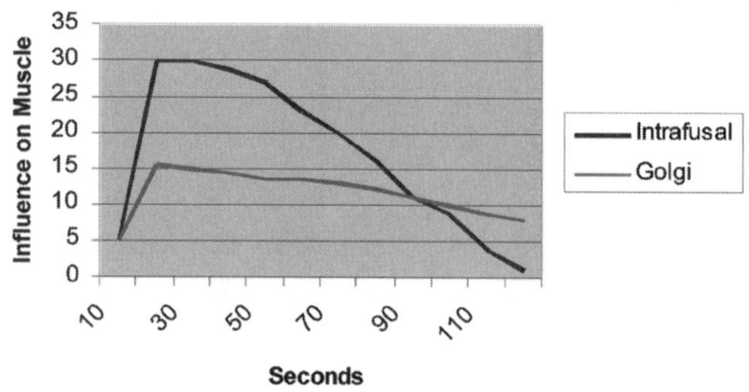

Janusirsasana

Head-to-the-Knee Pose

1. Seated with both ischial tuberosities on a flat surface, the left leg is extended completely, and the left foot firmly, but not rigidly, vertical and in neutral. The right knee is bent, and the entire leg brought laterally so that the lateral thigh and calf rest on the flat surface.

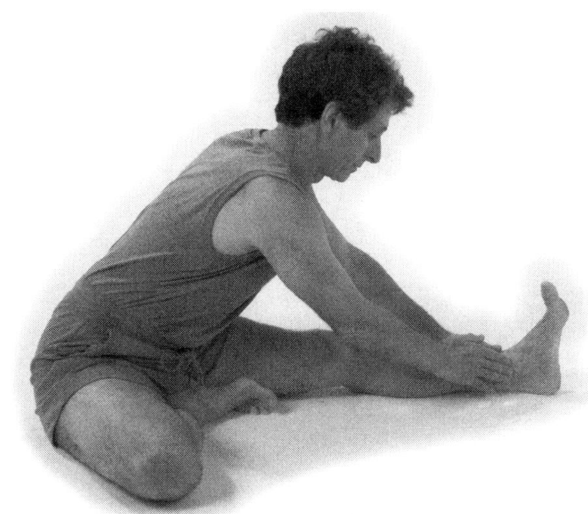

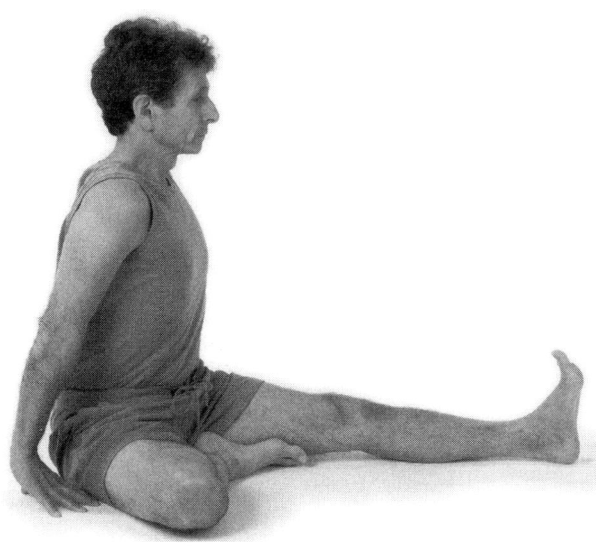

2. The arms stretch toward the left foot. The chest descends and advances toward the foot symmetrically.

3. The cervical and thoracic spine are retained in mild extension. All the flexion takes place at the lowest levels of the lumbar spine, and at the hips.

4. The left hand should grasp the right wrist just past the sole of the left foot. However, if one cannot reach behind to the sole of the foot, then it's all right to hold the left ankle or calf or knee. What is essential is to stretch the hamstring muscles, and maintain the right knee in total (180 degree) extension. If the knee is bent, the reflex inhibition and relaxation response will not occur.

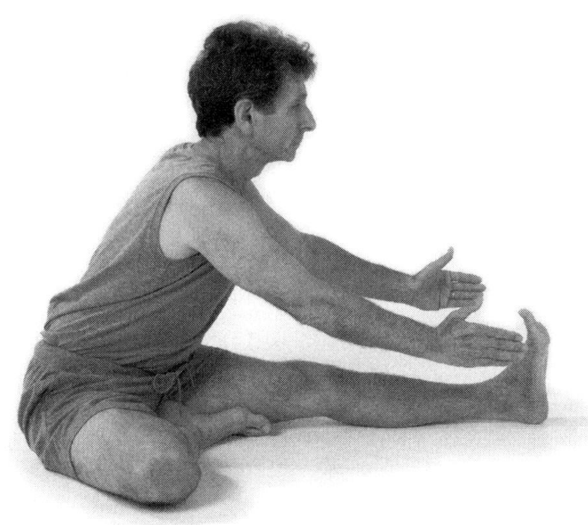

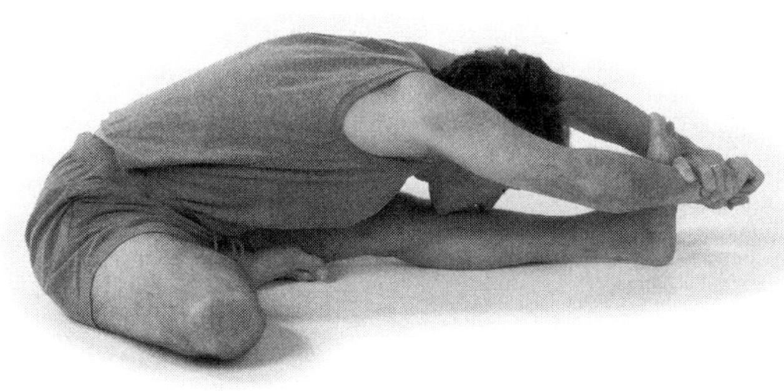

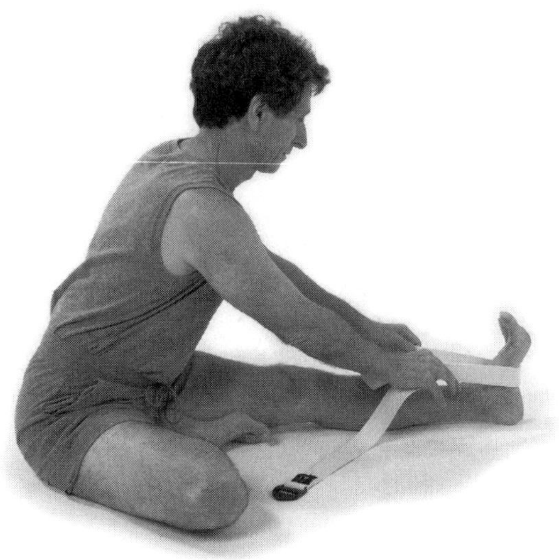

5. The pose is to be maintained for up to one minute on each side. Naturally, at first the time may be abbreviated.

6. Starting at 10-20 seconds per side is not unreasonable. Other means of easing into this position use a strap.

7. The person doing the pose then grasps the two sides of the strap and gradually "walks in" with the fingers to stretch the extensor muscles of the buttocks and the thighs.

8. The torso will gradually descend over months of practice, and less and less of the strap will be necessary.

This pose improves cervical, thoracic, and higher lumbar dorsal muscular flexion, and stretches hamstrings on the straight leg, and adductors of both legs, each in a different way. The straight leg revolves inwardly by virtue of the gluteus minimus and medius and gracilis, while the obturator externus, pectineus, gluteus maximus, piriformis, obturator internus, and gemelli superior and inferior, and quadratus femoris all laterally rotate the thigh. The adductor magnus's adductor part also flexes the thigh while its hamstring part extends it. Therefore the hamstring part of the adductor magnus is stretched in both legs, while both parts are stretched in the bent leg of this forward bend. Janusirsana also seems to promote these muscles' coordinated contraction, and, more important in multiple sclerosis, their coordinated relaxation and eccentric contraction. In this manner it effectively lengthens and strengthens the lowest trunk muscles, contributing to well-controlled trunkal support, while increasing hip range of motion in flexion. Thereby this pose gives the spine a wider range of painless and safe movement. It is useful in low back pain, the spasms and muscular pains of everyday living, for remediable contractures occurring in the exacerbations and remissions of multiple sclerosis, and in prolonged convalescence.

There is reciprocal front-to-back contraction here: As the extensors of the cervical, thoracic and upper lumbar spine contract, the sternocleidomastoid and other ventral cervical musculature, and the intercostal muscles, and the superior abdominal "sixpack" relax. The lower lumbar extensors, including the paraspinals and the sacral muscles relax, and the iliopsoas and very lowest abdominal muscles contract.

As the patient comes forward in the pose, the ischial tuberosities and inferior rami of the pubic bones move dorsally, stretching the hamstrings and adductors of the leg. In order to be sure to stretch the adductors, inversion of the legs and feet is minimized. This brings the external rotators such as the tensa fascie latae into play.

Through the gradual, persistent elongation of the hamstrings, flexion of the lowest lumbar spine, and extension of the rest of the spine, this pose is also a potent means to prevent or at least curtail chronic low back pain. Standard kinesiological reasoning applies here: greater range of motion at the hips, especially combined with reduced lordosis, makes a major difference in frequency, severity and duration of episodes of musculoskeletal low back pain.

The parkinsonian patient, the college athlete and the elderly post total knee replacement patient share this same problem and therefore have need of this same pose...but they do not go about it at the same level of intensity. One great beauty of Yoga is its adaptability. One person may perform Janusirsana by placing his hands at the straight leg's knee; another may grasp a wrist behind the sole of the foot. Each is still capable of progressing to the same ultimate goal; each is benefiting in the present from the posture.

But there are other, more specific adaptations for this pose in Rehabilitation Medicine. In spinal cord injury, and after ablation procedures, splanchnic pooling is a major circulatory concern, leading at times to sympathetic dysreflexic crises. This pose, and every Yoga pose, can be performed in gradual increments over time, beginning with positions that barely resemble the classical one. This process can take months, even years of mainly solitary or class practice, punctuated by weekly or monthly visits to a rehabilitation specialist that uses yoga, or a yoga teacher that is therapeutically oriented. However, once reasonably perfected, the pose can be used by the patient him- or herself to redistribute circulatory volume almost instantly.

The problem is getting started. Many people with more severe multiple sclerosis might consider the last few pages on a par with Alice in Wonderland. But the first step is half the journey; one can begin in a wheelchair, or in bed. It certainly can take assistants at the early phases of Yoga practice. That goes for every student, regardless of when and where he or she starts.

Janusirsasana may commence with simply straightening the leg. And to get there, one may need to stretch for some time with the leg bent!

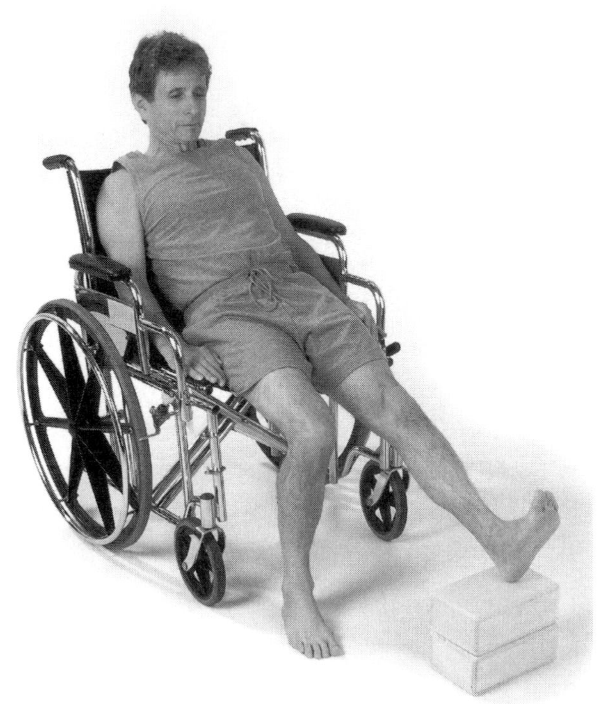

Is one doing Yoga at this point? No, and yes. One is not doing a known and practiced pose, one is not taking full advantage of the stretch reflex nor the intrafusal-golgi interaction, one is probably not physiologically inducing very much calm.

But one is applying self-management techniques, and may be totally in accord with Yama and Niyama as outlined above, by striving for a neutral and unattached consciousness. One may be approaching a serene and peaceful state more efficiently than the neatly hair-combed and lipsticked who do "beautiful" poses to hip-hop at health clubs.

There is a point at which Ludwig Wittgenstein asks: "Can one play chess without the queen?" (30) The answer there, as here, is that there are practices that come as close as you want to chess (and Yoga); they clearly resemble and derive from these known entities. The only thing at stake is that we know what we are doing.

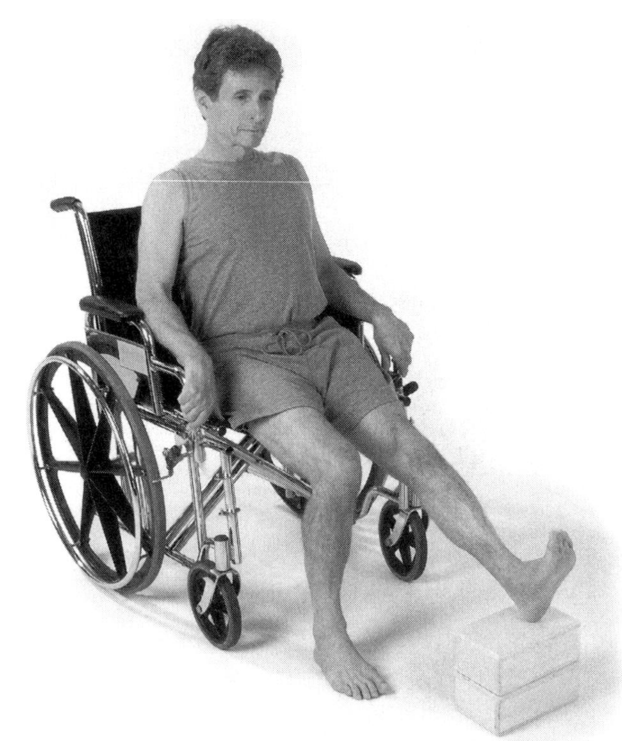

Entry-Level Janusirsana for People in Wheelchairs and in Bed

1. Come to the edge of the wheelchair. Lean back as far as you need to in order to make one leg straight.

2. Balance the straight leg on its heel, allowing the other leg to be in a comfortable, supportive position. Use blocks and/or pillows.

3. Now propping yourself up on the back or arms or seat of the wheelchair, gradually bend at the waist further and further, until you feel a pull, generally behind the knee. If there is no sensation from this location, you'll have to keep track of how hard your arms (or those of your care-giver) are working.

4. At first, let the stretch, or the muscular force from the arms that is pressing you forward, be very gradual. The most important thing is to keep the knee straight.

5. Work your way up from 10-20 seconds on each side to 30 seconds—one minute on each side.

6. After a week or two, you can start to progress, pressing ever so slightly more each time, each week. Barring changes in

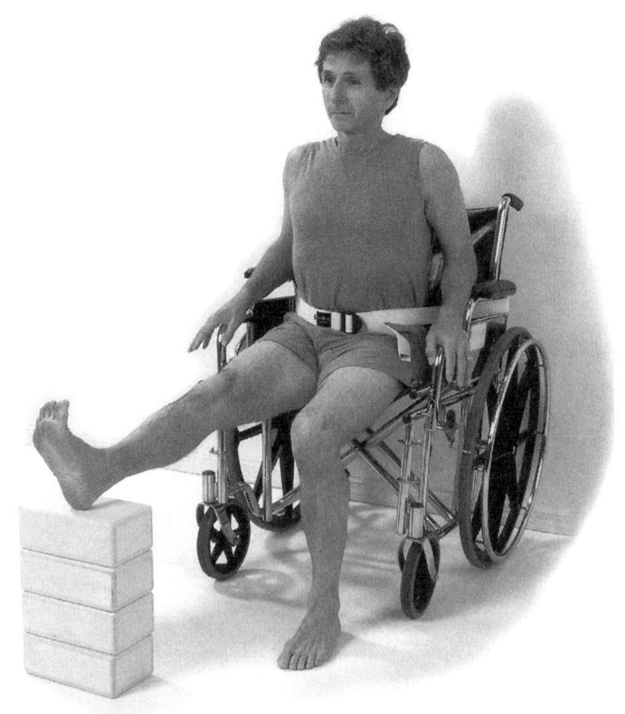

the underlying condition, people often move forward about 1/2 inch per month.

Janusirsasana for the Borderline Ambulatory Person

For individuals that are independent or minimally assisted in transferring, who are able to walk, but not very far, who are neurologically or otherwise compromised, an intermediate pose is available. It offers some of the benefits of Janusirsana, and it is "adjustable," bringing the practitioner closer and closer to the classical pose. This is true of all the intermediate postures in this book. For Janusirsana, it simply involves increasing the forward bend of the torso and the stretch of the muscles of the back of the leg.

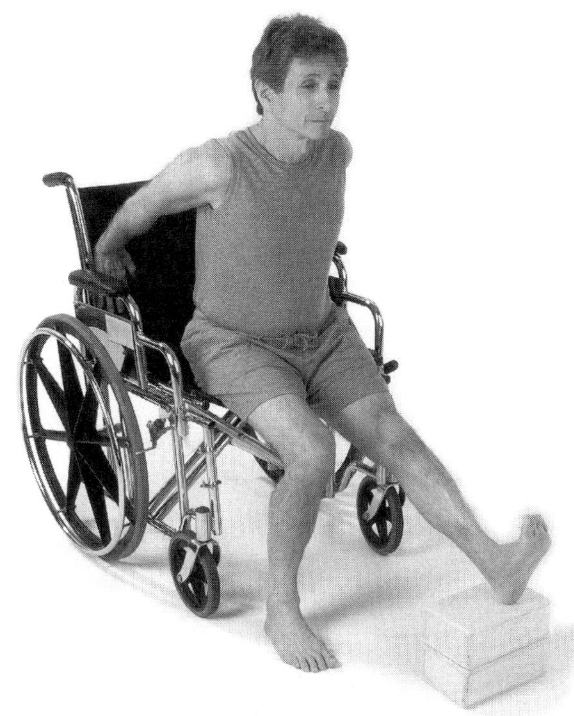

Reviewing this pose, several general advantages of Yoga as a treatment emerge: it is gradual and measured, and can be practiced alone and without almost any equipment. Therefore it is useful for safe long-term home exercise. It makes no noise, requires no medication and runs few risks. Another beauty of Yoga is that there are desirable "side-effects." A number of human and animal studies report that osteoporosis can be arrested and even reversed through the application of "'unusual' tugs by muscles' tendons on their origins and insertions." (31) Graded dynamic loads appear to function first, to inhibit boney reabsorption, and secondly to stimulate the activity of osteoblasts along the lines of force. (32) (Wolff's law).

The bones are not alone. The advantages of gradual and self-applied maneuvers to maximize the practical range of every joint are valuable in the focal degenerative joint disease that can follow compensatory overuse of certain joints. The glenoid fossae of wheelchair and crutch users, the cervicothoracic junction of a person with chronic torticollis, the feet of the on-point dancer are examples. As a safe and self-reliant promoter of calm, an enhancer of muscle length, bone strength and joint range, Yoga is fitting for the elderly people we all wish to become or remain, with neurological, orthopedic and functional clean bills of health.

PASCHIMOTTANASANA

West Pose

1. Sit on a flat surface with legs extended straight in front of you, palms on the floor, feet vertical.

2. After breathing quietly for a time, exhale and bring your entire torso forward, bending at

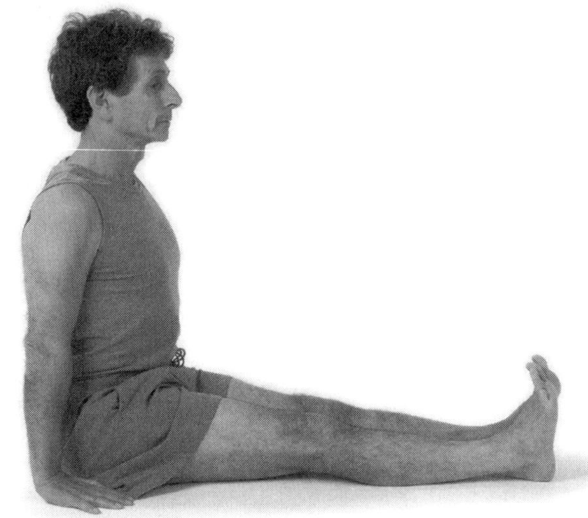

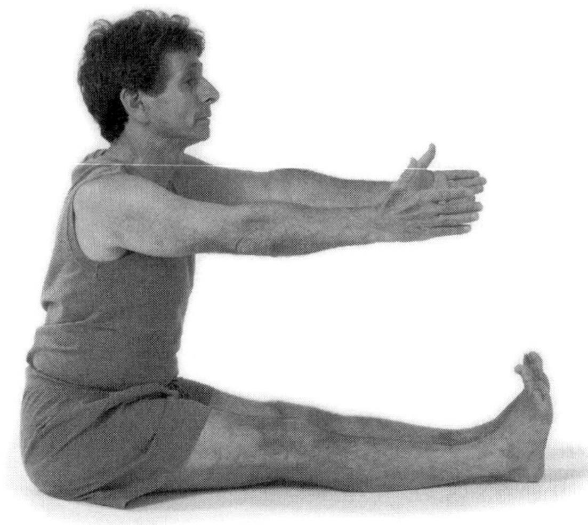

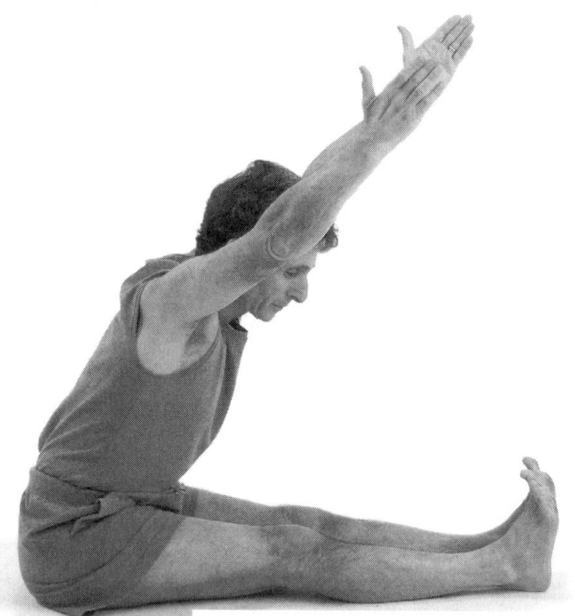

the lowest part of the waist, keeping the back straight, and aiming for a region a little above your toes.

3. This is a pose you can work with, possibly beginning with hands resting just below the knees, progressing through grasping the ankles, the outsides of the feet or great toes, palms on the soles of the feet, fingers interlaced behind the feet, to one hand holding the opposite wrist. At that point there is so little resistance that the chin rests on the shins.

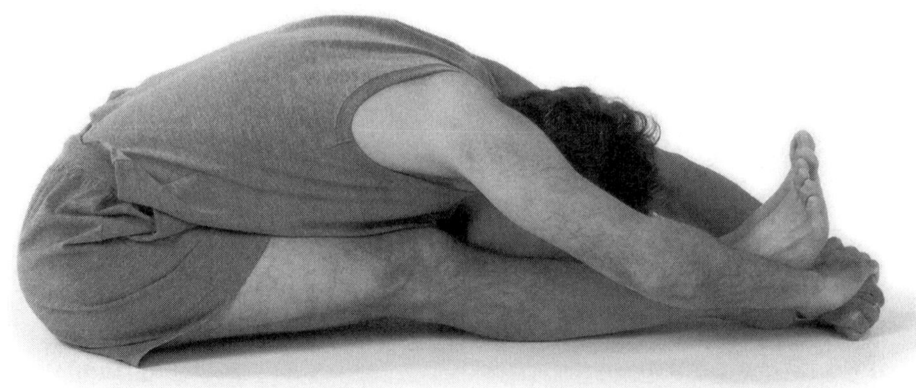

Entry-Level Paschimottanasana

1. Move to the edge of the wheelchair or the bed. Lean backward until you can straighten both legs maximally, with the knees touching each other, and the ankles as close together as possible.

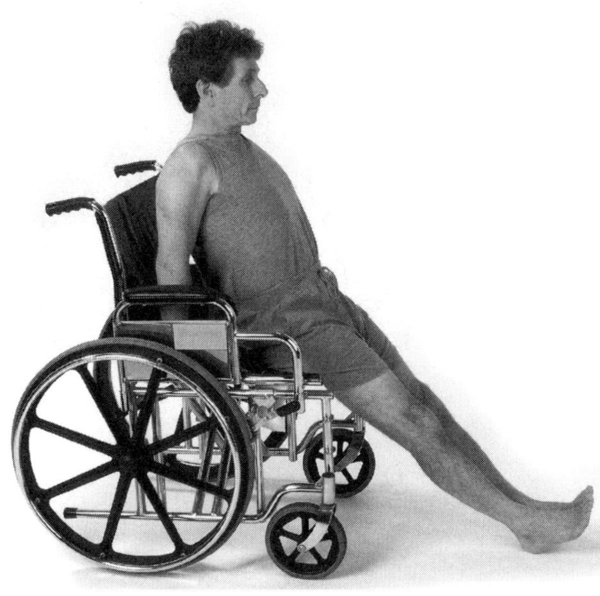

2. If you're leaning back as far as you comfortably can, and the knees still aren't straight, then start the pose from there.

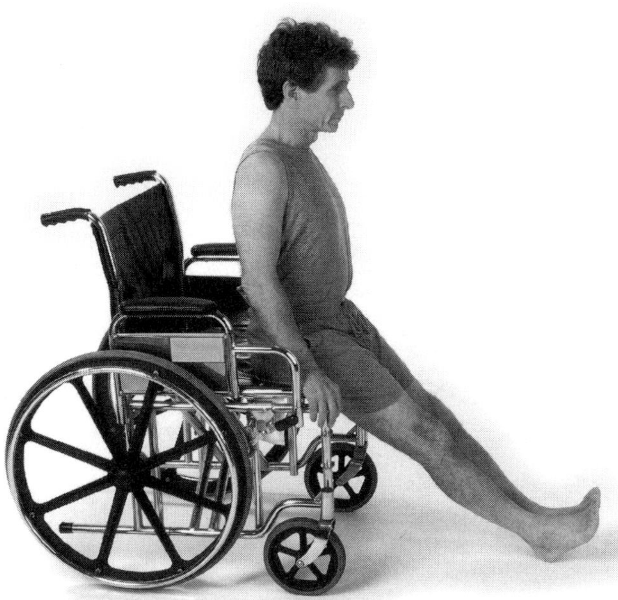

3. Pay attention to the weight on your palms, and breathe calmly for a minute or two. Then gradually increase the weight on your palms, raising your torso without bending the knees any further.

4. Apply moderate pressure to the hamstrings, by putting moderate pressure onto the palms, lifting the torso upward.

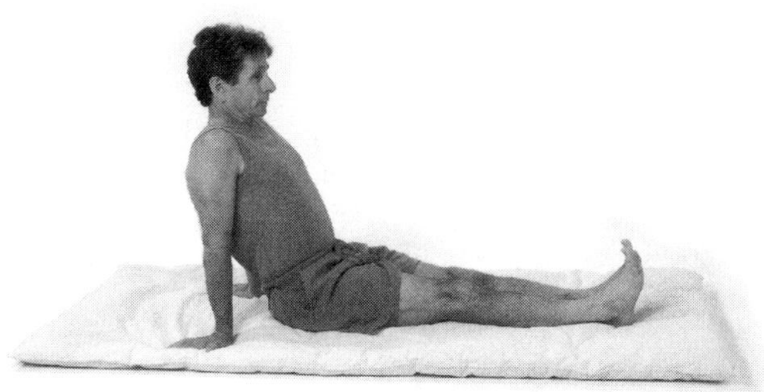

5. As you work with this pose, and rise up higher each week, the angle between your thighs and torso will gradually decrease. Then the same amount of "push," either from pulling on your legs or pushing downward with your palms will go more toward stretching the muscles of the legs, and less to countering the force of gravity.

6. When you can reach a point on your legs that you can pull forward from, you're ready for the intermediate pose.

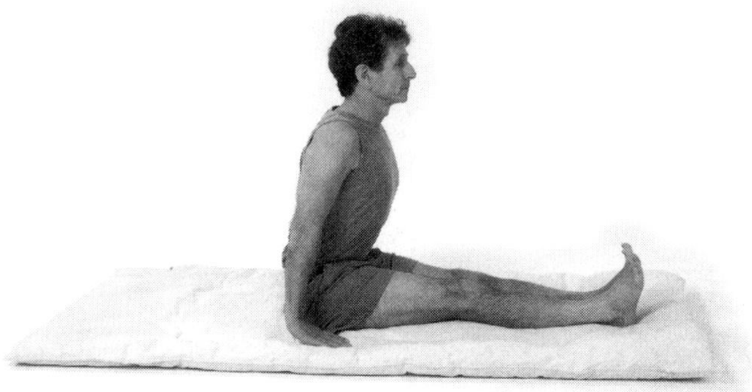

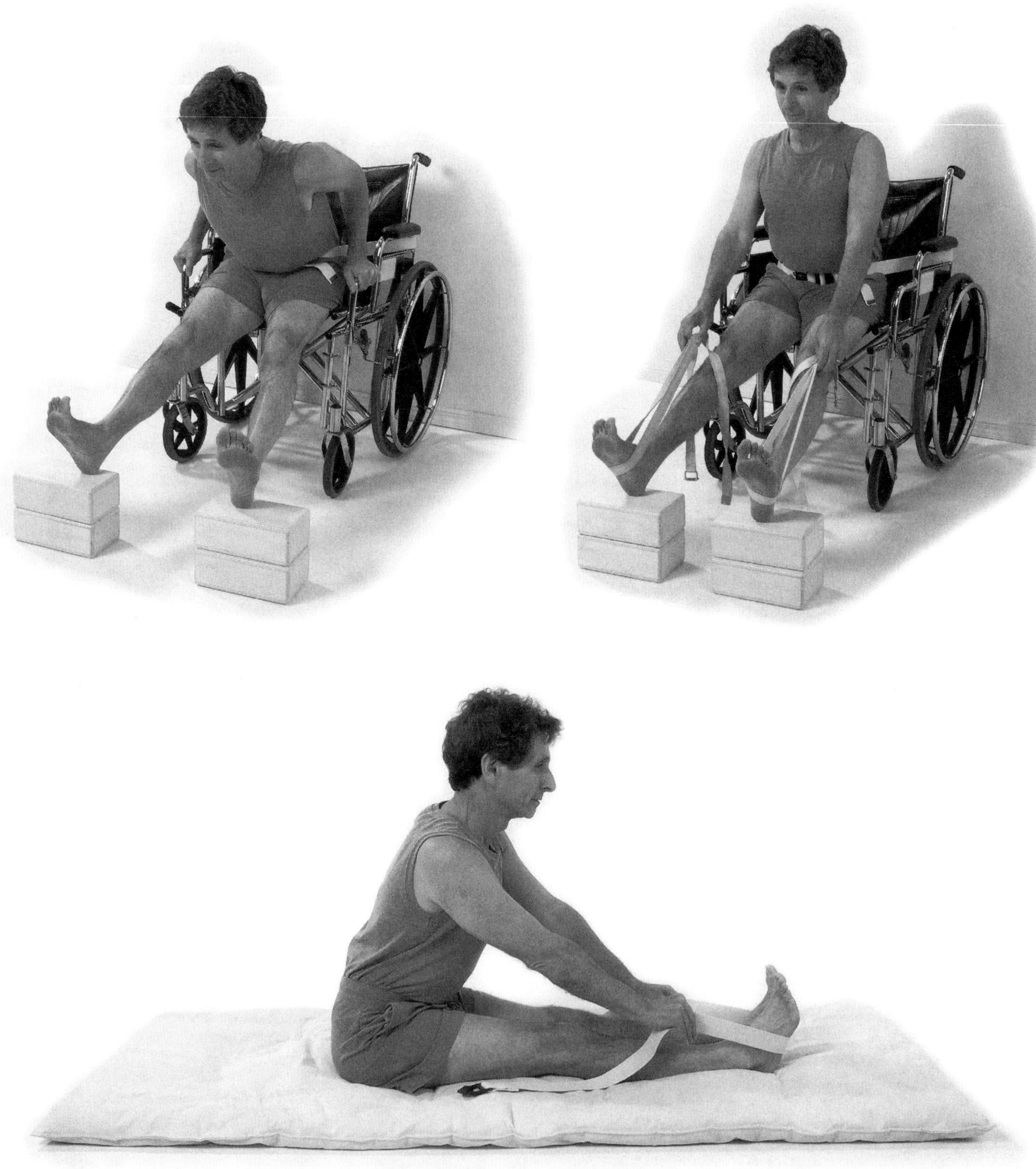

PARVATASANA

Daughter of the Himalayas (Parvati was a consort of Siva's)

This pose is classically done in padmasana, the lotus position. That aspect of it is rarely possible in the presence of any significant lower extremity spasticity. Any comfortable position, sitting or standing, is compatible with what follows.

Unduly forcing the hips and knees into this position is clearly dangerous and should not be undertaken. However, if there is sufficient safe range of motion, the lotus position can be attained while sitting on a flat surface or a pillow.

1. Bend the right knee and manually bring the right foot as high up on the left thigh as possible. The right heel is as close as possible to the navel.
2. Cradle the left foot in both hands and raise it up to the origins of the right thigh, approaching the navel with the left heel.
3. Lengthen the entire spine and lower the chin to horizontal. Balance your weight from left to right, and back to front.
4. The pose should also be practiced with the left foot placed first, to evenly lengthen the tendons, ligaments and joint capsules of each thigh and knee.

There are advantages to the lotus posture itself. It is often painful at first, but it becomes a reliable resource for comfortable, alert meditation, promoting intellectual and spiritual advancement.

Parvatasana continues from any stable and not sloppy sitting position:

5. The spine must be straight, the chin resting just below the adam's apple.
6. Interlock the fingers and stretch the arms vertically with palms facing directly upward, maintaining the straight spine, middle and upper chest forward, arms from the deltoid to the little finger, back. The biceps should be behind your ears.
7. Breathe evenly and calmly for a few minutes.
8. Then change the interlocking of the fingers, as one will change the legs in the lotus or other asymmetrical position, and repeat the pose and the breathing.

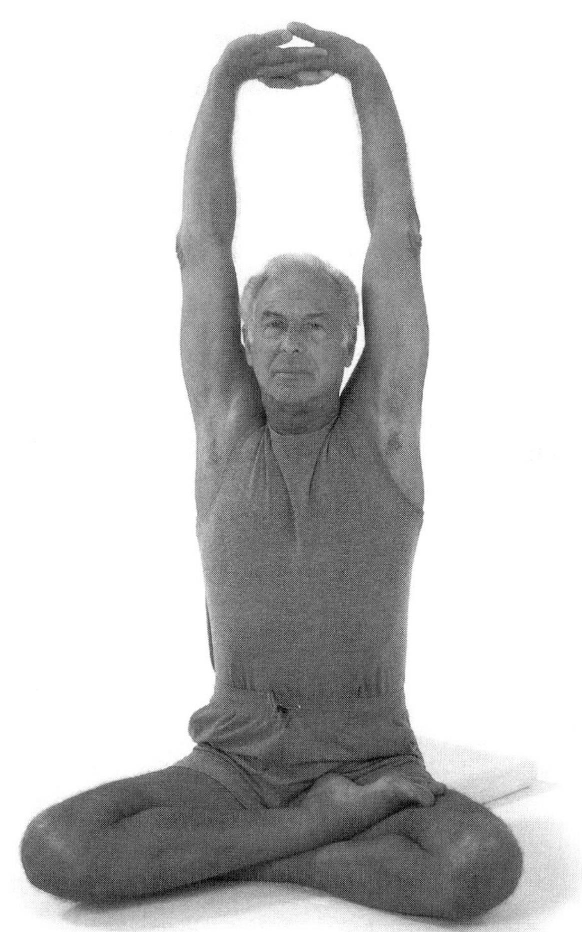

Entry-Level Parvatasana

This pose adapts itself extremely well to wheelchair use, and anyone who can be propped to sit position in bed.

1. It may begin with one arm, with less than vertical or fully extended positioning, and may even begin in supine or prone. The breathing aspect should not be omitted.

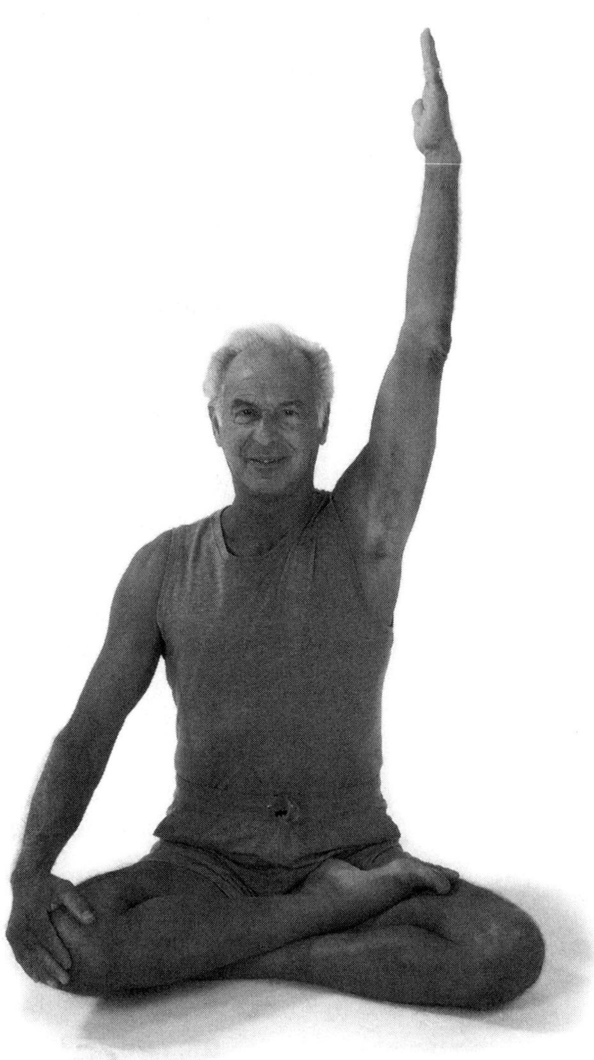

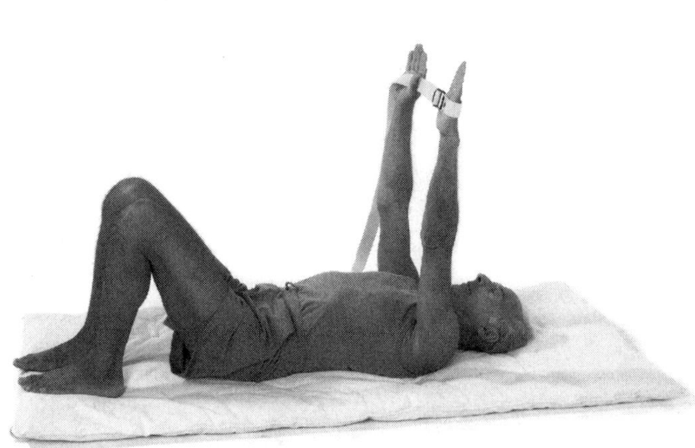

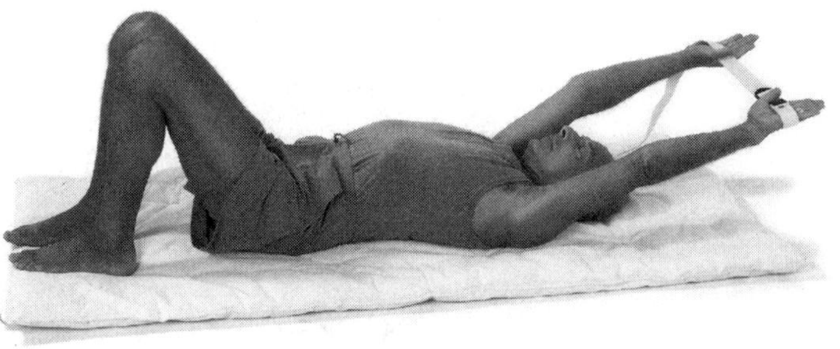

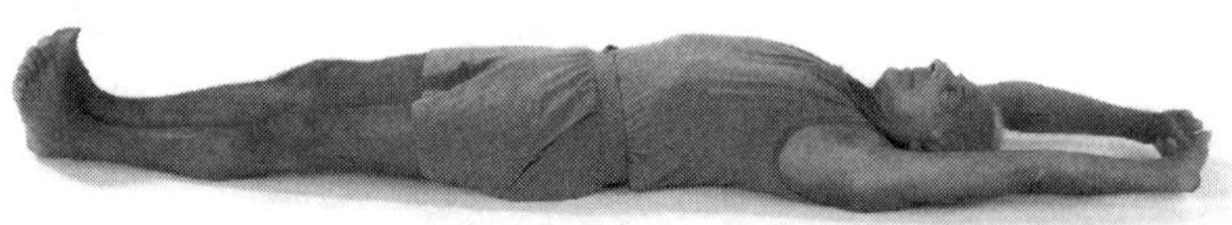

Intermediate Parvatanasana

The possible intermediates here almost defy description: one can alter the positions of the legs, the trunk and the arms... even when one or both arms are weakened. Parvatasana essentially refers to the world's highest mountains; any version should stress a firm foundation, a maximal stretch, and the best spinal extension that is achievable.

MARICHYASANA III

Marichi was a sage, and son of the creator, Brahma.

1. Sitting on a flat surface, extend the right leg and flex the left thigh until the shin is vertical. The left ankle should press against the inside of the right thigh.

2. Take a breath in.

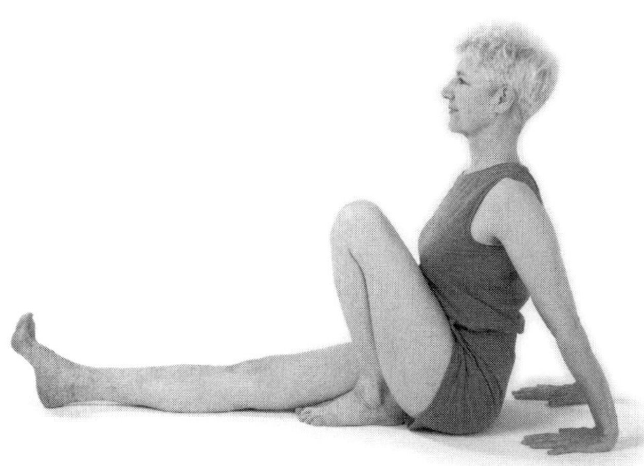

3. Upon exhalation, revolve the torso 90 degrees to the left, the right arm sliding past the outside of the left thigh, the back of the right armpit resting against the outside of the left knee and thigh.

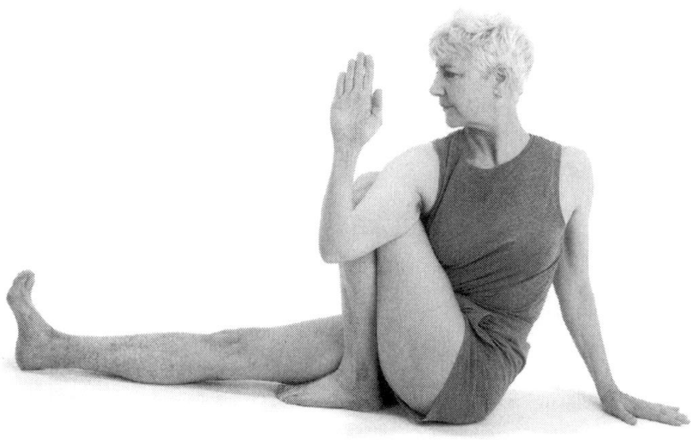

4. Cushions may be helpful to retain the bent knee.

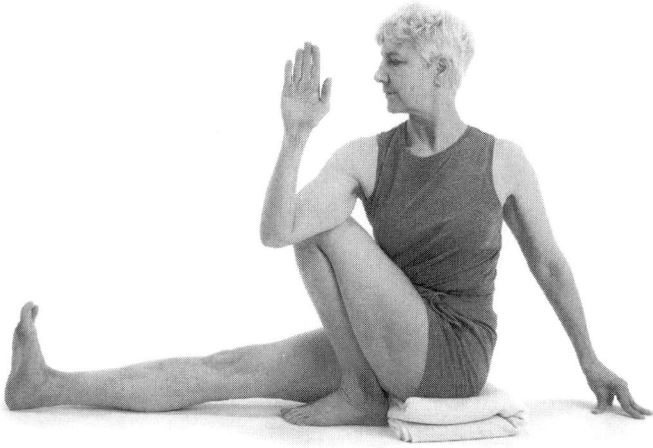

5. Walk behind (toward the right) with the left hand. Bring the right palm to the outside of the right calf.

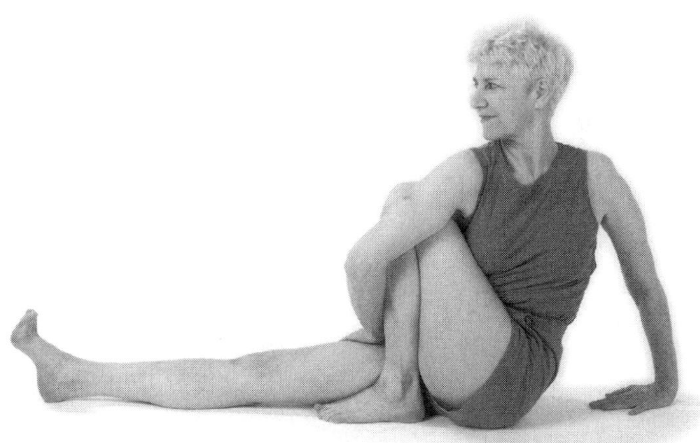

6. Move the left shoulder back by "walking" your left hand behind you; press the right chest forward and to the left by pulling the right shoulder blade back toward the spine, and downward toward the pelvis.

7. From its position near the spine the right shoulder blade impels the right chest

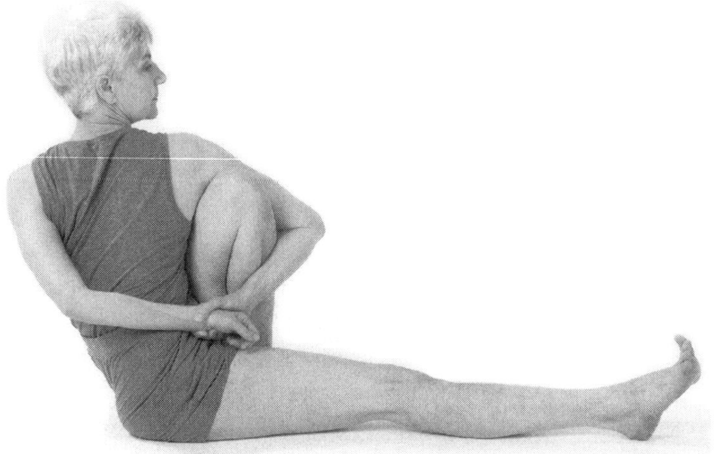

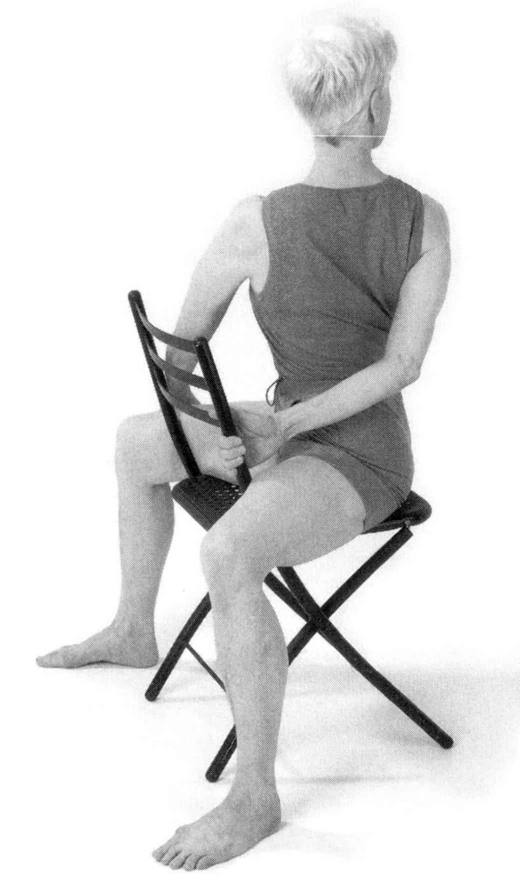

forward beyond the right shoulder. Gaze at the right foot, which should be firmly vertical, but not stiff.

8. Breathe calmly for 10 – 20 seconds.

9. Then repeat the entire pose and breathing on the other side. Gradually extend the time to 1 minute on each side.

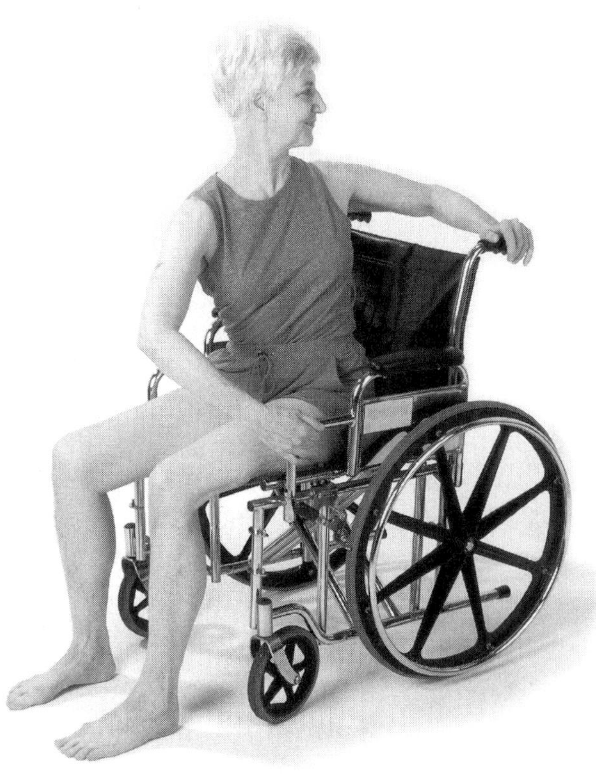

Entry-Level Marichyasana

1. Sitting in a wheelchair, or any chair with arms, work the left arm around behind the back of the chair, reaching to the right as much as possible.
2. Grasp the left arm of the chair with the right hand, bending the right elbow while keeping the upper arm by the side of the chest.
3. Revolve the entire right chest to the left, not just the shoulder.
4. Look to the left, aligning the head parallel to the back of the chair.
5. Reach with the left arm and pull with the right until a satisfying twist is obtained.

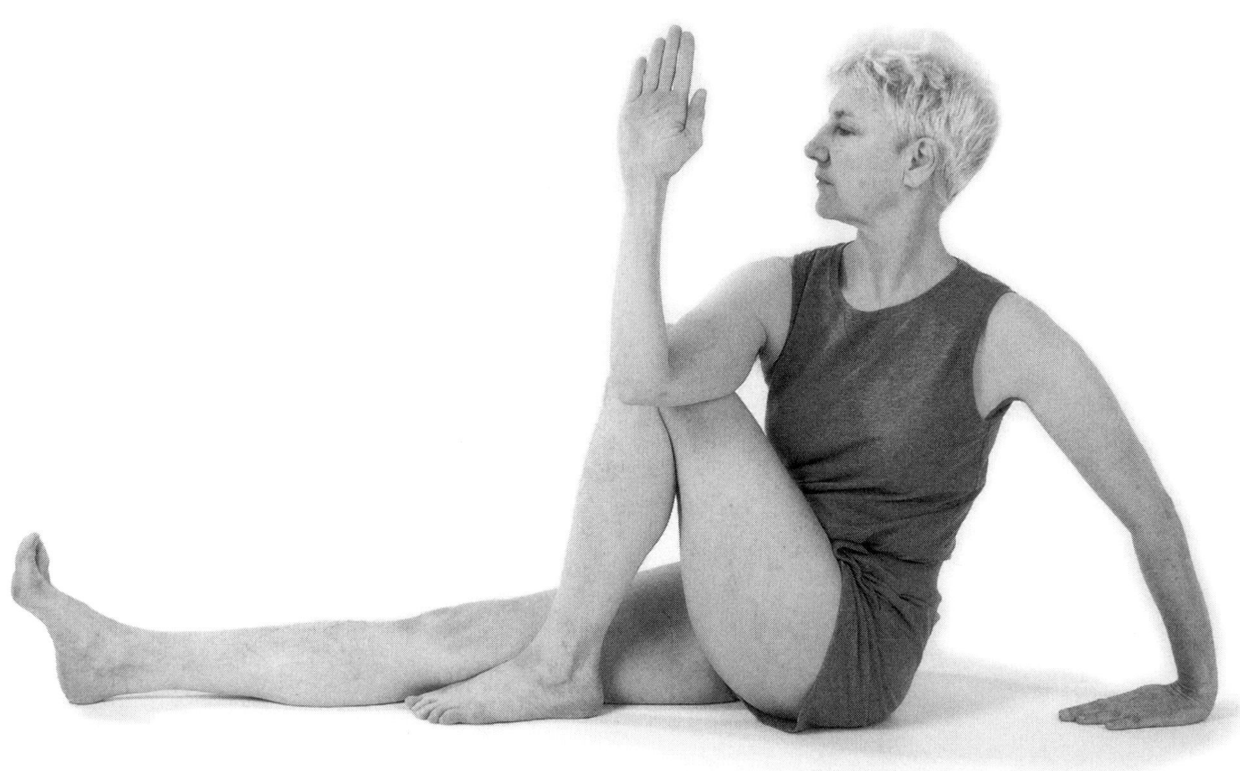

6. Then pay attention to breathing calmly and evenly, attempting to bring air to both sides of the asymmetrical chest as symmetrically as the position allows.

Intermediate Marichyasana

1. Sitting on a flat surface, extend the right leg, flex the left thigh and knee vertically, keeping the thigh and knee close to the left chest, and the shin as close to vertical as possible. The left ankle should press against the inside of the right thigh.
2. Take a breath in.
3. Upon exhalation, revolve the torso to the left, the right arm coming over the left thigh, so that the back of the right armpit approaches the outside of the left knee and thigh.
4. Walk behind (toward the right) with the left hand.
5. Bend the right elbow and stretch the right palm upward.
6. Let the right shoulder blade and the right chest move to the left.
7. Look to the left, keeping the right foot firm but not stiff.
8. Your arm is the lever, the knee is the fulcrum. You can increase the pressure by using the lever. Use it to revolve the chest, not the shoulder.
9. Breathe calmly for up to one minute.
10. Then repeat the pose and breathing on the other side.

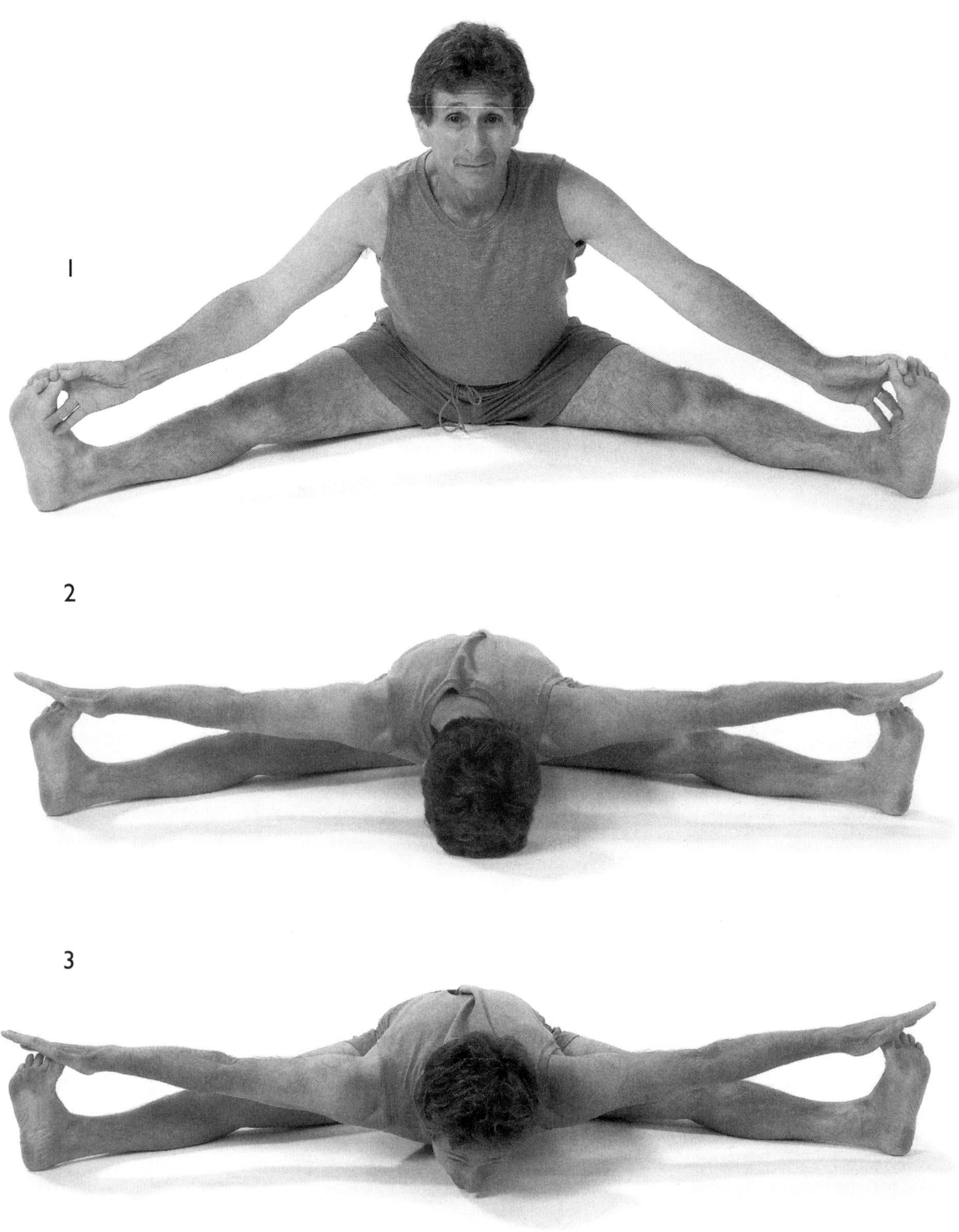
1
2
3

UPAVISTA KONASANA

Seated Angle Pose

1. Sit on a flat surface.

2. Spread your legs as far apart as possible. Keep the knees fully straight. Your weight should be on the ischial tuberosities or "sit-bones."

3. Hold the great toes between the thumbs and the next two fingers of each hand, straighten the spine maximally, open the chest with a full breath and pull in the abdomen. **[1]**

4. Exhale and bring the entire torso, from below the navel to the sternum, down to the surface, keeping the spine as straight as possible. The head and shoulders come down only insofar as the hips and torso descend. **[2]**

5. Eventually the chin should join the torso on the flat surface. Now your weight should be evenly balanced on the thick muscles of the back of the thighs, and the abdomen and chest. The head's 13-16 pounds are supported by the chin. **[3]**

6. Remain in the pose for 10-20 seconds, slowly increasing the time to 1 minute.

Entry-Level Upavista Konasana

This pose is best begun in bed.

1. Sit with legs as far apart and as straight as possible. Make sure the heels and buttocks are firmly "planted" in their spots.

2. Raise the chest and neck and head so that they are as close to vertical as can be, without changing the placement of the heels and buttocks. Palms should be placed on the thighs, fingers pointing toward the feet.

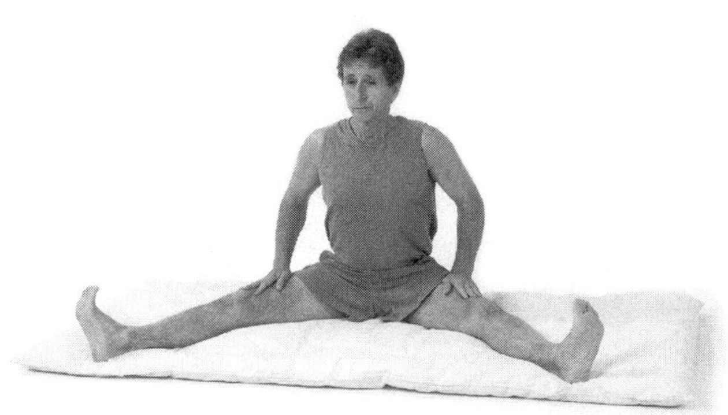

3. Pushing on the thighs will straighten the spine still further.

4. Take a minute or two; calmly breathe normal-sized breaths.

5. Now reach along the underside of the thighs as far as is practicable without bending the knees any further, pressing the palms against e.g., the backs of the knees, or closer in toward the hips. Bend as symmetrically as possible.

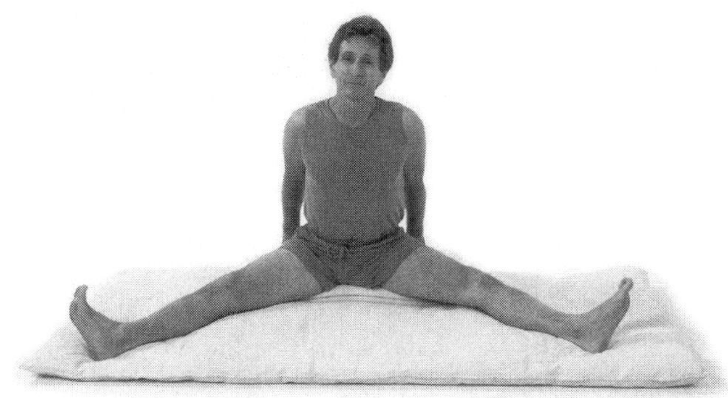

6. Holding the backs of the legs this way, bend the elbows to bring the torso down toward the bed. Let the whole torso move as one piece, resisting the temptation for head or shoulders to stoop forward.

It may be necessary to recline against the headboard, and with palms on the bed behind

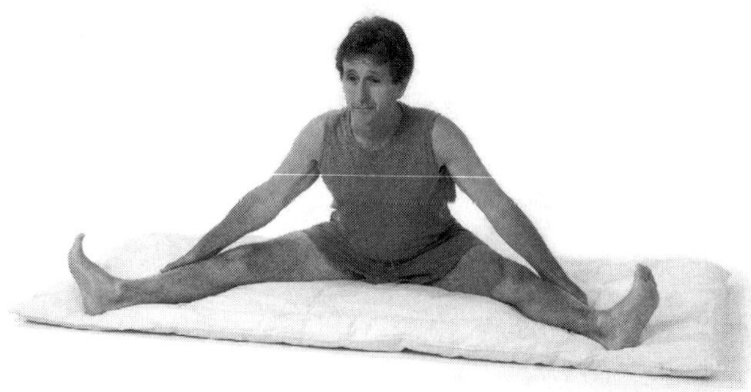

the back, pushing gradually into greater and greater flexion of the torso on the hips.

When one approaches the end of the range for such pushing, it's time to bring the hands in front, to the undersides of the thighs, with straps, or as described in Part I, using chairs.

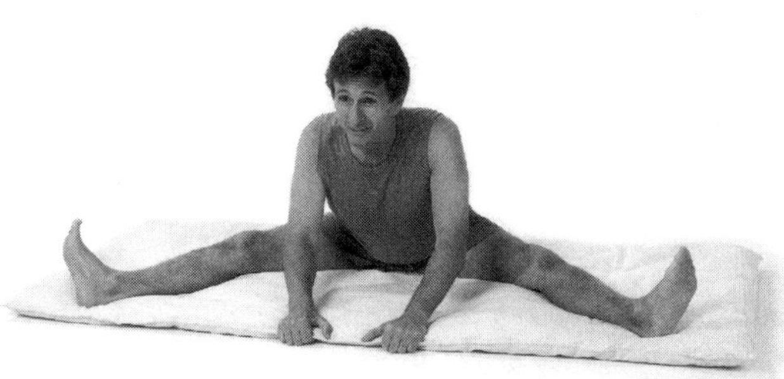

On the other hand, if one can reach forward beyond the knees, then straighten them more, so that one can still usefully place the hands above the knees, or go to the intermediate pose. If this pose is suitable, descend (or if one is using the headboard, ascend) as much as one can without bending the knees further. Breathe calmly for 10-20 seconds. Gradually increase your forward bending, and gradually hold the pose up to 1 minute.

Intermediate Upavista Konasana

1. Sit on the edge of a sturdy armchair or locked wheelchair with safety belt in place.
2. Holding on to the fronts of the arms, spread the legs as far apart as possible, keeping the knees as straight as possible.
3. Straighten the entire spine, from the coccyx to the nape of the neck. Take a few deep breaths, enlarging the front of the chest while pulling in the abdomen. Straighten the back as much as possible.
4. Exhale and pull the shoulders and chest forward together without changing the seating at all, or the position of the heels.
5. Use the front of the arms of the chair to pull the whole torso forward as much as possible without bending the knees or hunching over the back.
6. Breathe quietly for 10-20 seconds at first, and gradually extend the time-period to 1 minute. Over time the chest and shoulders will come down further and further.

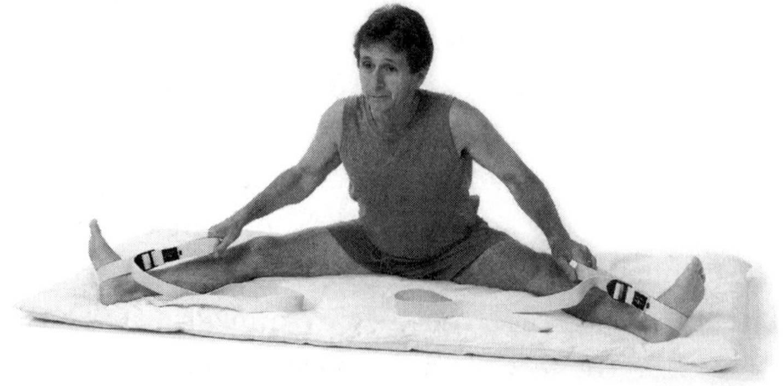

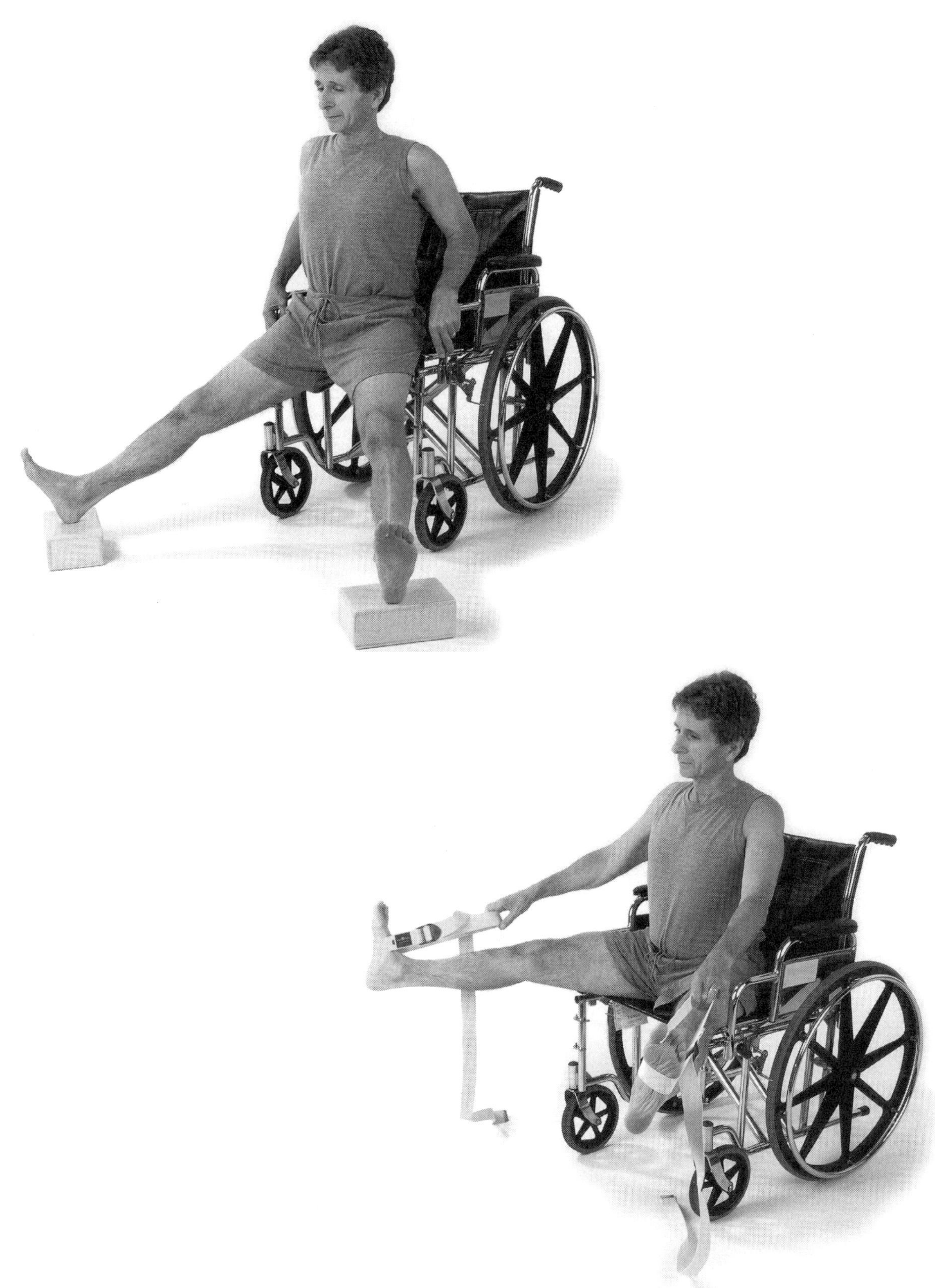

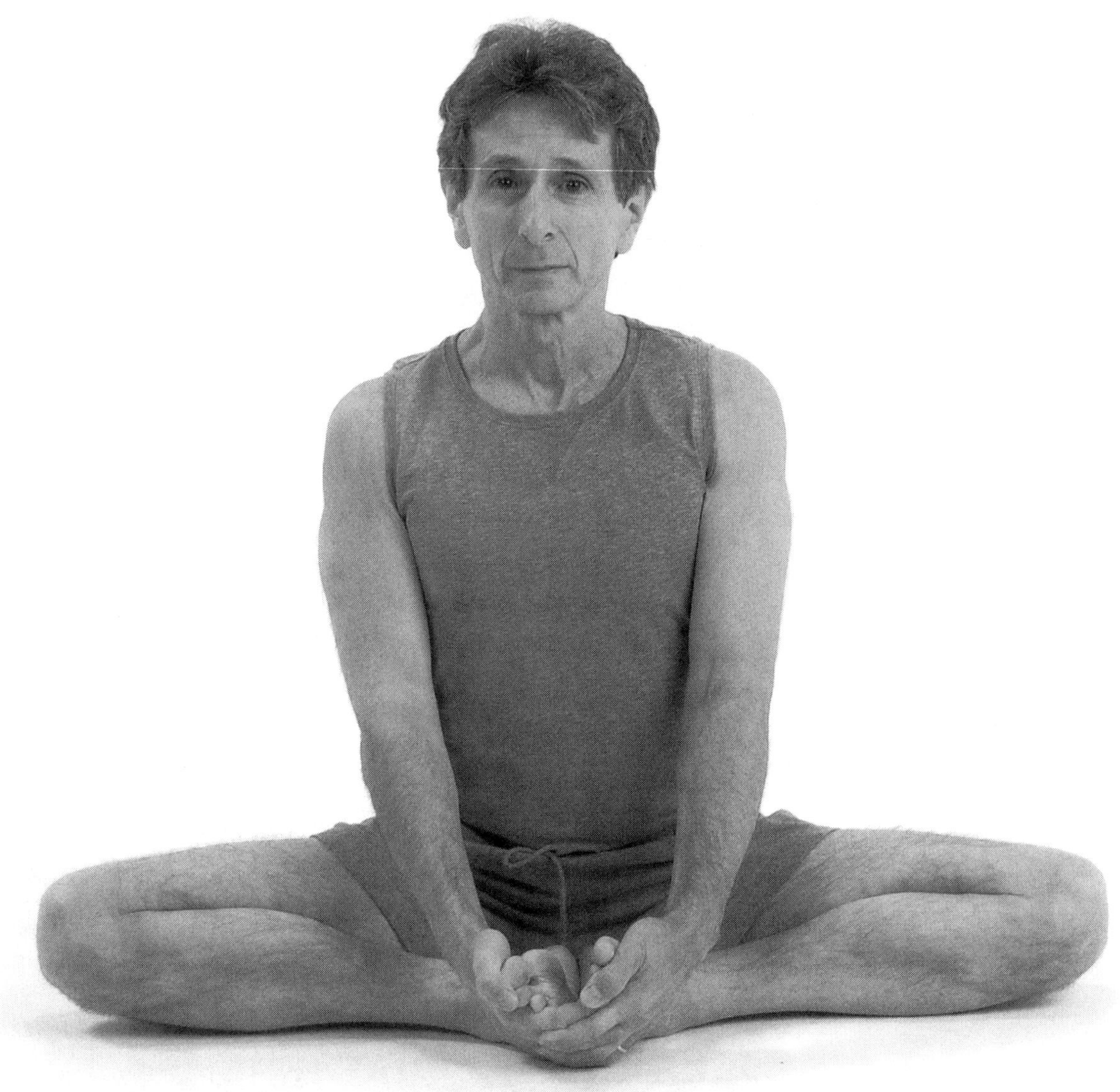

BADDHA KONASANA

Bound Angle Pose

The adductor muscles often become spastic. This is particularly disabling when they respond to the flexion and extension that occurs during walking. MS patients are particularly susceptible to "scissor gait," where tripping occurs during walking. When the leg being brought forward for the next step is adducted, its foot catches behind the leg on which the person is currently standing.

Baddha Konasana, the bound-angle pose, works to stretch the adductors, reduce spasticity, and improve practitioners' control of these muscles.

1. Begin just as in Konasana: Sitting on a flat surface, spread your legs as far apart as possible.

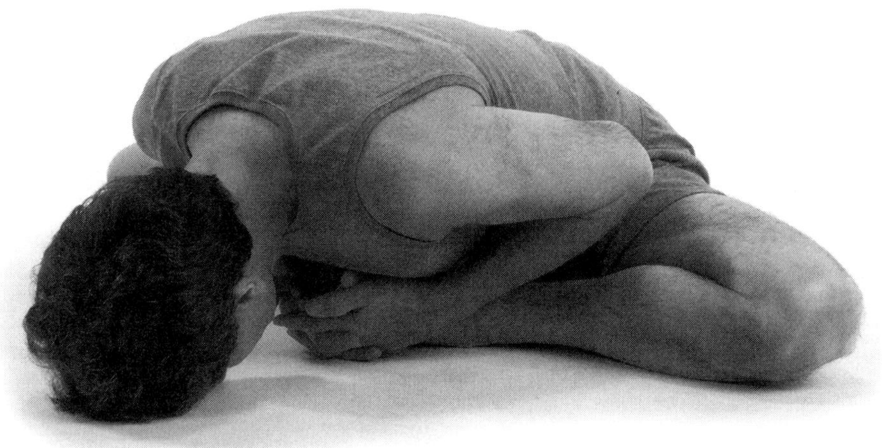

2. However, in Baddha Konasana, bend your knees until the soles of the feet are pressed together, the outer ankles are against the surface, and the heels are pressed inward to the perineum as much as possible. The outer aspects of the shins, knees and thighs should rest on the surface. Your weight should be mainly on the ischial tuberosities or "sit-bones." The ankles are supporting only the weight of the feet.

3. Hold the great toes between the thumbs and the next two fingers of each hand, straighten the spine maximally, open the chest with a full breath and pull in the abdomen.

4. Exhale and bring the lower abdomen, from below the navel to the sternum, down to the inner ankles, keeping the spine as straight as possible. Your weight now should be distributed symmetrically on the outer thighs, calves, and ankles. The head and shoulders come down only insofar as the hips and torso descend.

5. Eventually the chin should rest on the flat surface.

The entry-level and intermediate versions of Baddha Konasana have been described earlier in the book.

PARSVOTTANASANA

Intense Flank Stretch

1. Standing still with feet together, bring the palms back and together with little fingers touching the spine.

2. Pull the shoulders and elbows back as well, and urge the upward pointing fingers upward, until they are between the shoulder blades.

3. Spring so that 3 1/2 feet separate the feet, and turn the right foot 90 degrees outward, and the left 30 degrees inward.

4. Inhale and revolve the torso 90 degrees to the right, straightening the back, opening the chest, pulling in the abdomen and thrusting the head back so that the face is nearly horizontal.

5. Finally, exhale, bending at the lowest waist, pressing the navel to the thigh, the

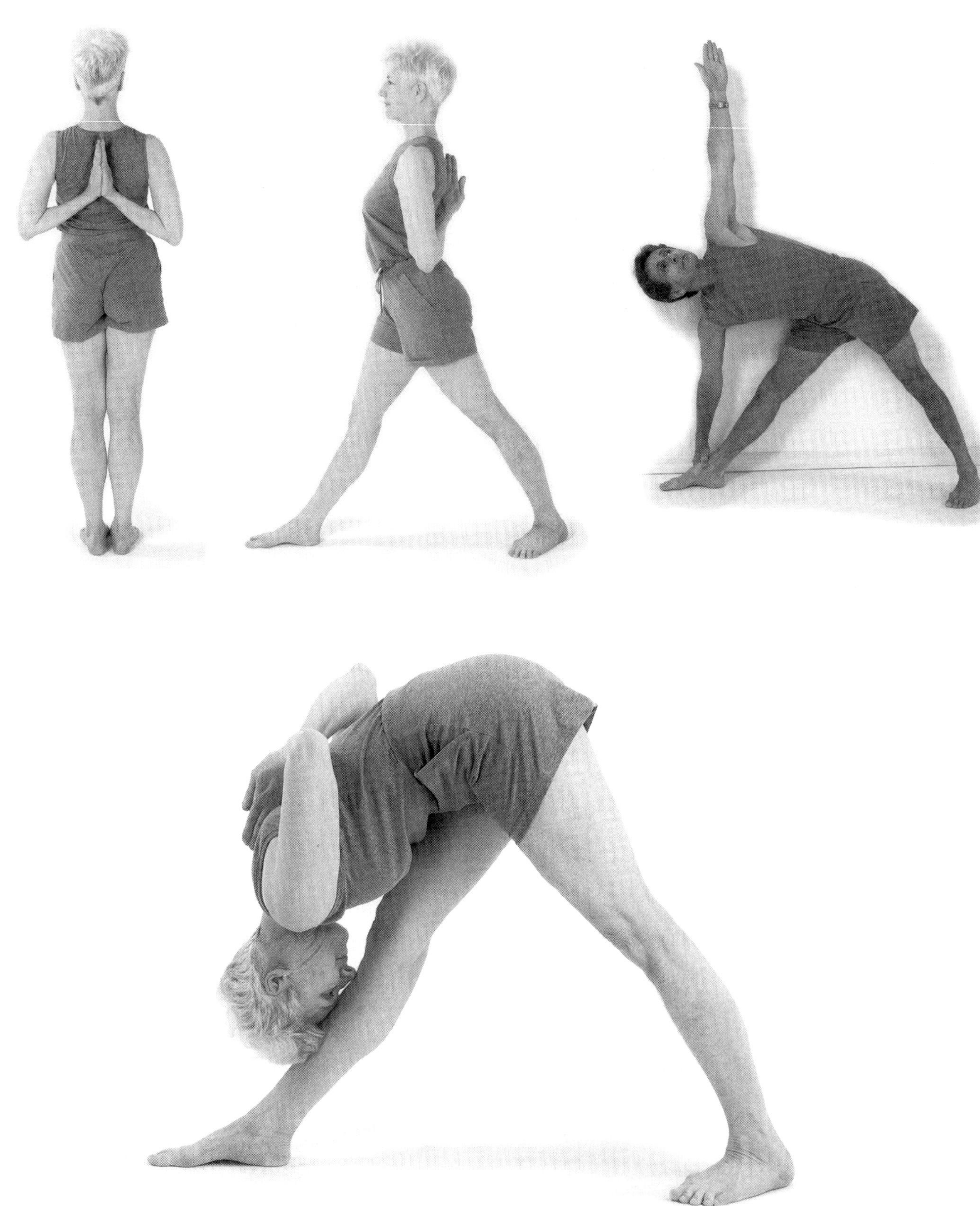

chest to the lower thigh and knee, and first the nose, then the lips, then the chin to the tibial region below the patella.

6. Splay apart the toes of both feet, keep knees poker straight.

7. Breathe calmly for 10-20 seconds, gradually extending the time to 1 minute. Repeat on the other side.

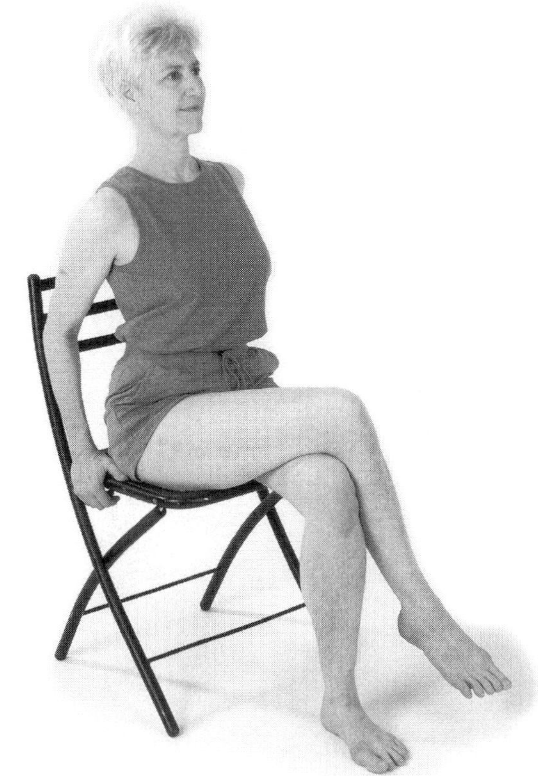

Entry-Level Parsvottanasana

1. Sit squarely in a solid armchair or wheelchair.

2. Cross the right leg over the left, clasping the seat of the chair with fingers facing backwards. Bring the shoulder blades back, down and together.

3. Straighten the spine, pulling the entire torso forward with both hands' pressure against the seat of the chair.

4. Breathe normally during the pose, gradually increasing the time spent in it from 10-20 seconds to 1 minute.

5. Then repeat the procedure crossing the left leg over the right.

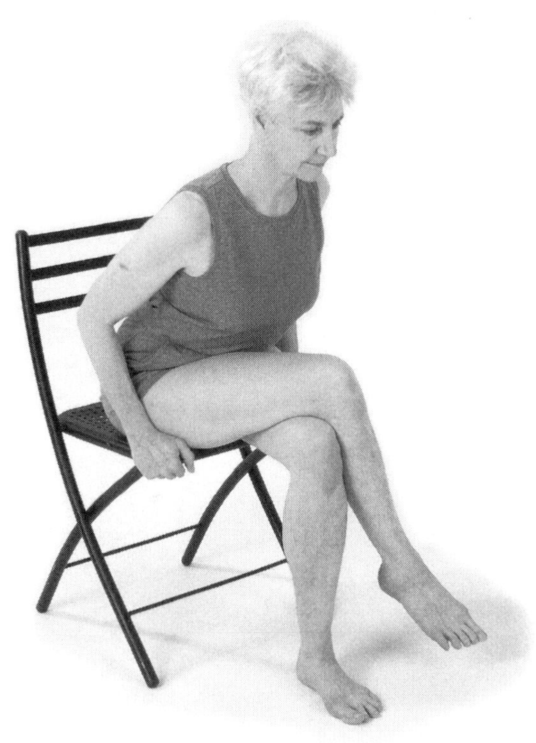

Intermediate-Level Parsvottanasana

1. Stand with the feet three feet apart and facing forward.

2. Interlace your fingers behind your back. If there are difficulties balancing, stand with one side in contact with a wall.

3. Bring the shoulders back, down and together and pull in the abdomen while taking a deep breath and sliding the hands down as far as possible toward the floor.

4. Now exhale and descend down with the shoulders staying back.

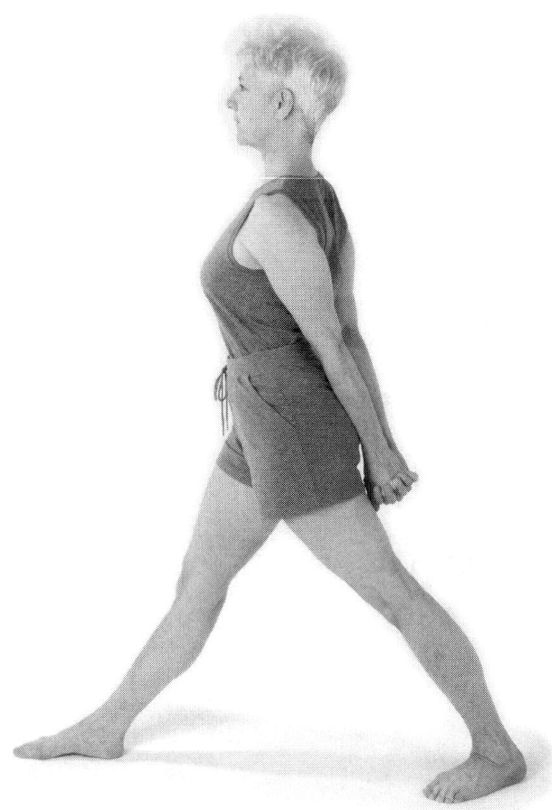
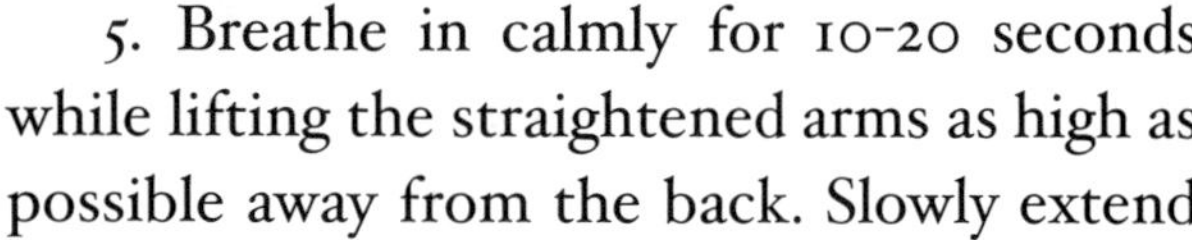
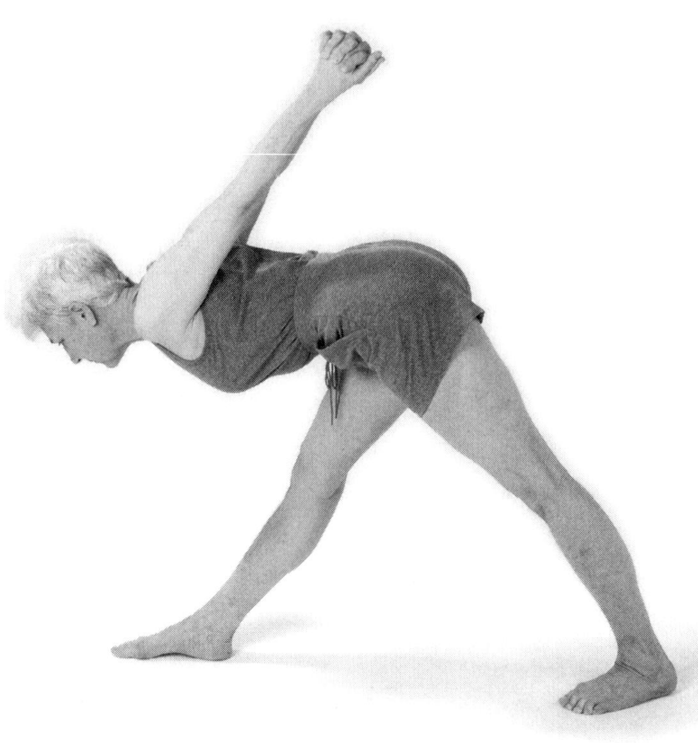

5. Breathe in calmly for 10-20 seconds while lifting the straightened arms as high as possible away from the back. Slowly extend the period of time in the descended position up to 1 minute.

6. To leave the pose, first raise the torso up during inhalation, then release the arms.

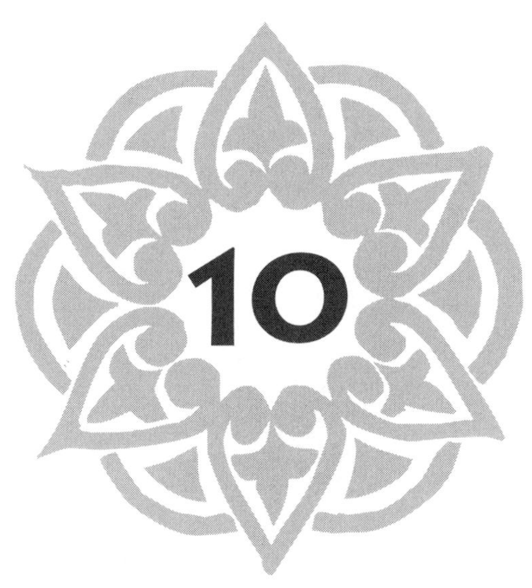

Strength

Yoga poses are generally stable. The practitioner gets him- or herself into a position, and then stays there for a length of time. This serves three purposes very directly, and two more besides. First, as we have already emphasized, it stretches the soft tissues that limit the range of motion of every joint, and secondly, it quiets painfully spastic muscles that restrict the activities and trouble the lives of neurologically compromised patients. Simple as that.

Third, although it involves no weights or equipment apart from ones own body, strength increases in the Yoga practitioner: Standing poses, arm balances and twists require protracted muscular efforts.

Holding any of these groups of poses for more than a few seconds requires isometric effort that has been proven to increase strength in a very efficient way. A muscle's active range of motion is defined by the limits of its effective functioning. Therefore, in a real, practical, and immediate sense, raising strength increases range of motion.

Strengthening

Examining strength may be the best way to see the tension between conscious, intended action and the involuntary physiology that supports it. A strong muscle is a great resource, but that same muscle, contracting in a way that

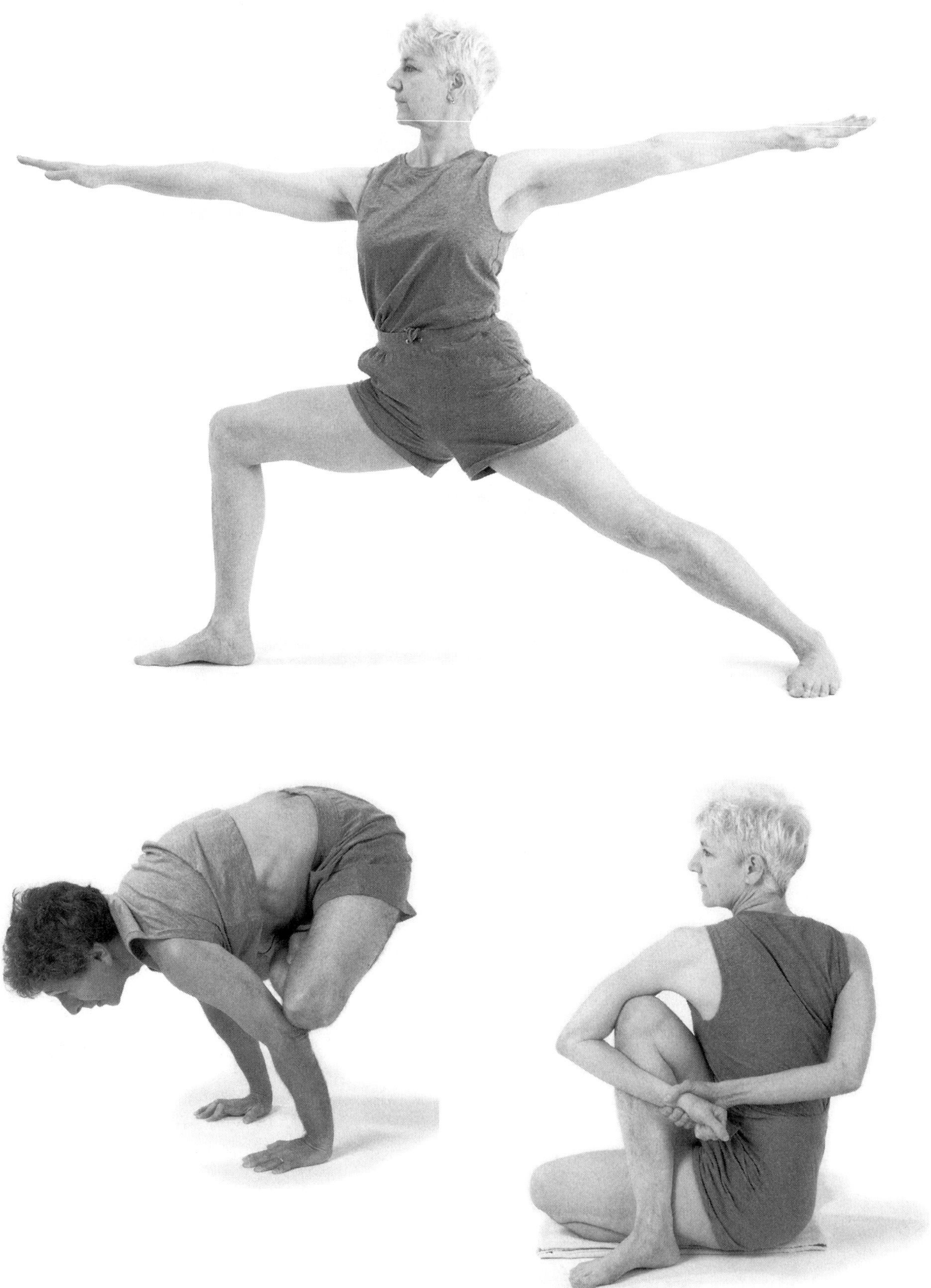

impedes you in what you're trying to do, becomes a formidable adversary. The spastic muscle is a painful reminder that strength without control is a two-edged thing at best. Our idea of a strong man or woman is one that can perform feats that require coordination and teamwork between powerful muscle groups.

I suppose we could say a given muscle is strong because it can generate a certain amount of pull with its contraction. But the person that has that muscle is not strong unless it can be applied intentionally. It is difficult or impossible to measure strength in the presence of spasticity, and impossible to utilize the strength of spastic muscles in most circumstances. This is why strength, as we generally recognize it, logically comes after spasticity.

Yet there are circumstances every hour, such as getting out of bed, or walking up stairs, in which hundreds of pounds of force are generated nearly without our consent usually not really consciously. And there are times that nerve blocks and other weakening measures, applied to spastic muscles of the legs, actually help people's efforts to walk, turn and transfer.

First, we learn to walk or stand, and many other complex but standard applications of muscle strength. Then, over time, we learn to instigate and modify these patterns of muscle activation, paying almost no attention to what had previously been a major challenge. It is the basic necessity of creatures with limited breadth of attention: if we could not relegate learned actions to "auto pilot," we could not keep advancing, given the finite number of things we can attend to at the same time.

Yoga reverses the process, bringing into consciousness, and under intentional control, what has been dropped from the spotlight, or had never been there at all. In MS, and many neurological conditions, yoga gets help, paradoxically, from the illness: weakness is the opposite of strength, but the twin of spasticity. Both stop us from doing what we purpose to do. But both come to our attention on their own. This section focuses on returning strength to the essential and delightful attribute it is in the largely human realm of intentional action.

NAVASANA

The Boat

1. Sit in Dandasana.

2. Raise your legs up thirty degrees; the trunk will recline backwards to maintain balance. Your feet should be above eye-level. Keep both legs and back straight.

3. Raise both straightened arms to horizontal, palms facing one another.

4. Remain in the pose breathing regularly for 10-20 seconds.

5. Now inhale, bend the knees, interlock your fingers behind them, and straighten the legs again, pulling the legs and torso together with exhalation. Retain the straight back, keep shoulder blades close to each other and the spine.

6. Remain in this pose, forehead or face in contact with the shins, breathing quietly for 10-20 seconds.

7. Gradually, as balance and stamina permit, increase the time to 1 minute.

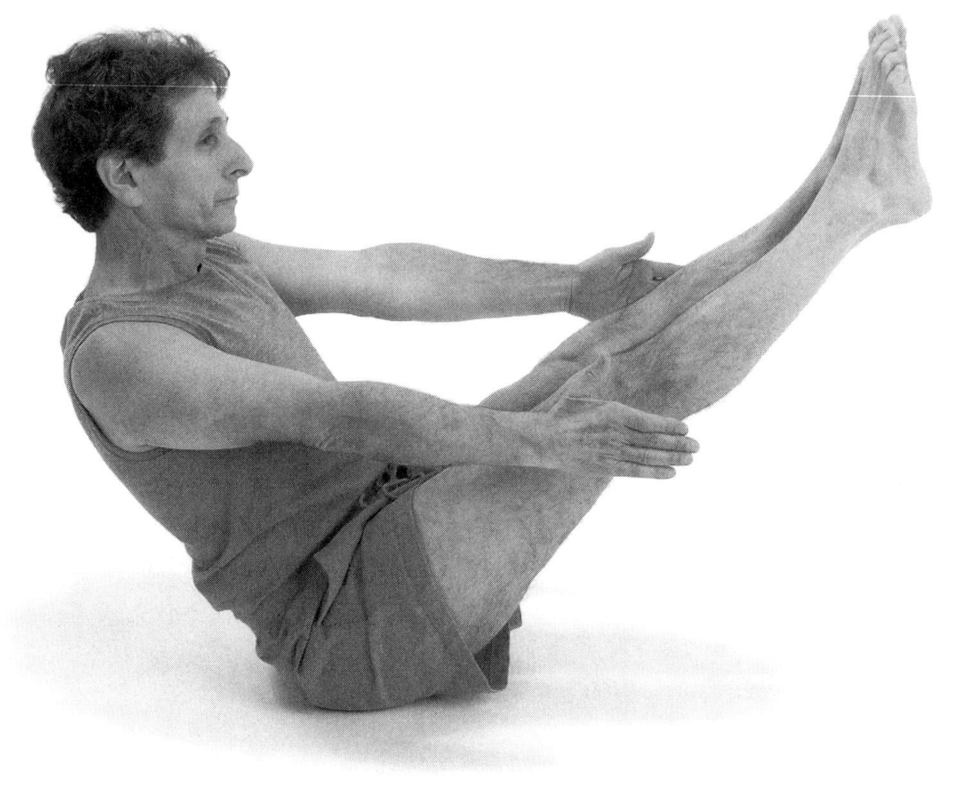

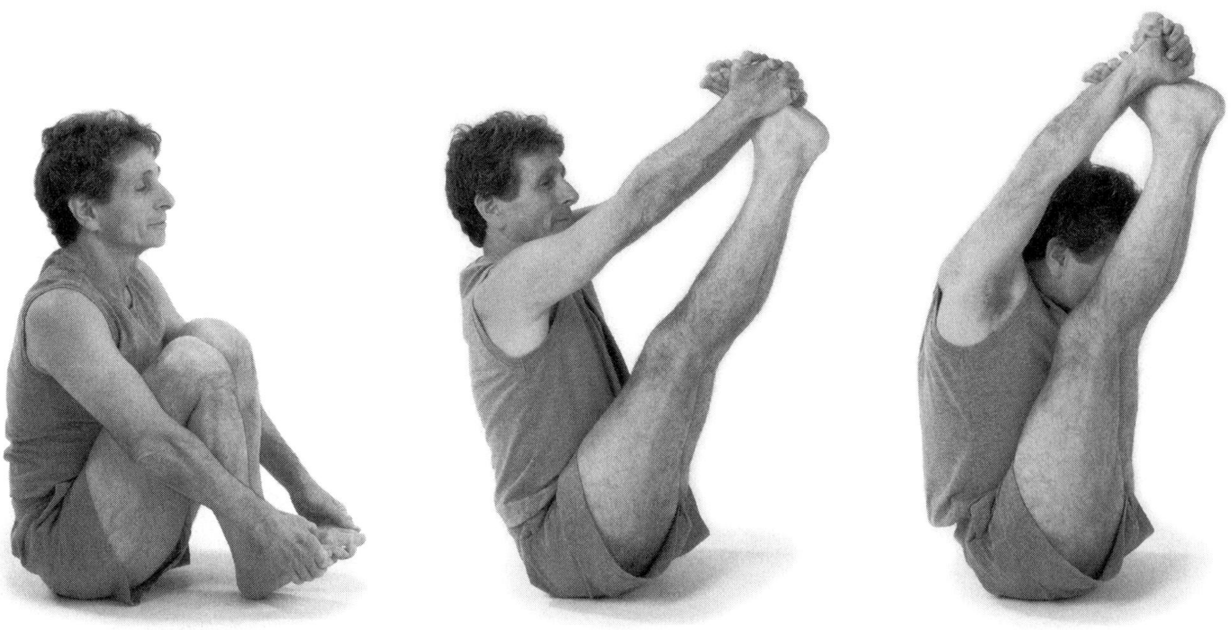

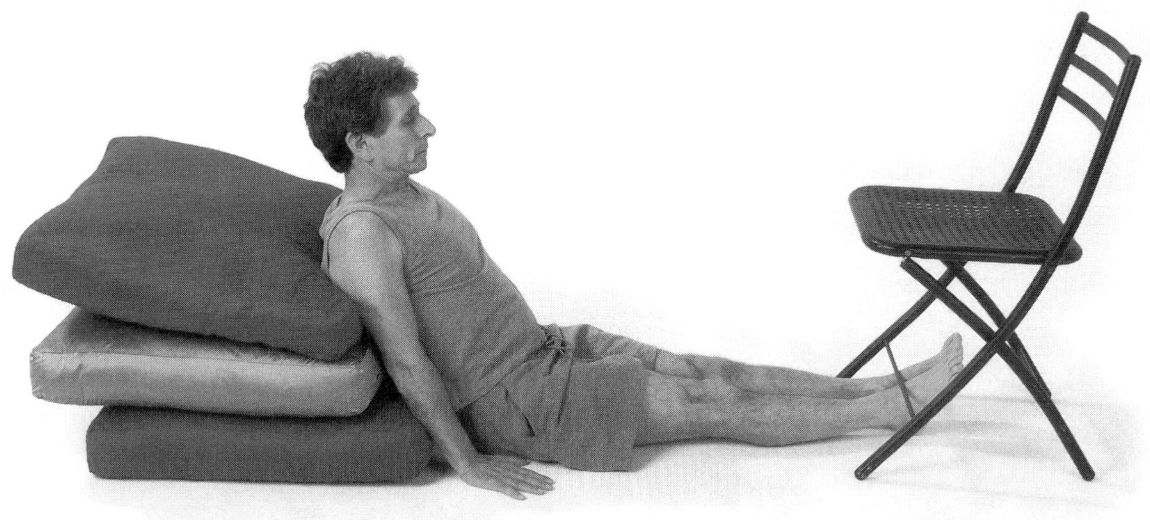

Entry-Level Navasana

1. Lie supine on a flat surface with torso elevated to 30 degrees by supports, and palms down, fingers pointing toward the feet.

2. Hook your ankles under a heavy piece of furniture, or have another person hold them down. Take two quiet breaths.

3. With the second exhalation raise the torso a few inches off the support. The higher the torso supports, the easier this will be. Use your hands' pressure against the surface to help raise your torso.

4. Breathe quietly for 10-20 seconds.

5. Gradually, over weeks, attempt to perform the pose with less and less help from the arms. Then work to reduce the height of the torso supports.

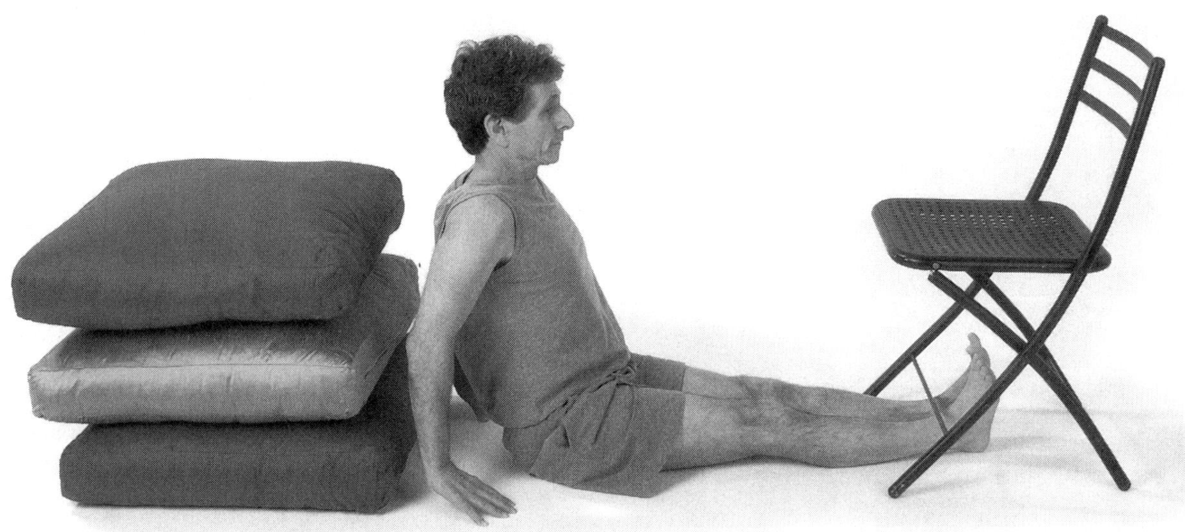

Intermediate-Level Navasana

Perform the first part of Navasana without interlocking the fingers behind the feet. If balance is not up to the task, begin with one arm supporting, the other horizontal, and/or only one leg elevated.

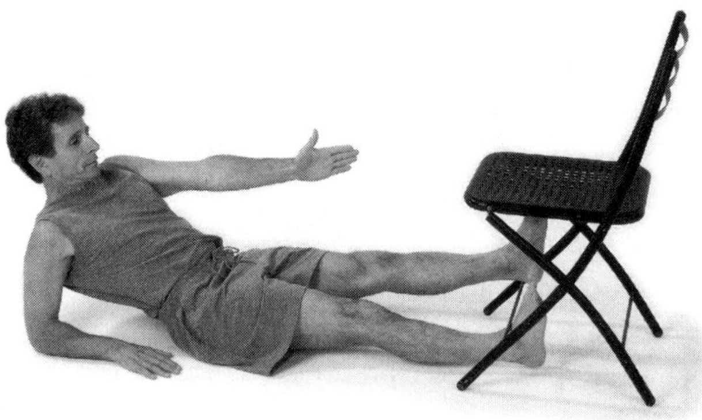

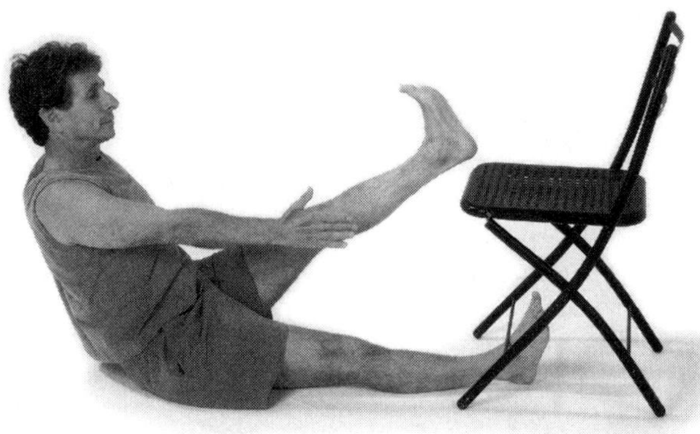

UTTHITA AND PARIVRITTA PARSVAKONASANA

Extended and Revolving Lateral Angle Pose

1. Both poses begin in Tadasana. Spend a full minute equilibrating weight on the two feet, and balancing finely enough so that the act of breathing causes no sway in any plane.

2. Now rapidly draw the feet apart, jumping up vertically as little as possible in order to land with the feet 4-5 feet apart without jostling the internal organs. Raise the arms to horizontal.

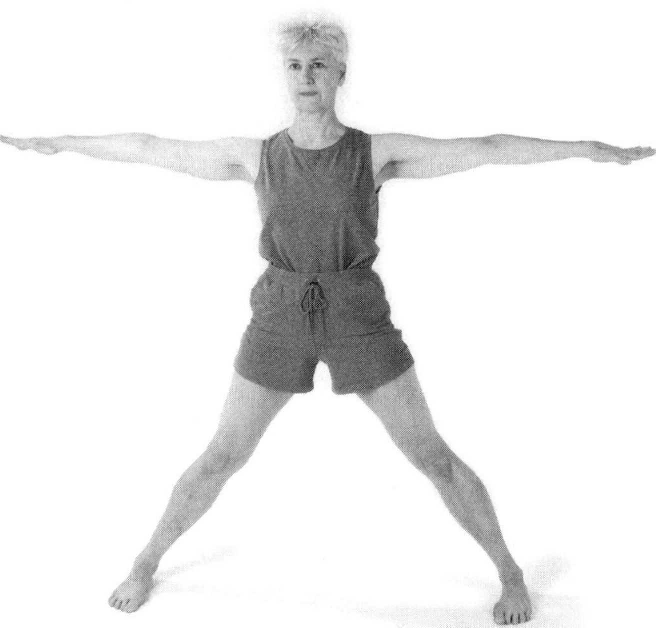

3. Turn the right foot outward 90 degrees, the left foot inward 30 degrees, then descend, retaining an entirely straight left leg while the right knee bends to 90 degrees. Keep the little toe side of the left foot on the floor.

4. Take a quiet breath.

The two poses are alike up to this point. After starting out the same way, they go separate ways from here on. They are presented one after the other.

5. For Utthita Parsvakonasana incline the trunk to the right as you exhale, and place the right palm at the little toe side

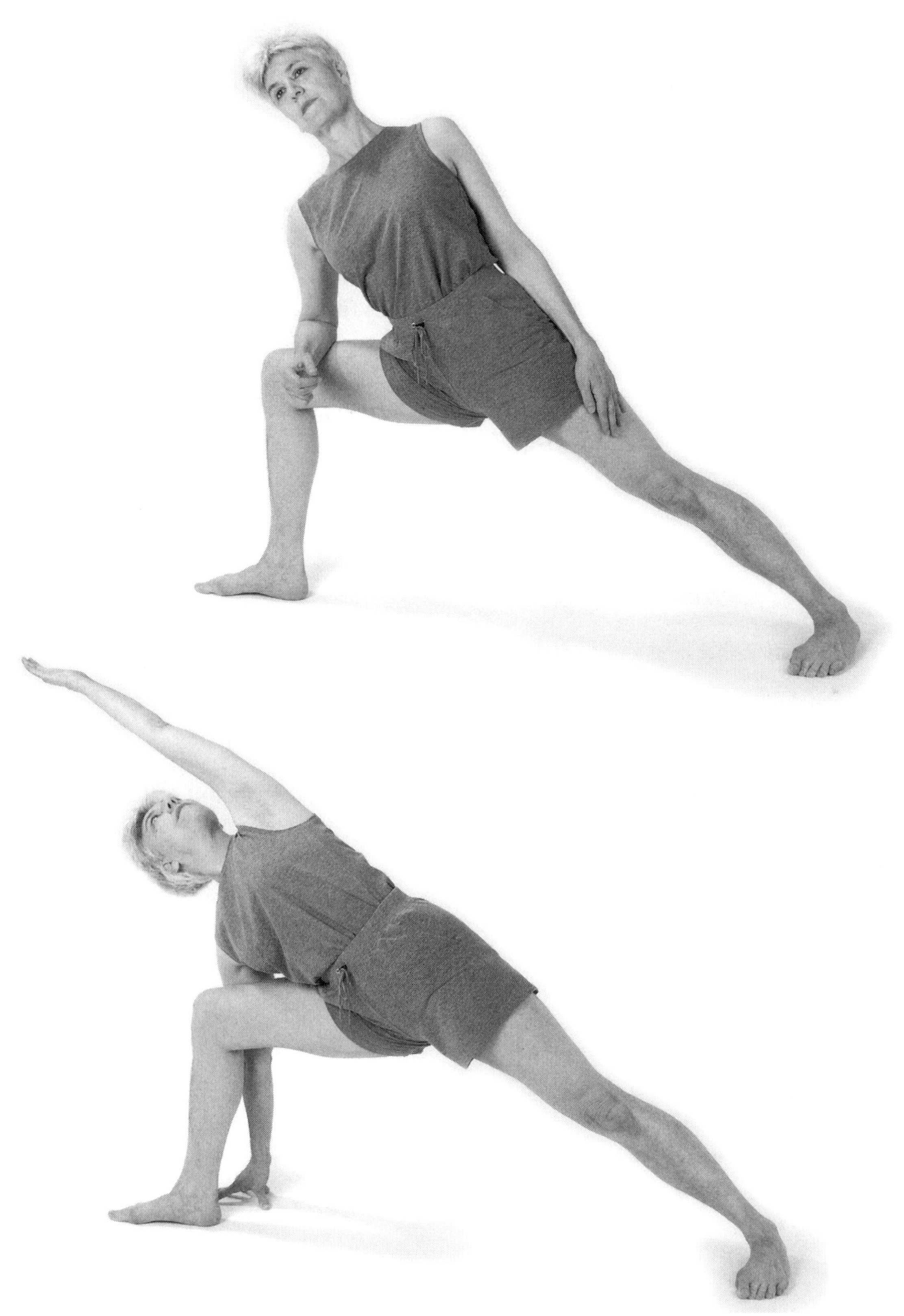

of the right foot, parallel with it. The right forearm and shin should be vertical, and in line.

6. Revolve the torso, the left flank, and the left shoulder upward. Keep the left knee straight. Extend the left arm behind the ear and over the head. The slanting line from the back of the left hand to the left outer foot should be straight.

7. Press the right biceps in against the right knee; press the knee outward against the biceps. These two forces, and the pressure they generate at their meeting point, serve as the fulcrum for rotating the left torso and hip upward.

8. Stretch the left fingertips forward and the little toe side of the left foot backward, maximally elongating and maximally revolving.

9. Breathe smoothly and symmetrically for 10-20 seconds.

10. Then return, retracing the steps back to Tadasana, and perform the pose on the other side. Each side should be built up gradually to 1 minute.

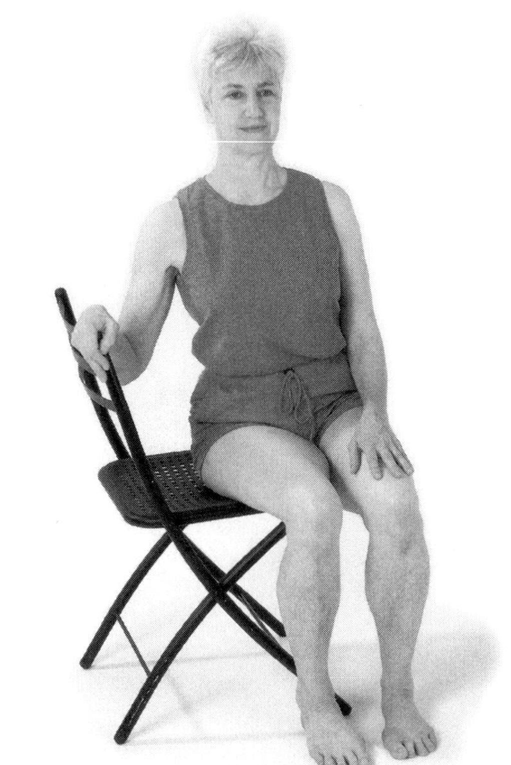

Entry-Level Utthita Parsvakonasana

1. Sit crosswise on a card chair with the right buttock and thigh.

2. Bend the right knee to 90 degrees, so the shin is vertical and the thigh horizontal.

3. Extend the left leg out behind you.

4. Straighten the knee as much as possible and invert the left foot to sustain the little toe on the floor. Use your hands for balance.

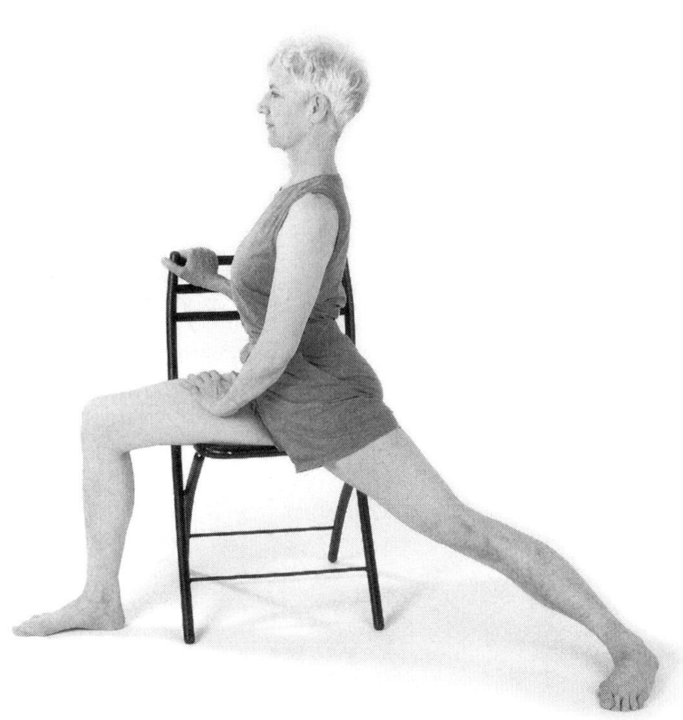

5. Incline your torso forward to the right, and lean on your right thigh with your right forearm. Raise your left arm over your head behind your ear, making as straight a line as possible from the back of the left hand to the outside of the left foot. Press the right elbow into the inside of the right thigh. Press the thigh forward against the elbow. This will help to revolve the right chest forward and raise the left shoulder.

6. Breathe smoothly and symmetrically for 10-20 seconds.

7. Then reverse the sequence, sit on the chair with the left buttock and thigh, and repeat the pose.

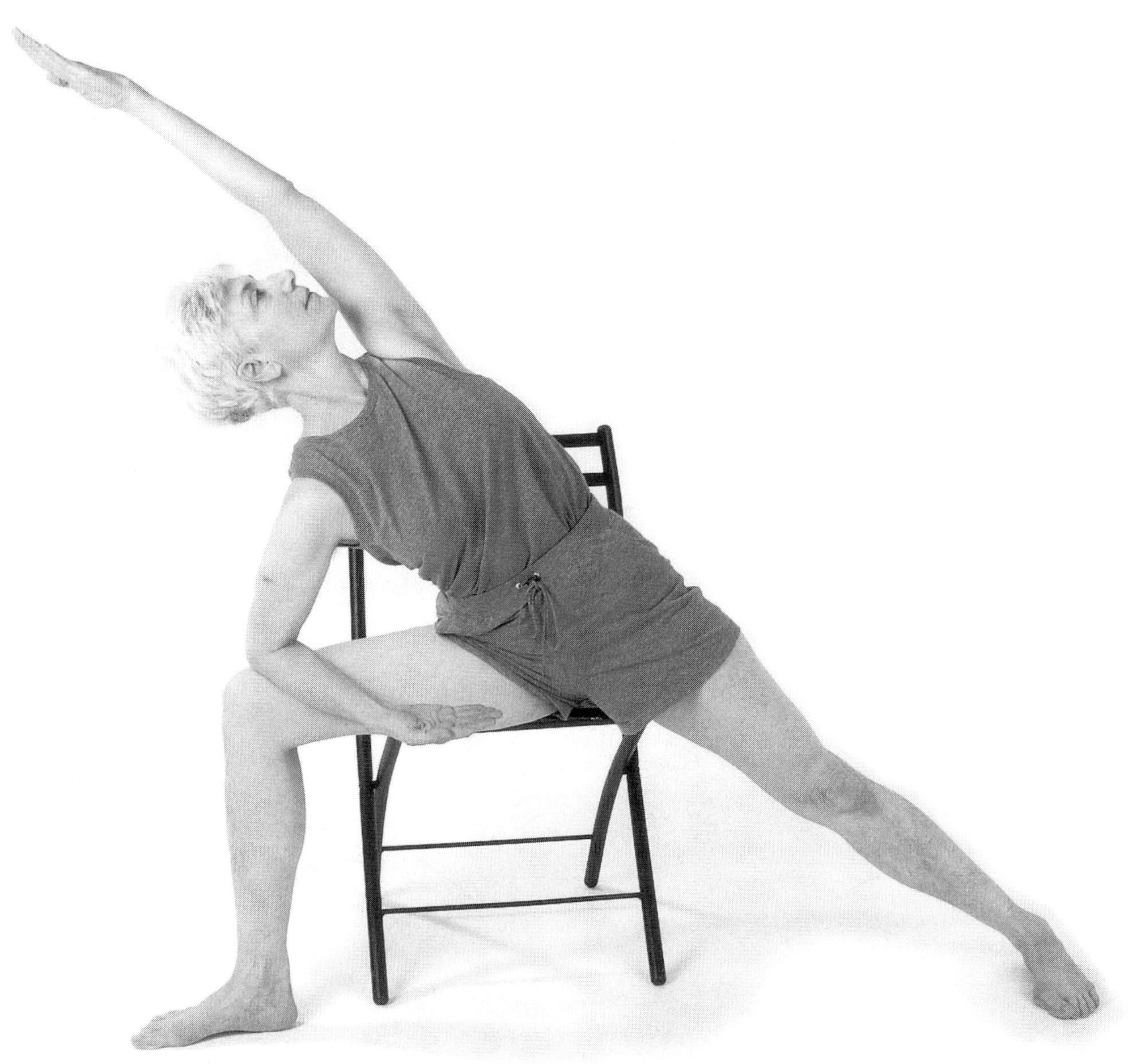

Intermediate
Utthita Parsvakonasana

1. Stand facing a wall with feet 4-5 feet apart, the right foot parallel to the wall and 5-6 inches away from it.

2. Turn the left foot inward 30 degrees. Raise the arms to horizontal.

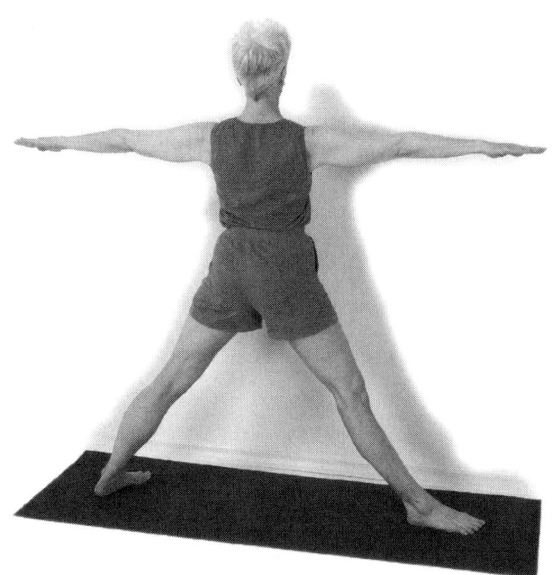

3. Breathe calmly for 20-30 seconds, then descend, retaining the straight left leg, but bending the right knee to 90 degrees, or as far down as your muscular strength allows.

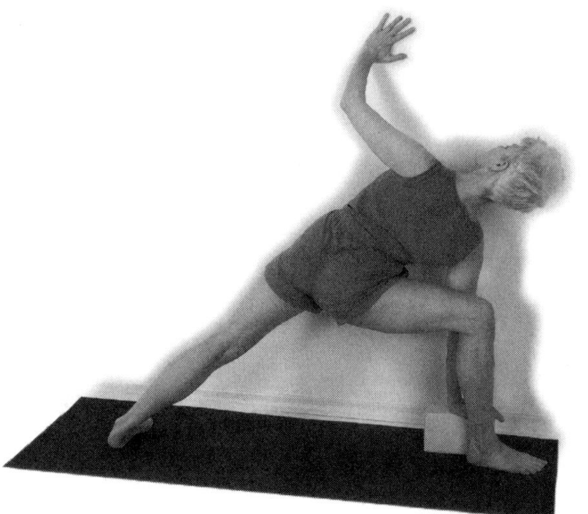

4. Place your right palm parallel to the right foot between it and the wall, with forearm parallel to the right calf. Press against the wall with your left hand, revolving the torso as much as possible.

5. Stay in the position for 10-20 seconds at first, gradually working up to 1 minute.

6. Repeat the pose on the other side.

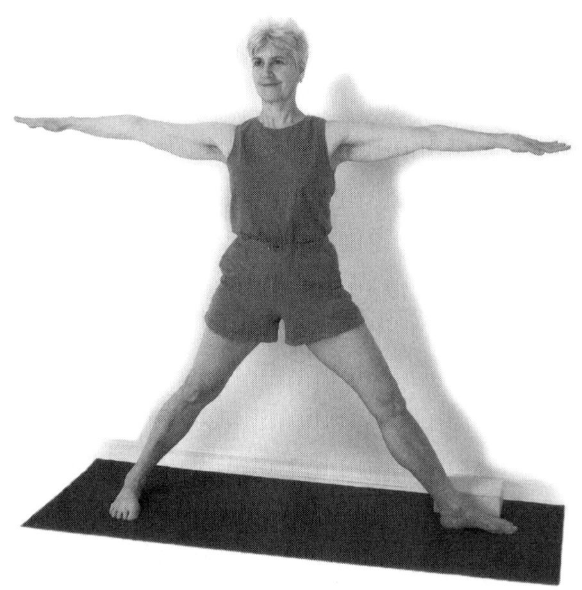

7. This pose may also be done with your back to the wall if balance is a greater problem than mobility.

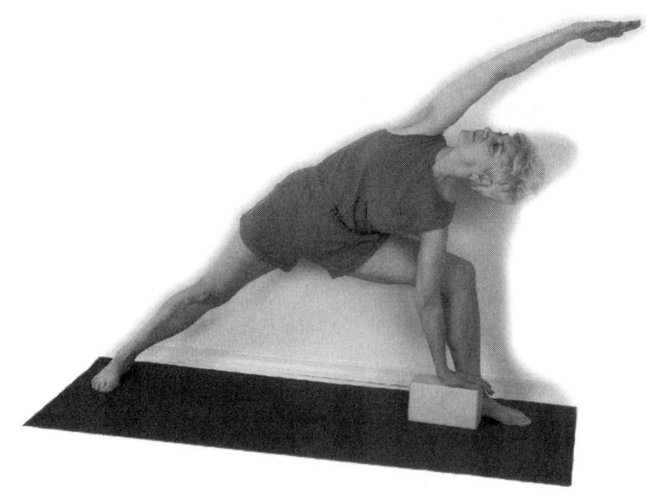

Parivrtta Parsvakonasana

For Parivrtta Parsvakonasana, proceed through the first three directions, as in Utthita Parsvakonasana. Then revolve the trunk to the right while exhaling.

1. Bring the left shoulder over the outside of the right knee, and the left hand to the floor beside the fifth toe, left hand parallel to the right foot, left forearm parallel to the right shin.
2. The right arm extends in a line with the left leg, and in the same plane as the right thigh, knee, and right lateral torso.
3. Use the left arm as a lever, the outer right knee as a fulcrum to move the chest, not the shoulder, to the right of the right leg.

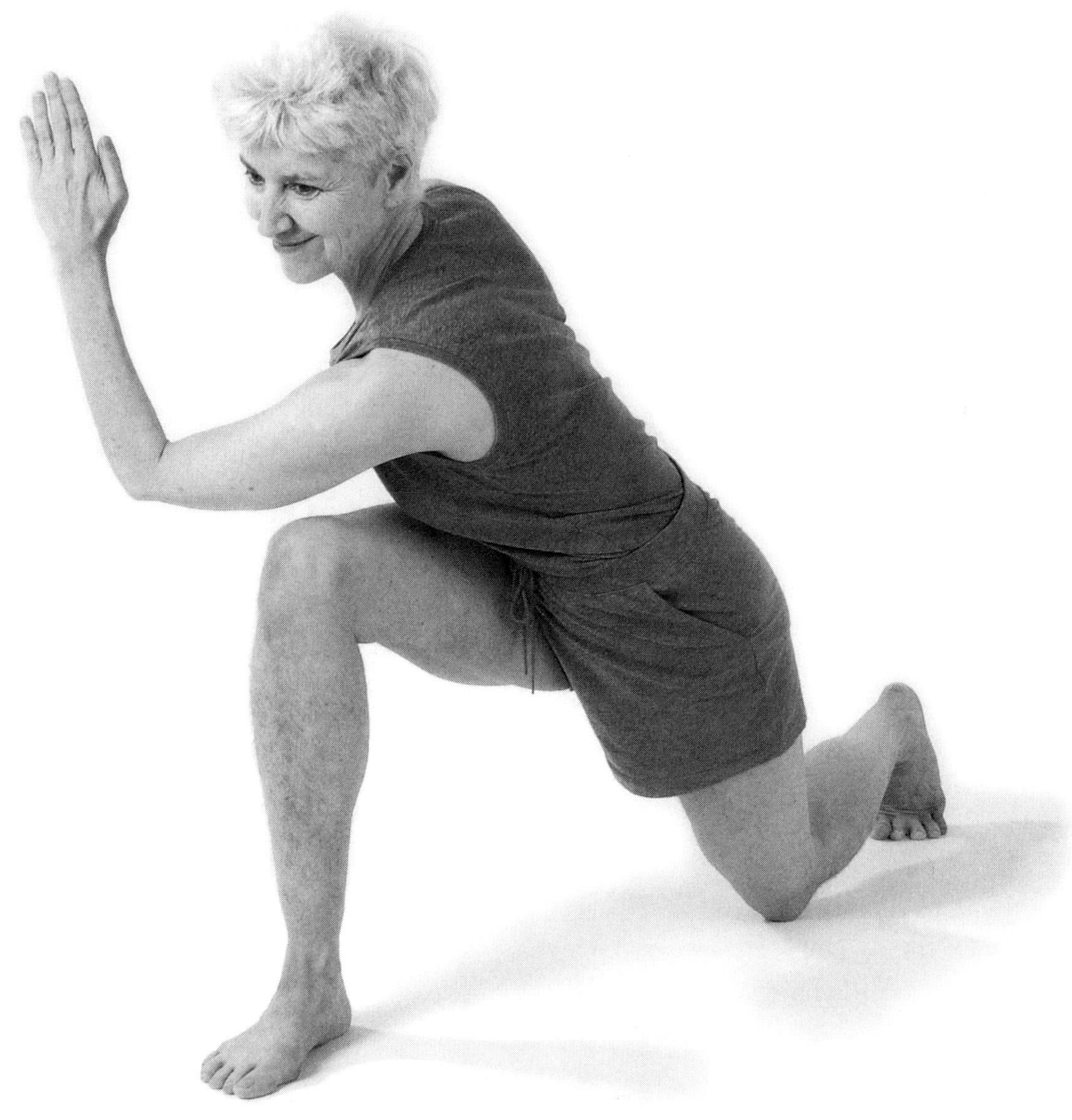

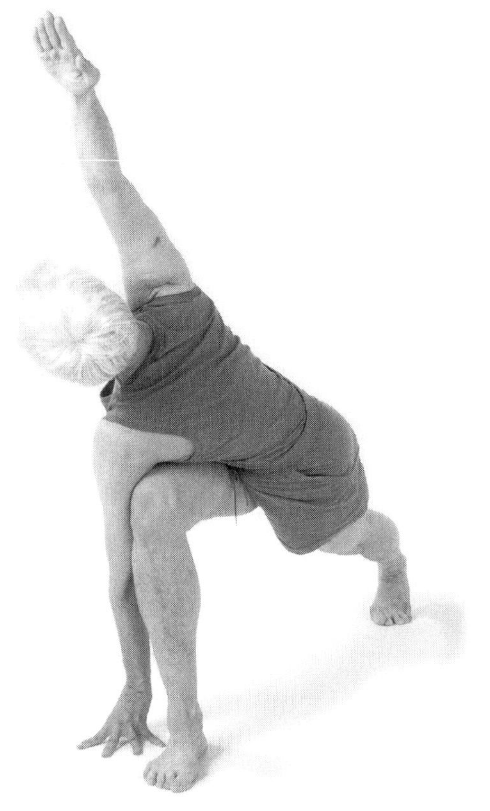

7. Breathe calmly, without force and as symmetrically as possible for 10-20 seconds.

Here the fulcrum is the outside of the left arm, above the elbow, and the outside of the right knee. The opposition is quite natural, and working with it increases the twist of the torso strengthens both upper and lower extremities while improving just aboiut every major joint's range of motion.

Entry-Level Parivritta Parsvakonasana

1. Straddle a card chair. **[1]**

2. Flex the right knee to 90 degrees, making the shin vertical and thigh as close to horizontal as the height of the chair allows.

3. Straighten the left knee behind you, turning the foot inward sufficiently to put some weight on the little toe side of the left foot. **[2]**

4. Distribute your weight to both feet equally and breathe calmly for 1 minute.

5. Then reach the left hand over to the left side of the chair back, and the right hand behind until it rests on the right chair support **[3]**

6. The positions of the arms and legs may be modified for wheelchair use and according to patients' capacities. **[4]**

7. Use the left hand to revolve and incline the torso to the right. If possible, move the left hand onto the outside of the right thigh just above the knee and apply twisting pressure from there. The idea is to move the left chest past the chair back, and the left shoulder is just the right means to accomplish this. Paradoxical as it may seem, it is best to keep the shoulder blade close to the spine, and fixed there. When you pull or push to the right with your left hand, the shoulder blade does not move relative to the chest, rather, the left side of the chest moves to the right, and naturally, the shoulder blade moves with it. The left shoulder will move, of course, but the focus is on the left chest.

8. Once in the position, breathe slowly and carefully for 10-20 seconds.

9. Then release the left arm, sit vertically again, and repeat the pose by flexing the left knee and straightening the right.

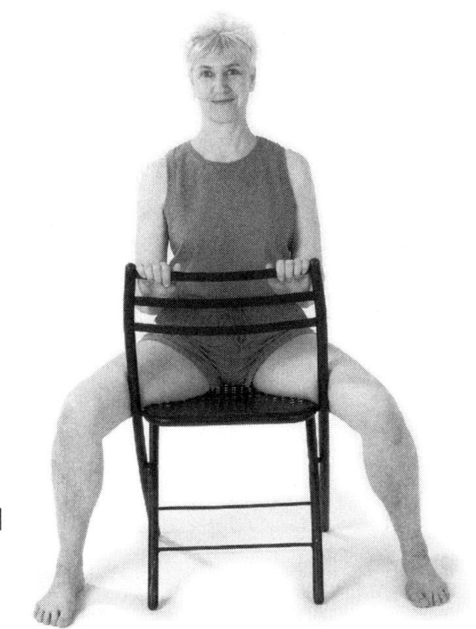
1

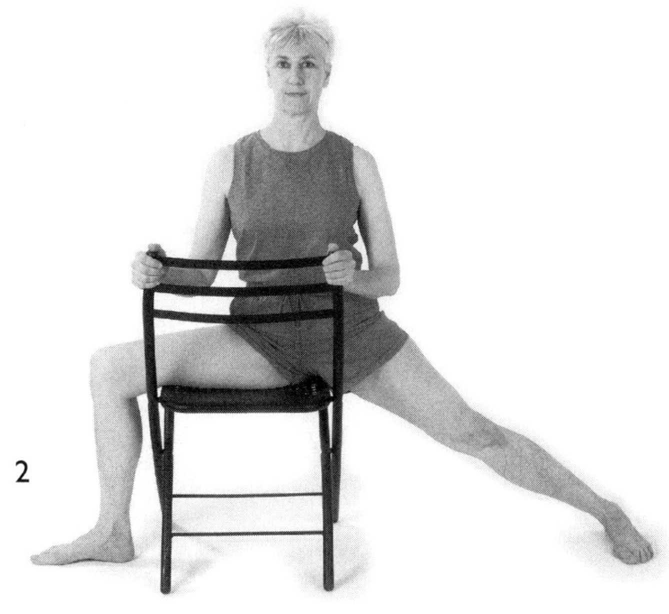
2

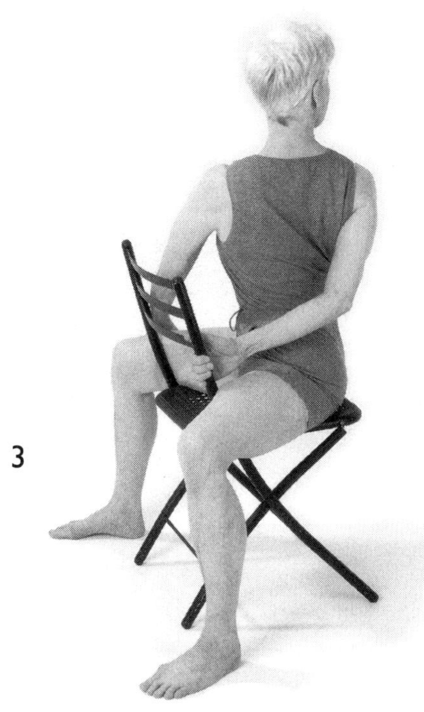
3

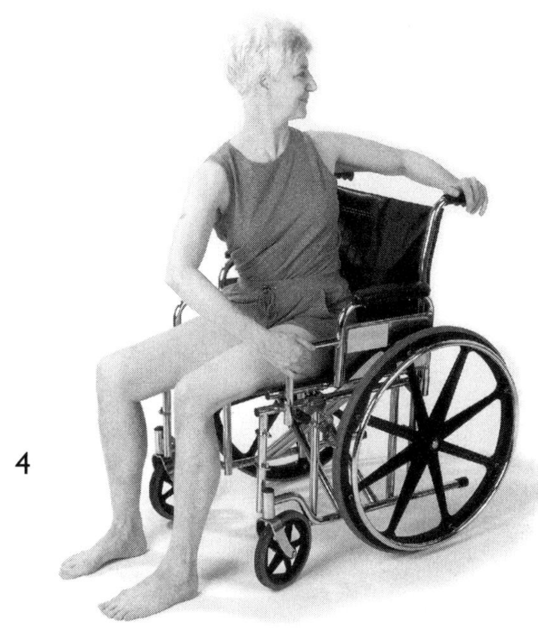
4

Intermediate Parivritta Parsvakonasana

1. Stand facing a wall with feet 4-5 feet apart, the right foot parallel to the wall and 5-6 inches away from it. Appropriately place a block, if needed.

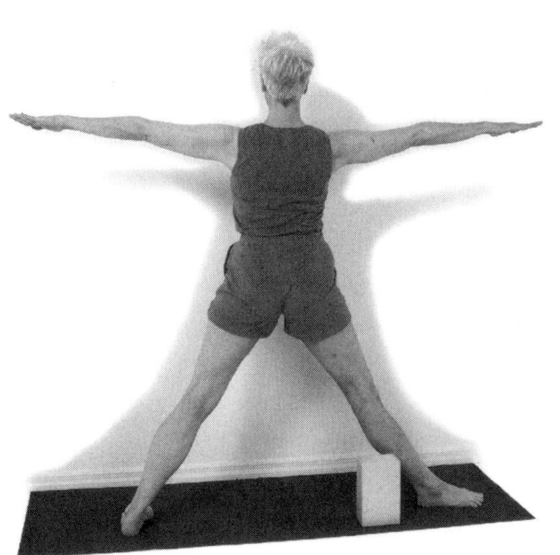

2. Turn the left foot inward 30 degrees. Raise the arms to horizontal.

3. Breathe calmly for 20-30 seconds, then descend, retaining an entirely straight left leg while the right knee bends to 90 degrees. Keep the little toe side of the left foot on the floor.

4. Take a quiet breath.

5. With exhalation revolve the trunk to the right, bringing the left shoulder over the outside of the right knee, sliding the left arm between the head and the knee.

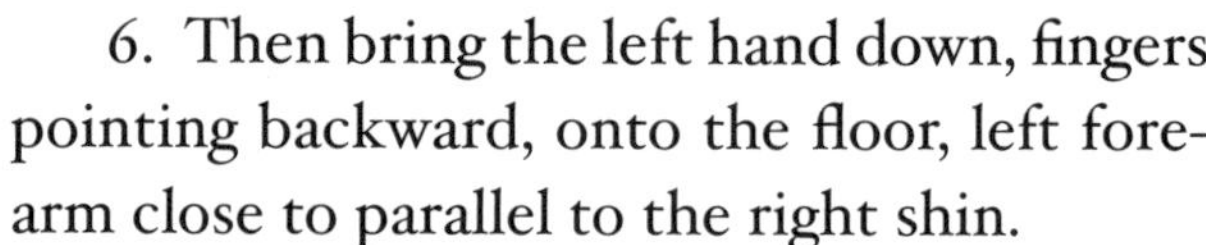

6. Then bring the left hand down, fingers pointing backward, onto the floor, left forearm close to parallel to the right shin.

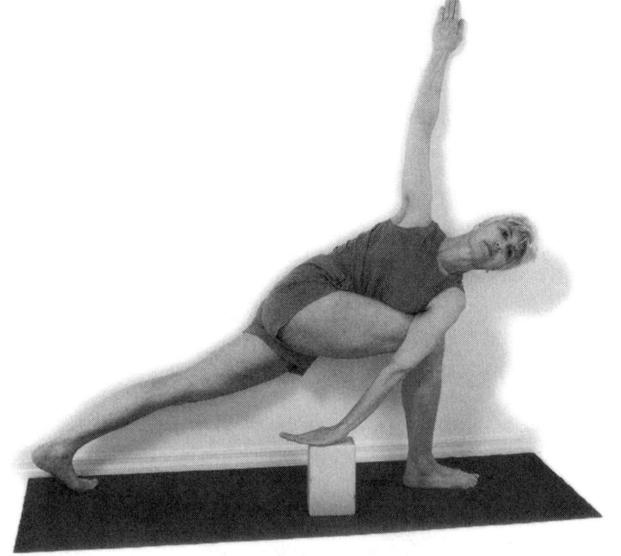

7. The right arm extends collinear with the right leg, in the same plane as the right torso.

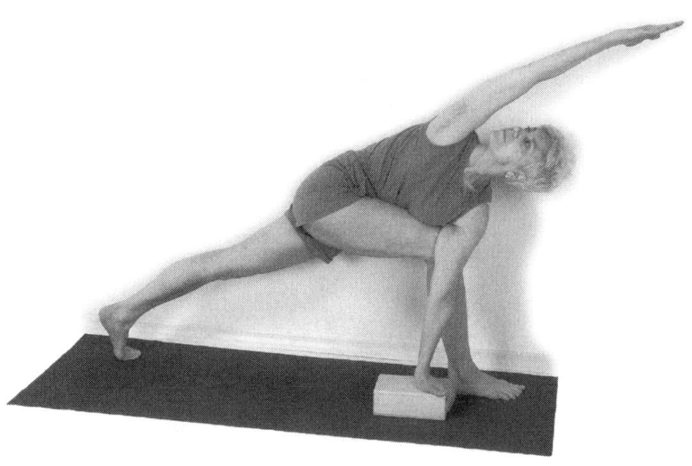

Alternative Parivritta Parsvakonasana

1. An alternate set begins with your back to the wall, with feet 4-5 feet apart.

2. Orient the left foot parallel to the wall. Turn the right foot 30 degrees inward.

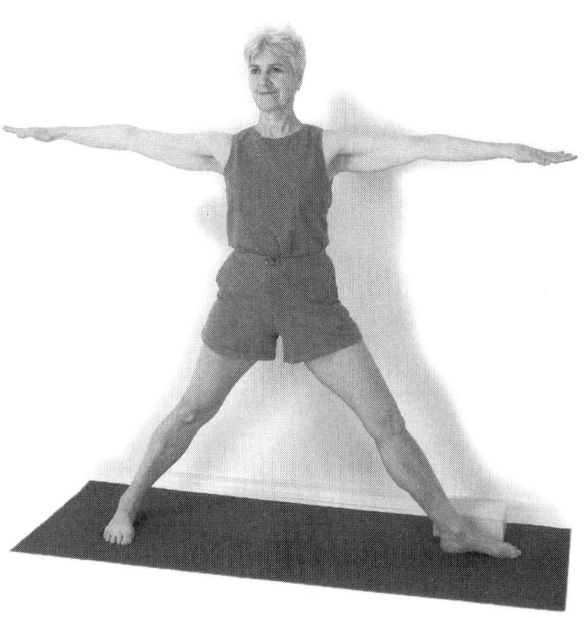

8. Use the left arm as a lever, the outer right knee as a fulcrum to move the chest, not the shoulder, to the right of the right leg.

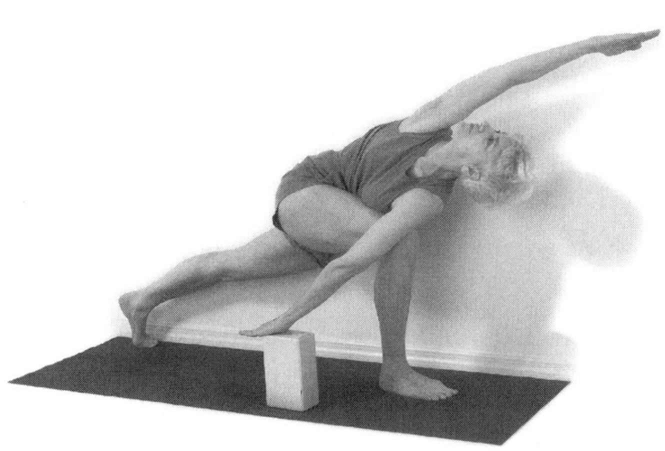

3. Bend the left knee 90 degrees. Lower the right knee to the floor while twisting toward the wall. This is the entry-level pose.

9. Breathe calmly and without force for 10-20 seconds.

10. Then release the left arm, return the torso to vertical, and repeat the pose with left leg bent to 90 degrees and right knee straight.

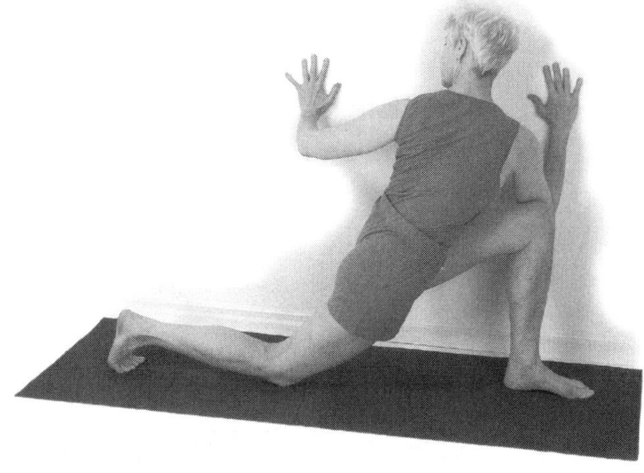

4. Place your right palm on the floor between your left foot and the wall. The back of your armpit should contact the outer left knee. Straighten the right knee.

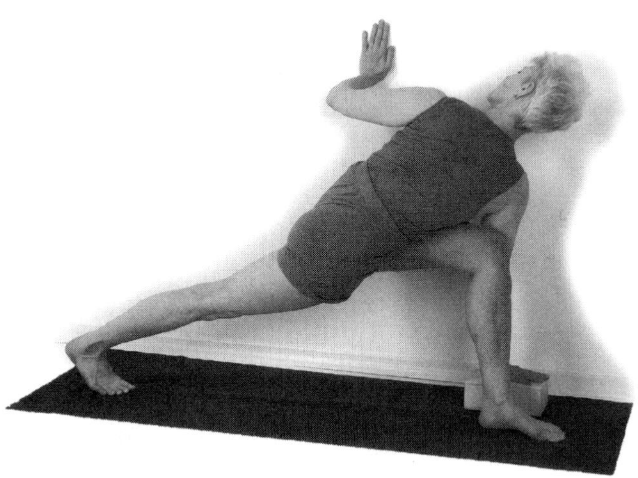

5. Press your left hand against the wall. Use it and your right shoulder to twist still further. Every part from the right ankle upward will revolve together.

6. Raise your left arm toward vertical, attempting to extend the entire left body in a straight line from outer ankle to fingertips. You may use the wall as shown. This is the intermediate pose.

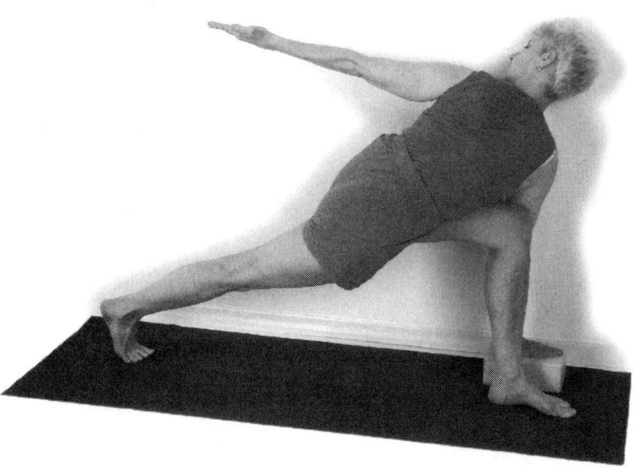

7. Stay in the pose 20-30 seconds.

8. Exit by bringing the right knee to the floor while sliding the right shoulder and arm away from the left knee.

9. Now repeat on the other side.

VIRABHADRASANA I, III

The Warrior Poses

Both poses start the same way.

1. From Tadasana, raise both arms laterally to vertical.

2. Step legs to 4-5 feet apart. Maintain a straightened spine from the sacrum to the base of the skull.

3. Exhale, turn your torso toward the left leg, and bring its foot 90 degrees to the right, while the right foot turns 30 degrees toward the left also. Your navel should point in the direction of the left great toe. **[1]**

4. During a few calm breaths, balance weight evenly between feet, and within each foot.

5. Bend the left knee to 90 degrees while exhaling. **[2]**

6. Still holding the spine erect, inhale and steady your hands in line with the entire spine.

7. Retain the straightened right knee and breathe calmly for 10-20 seconds.

8. Then straighten the left knee as the head returns forward, return to facing forward, lower the arms and breathe quietly for 1 minute.

9. Then reverse the legs. This is Virabhadrasana I.

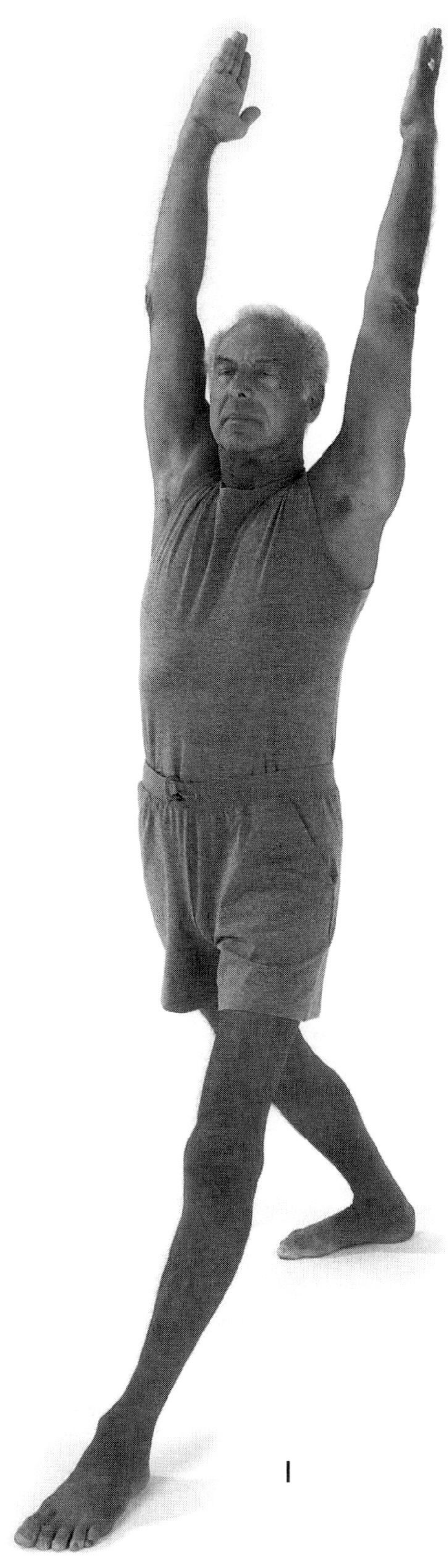

1

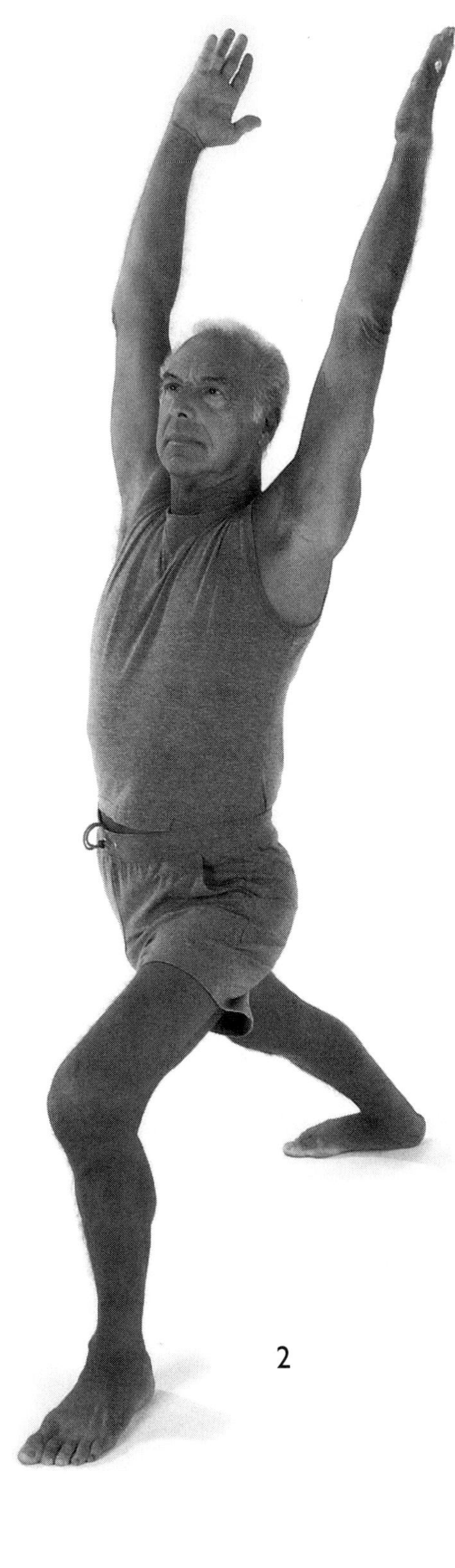

2

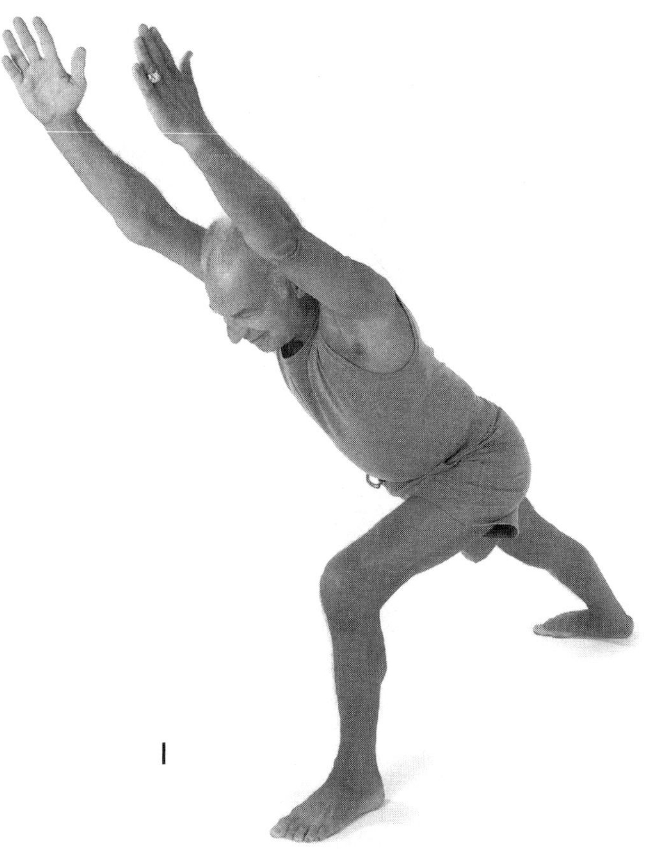

1

Virabhadrasana III

To perform Virabhadrasana III, continue through direction 7 in the last pose, but only hold it for 10 seconds.

10. Then draw the arms and torso forward at an angle of 45 degrees. **[1]**

11. Inhale and launch upward onto the left leg, bringing the right leg and buttock to horizontal and extending the arms fully horizontally as well. Lift, don't drag the right leg. **[2]**

At this point Mr. Iyengar suggests that one stretch "as if two persons were pulling you from either end."

12. Breathe calmly in the pose for 10-20 seconds, then descend in the opposite order and do the same steps with the opposite leg.

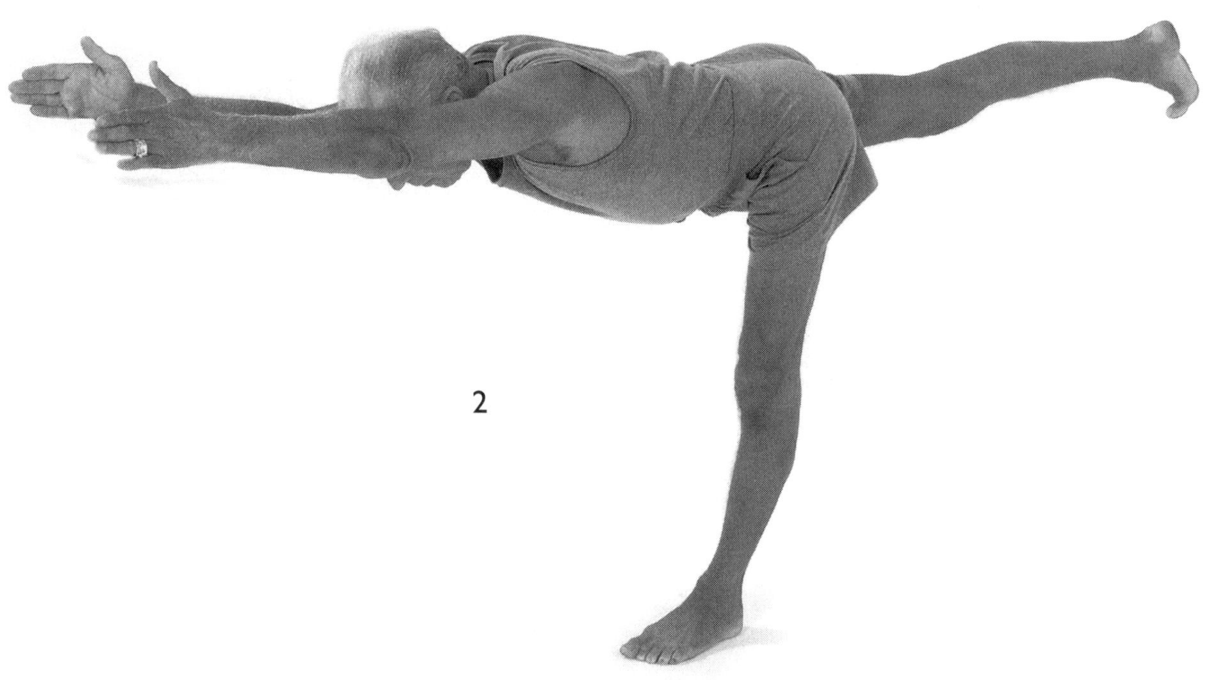

2

Entry-Level Virabhadrasana I

1. Sit well within a wheelchair or chair, balancing weight evenly between the ischial tuberosities.

2. Breathe in and straighten the spine from the coccyx to the top of the skull, making the torso as long as possible and looking straight ahead. Pull in the abdomen and open the chest.

3. Calmly take two breaths. Balance ischial weight-bearing once again.

4. Now inhale and bring the arms out to the sides and upward, elbows straight, until the palms and arms are parallel.

5. Breathe calmly for 10-20 seconds, then slowly return the arms to the armrests (if there are armrests).

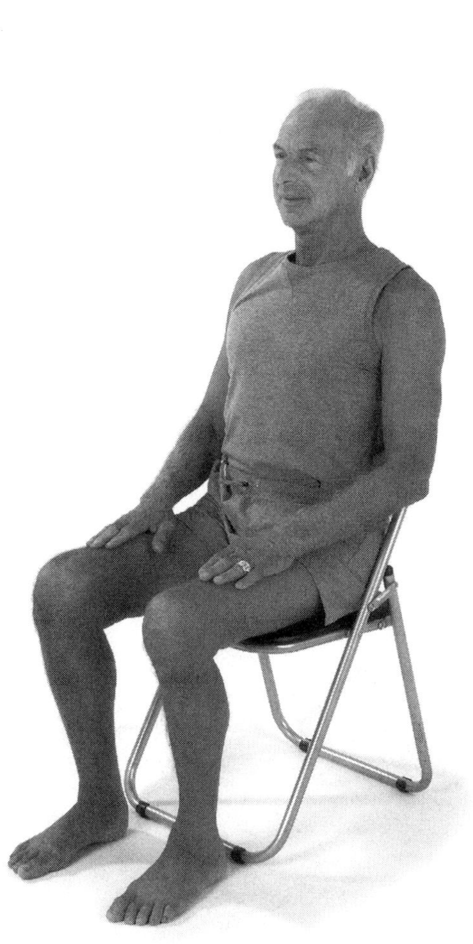

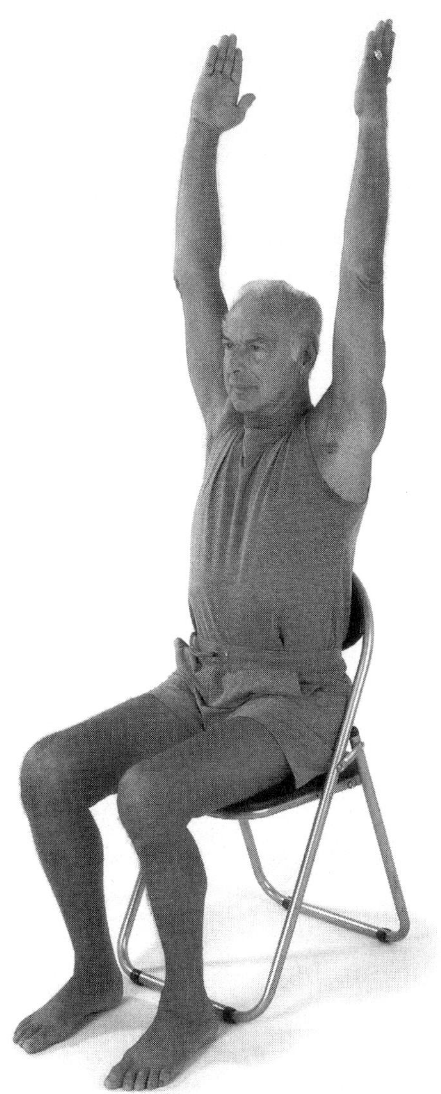

Intermediate Virabhadrasana I

1. Sit cross-wise on the seat of an armless chair with the left buttock and thigh.

2. Flex the left knee to 90 degrees, while placing the whole sole of the straightened right leg on the floor behind, on the other side of the chair, or straighten the right knee as much as possible (pictured).

3. Straighten the entire spine from its support at the left ischial tuberosity to the top of the head. Use your left hand for balance.

4. Breathe calmly for 1 minute.

5. Now bring the head back as far as possible, pulling in the abdomen and opening the chest. Straighten and slowly raise the right arm laterally, turning the palm until it is directly overhead and facing to the left.

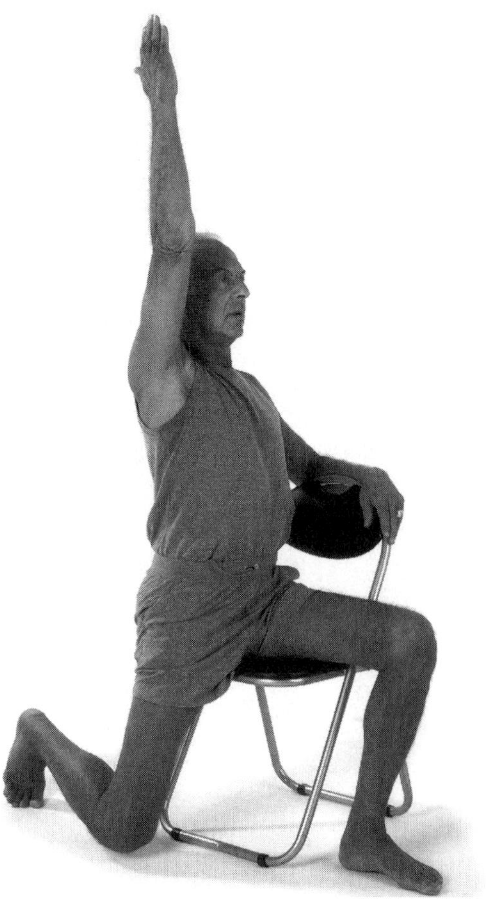

6. If balance permits, attempt to elevate the left arm in its mirror image, until the two palms are parallel. Keep the right little toe on the floor; put an equal and maximal amount of weight on each foot. Align the navel with the left thigh. In any case, stretch the torso and arms up as much as possible, without disturbing the breathing for 10-20 seconds.

Entry-Level Virabhadrasana III

1. Place a chair in front of your chair, as shown.

2. Follow entry level Virabhadrasana I through direction 4, the point at which the hands are parallel overhead and the head is extended backwards until the face is as close to horizontal as possible.

3. Calmly inhale, then exhale, bringing the entire torso forward as exhalation proceeds until the torso is as close to the thighs as possible, and the arms remaining fully extended. Move the arms and torso together, as though they were a single unjointed piece. Hold them as close as possible to a straight line.

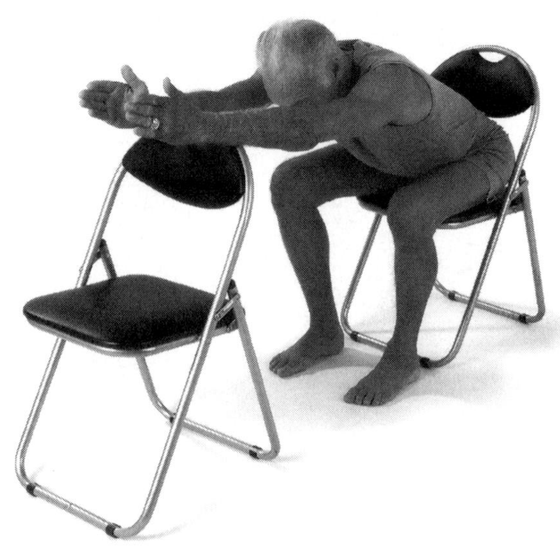

4. Breathe quietly for 10–20 seconds.

5. Then reverse these steps and return to Virabhadrasana I.

6. Then reverse the steps to leave this pose, and after a short rest, do the other side.

Intermediate Virabhadrasana III

1. Arrange two armless chairs facing in the same direction, approximately a body-length apart.

2. Stand midway between the two chairs in Tadasana facing the back of the foremost chair.

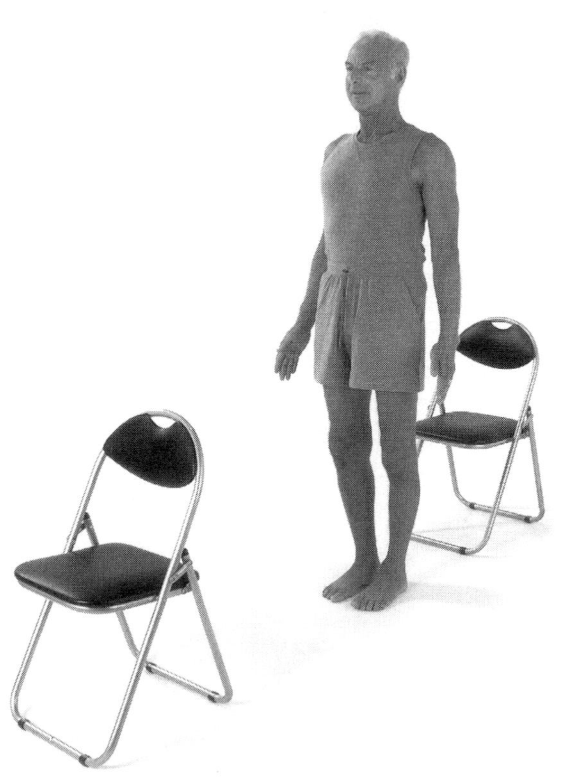

3. Take a calm breath.

4. Raise both arms laterally, palms parallel overhead, navel pointing toward the forward chair.

5. Step forward with the left leg and back with the right leg until your feet are 4-5 feet apart.

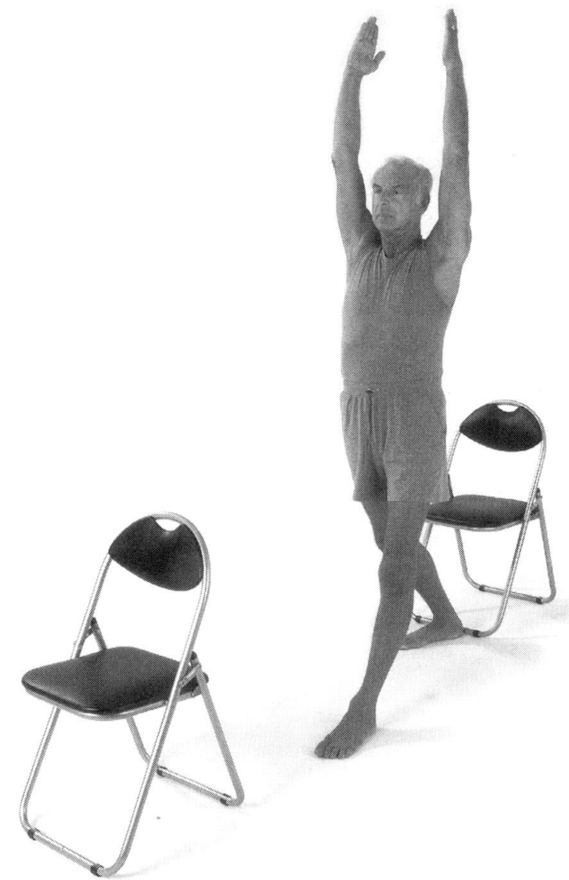

6. Maintaining a straightened spine from the sacrum to the base of the skull, turn the right foot 30 degrees toward the forward chair.

7. During a few calm breaths, balance weight evenly between feet, and within each foot.

8. Now bend the left knee to 90 degrees while exhaling.

9. Still holding the spine erect, inhale and bring the head back as far as possible, biceps close to the middle part of the jaw bone.

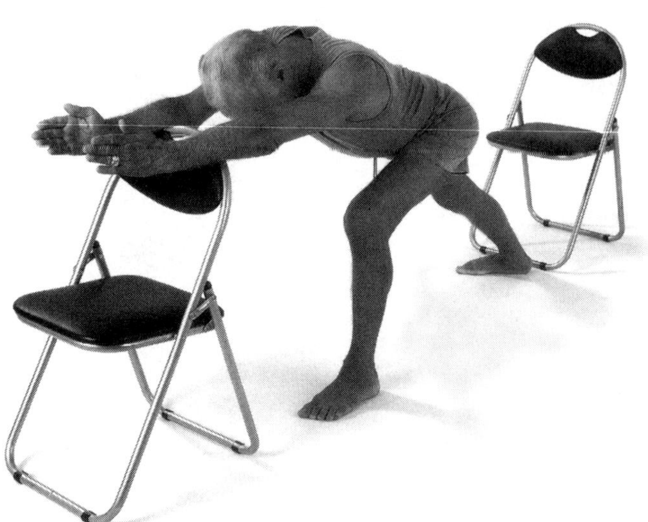

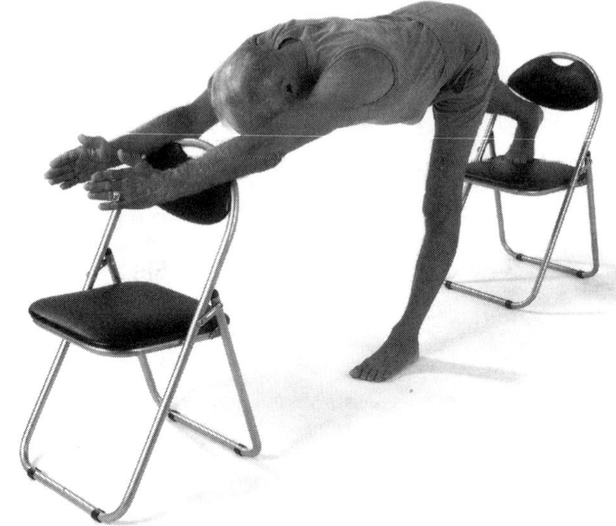

10. Retain the straightened right knee, keeping the little-toe side of the left foot on the floor and breathe calmly for 10-seconds. This is Virabhadrasana I.

11. Now tilt the arms and torso forward as a unit until they are inclined 45 degrees.

12. Bring your weight forward onto the left leg and straighten that leg, raising the right leg onto the chair placed behind, and resting the little finger sides of the arms on the back of the chair directly in front of you.

13. Stretch the back of the right leg and the entire back of the body including the wrists and thumbs maximally while breathing calmly for 10-20 seconds.

14. To deconstruct the pose, first place the right foot back on the floor, then return to Virabhadrasana I, then bringing the arms down.

15. Rest for 1-2 minutes before beginning again with the right leg forward.

11 Coordination and Balance

Yoga acclimates muscle groups to working together. Coordination and balance have a lot in common. Good balance in motion requires coordination. Coordination relates one muscle group to another, balance relates the entire person to his or her environment. The person doing one of Mr. Iyengar's standing poses gets used to balancing hamstrings with quadriceps; iliopsoas and adductors with glutei; maximally stretching the latissimus dorsi on one side and simultaneously contracting its contralateral partner. This is coordination.

At the same time he or she is equilibrating anterior and posterior deltoid groups, and all while maintaining forward-backward and left-right balance. This is what keeps us from falling. The stretching activates the complex check-system of the stretch reflex, the agonist-antagonist balance activates that reflex. Both of these serve, at the spinal cord level, to reduce spasticity. Both of these are integrated into the titration of one group's strength with all others', (coordination) and all groups' efforts against gravity and other forms of acceleration (balance).

Increasing range of motion is critical to mobility; reducing spasticity is a *sine qua non* for voluntary and intentional action. Holding the same pose for any length of time takes (and therefore builds) a safe and estimable degree of strength and endurance as well.

But unless these groups of muscles can work together in mutually supportive and jointly sensitive ways, each adjusting to the others, and then adjusting to the others' response to their adjustment, a recursive and continuous flow that still manages to focus on the goal of the action—unless they can do that—there is virtually no point in all our work—no point in muscle contractions at all!

It seems logical to start with our capacity to adjust muscles to each other's efforts, coordination. After that we'll examine how they attain one common goal: balance.

Coordination

These asana combine several different extreme positions and balance skills. Because of this they also build strength, endurance and grace in movement. It has been said that we sculpt our movements out of larger, often instinctual patterns by inhibiting (and thereby eliminating) unwanted movements or parts of the pattern. If so, then these poses may be seen as the sculptor's tools, helping one to leave parts of movements out of the picture, and only doing exactly what one intends.

Coordination is largely a matter of balancing the mixed intensity of contraction of some muscles with the varying degrees of relaxation of other muscles. As such it is the basis of good balance, ergonomic action and smooth movement, and the antithesis of spasticity. In particular acts, such as throwing or jumping, it can be practiced and learned. Yoga instills the general principles of coordination in the course of practicing some nearly universal examples of the differential contraction and relaxation of key muscle groups.

Bhujapidasana

Shoulder Pressure Pose

1. Sit on the floor. **[1]**

2 Starting with the legs two feet apart, one foot on the floor, the other leg kneeling, slide arms behind the bent knees, palms on the floor, fingers facing forward. The palms are behind and further apart than the feet. **[2]**

3. Take a few slow, even breaths.

4. Bring your weight backward onto the arms, resting the backs of the thighs on the arms behind the shoulders. **[3]**

5. Raise your thighs and pelvis by straightening the elbows somewhat.

6. Breathe calmly for 10-20 seconds, then transfer enough weight onto the shoulders that first the heels, then the toes can be raised off the floor.

7. Straighten the arms as much as possible, interlock the ankles, straighten the spine and lift the head. **[4]**

8. Relax the head and neck, and breathe evenly for 10-20 seconds.

9. Then release the legs one at a time, reverse the ankles for another 10 second.

10. Reverse the movement sequence to return to sitting on the floor.

1

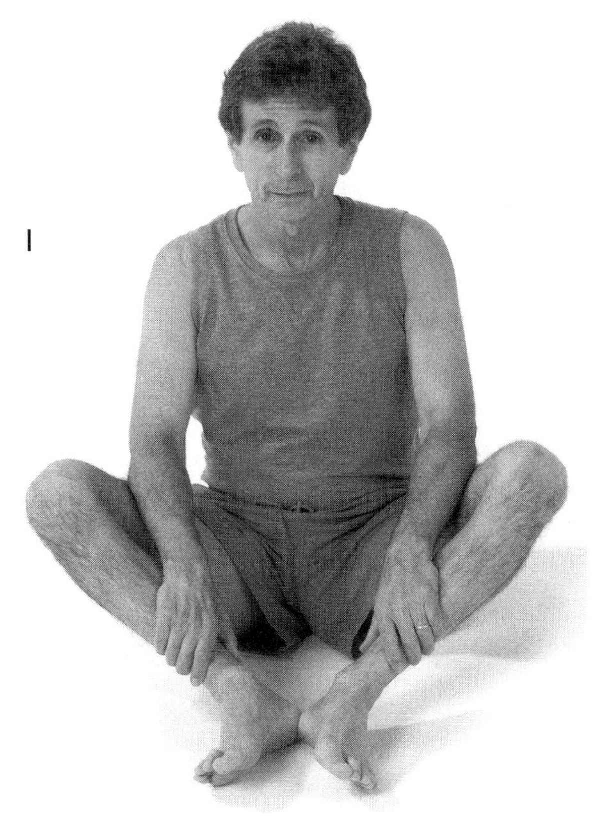

2

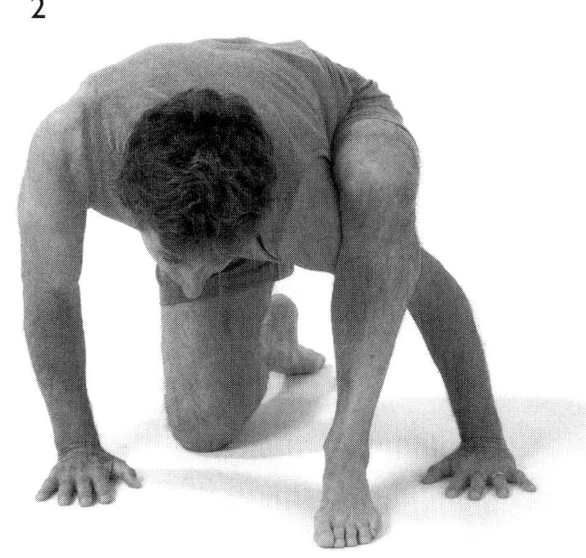

3

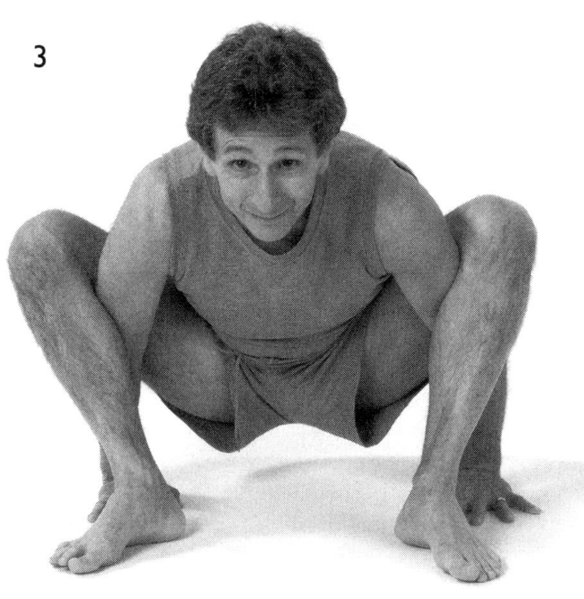

4

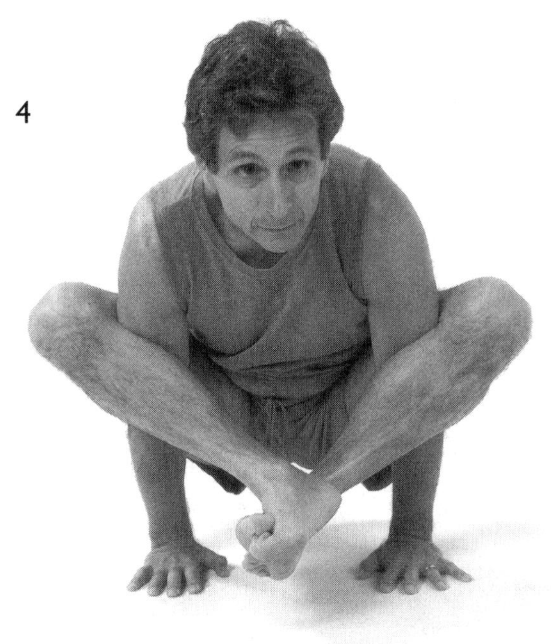

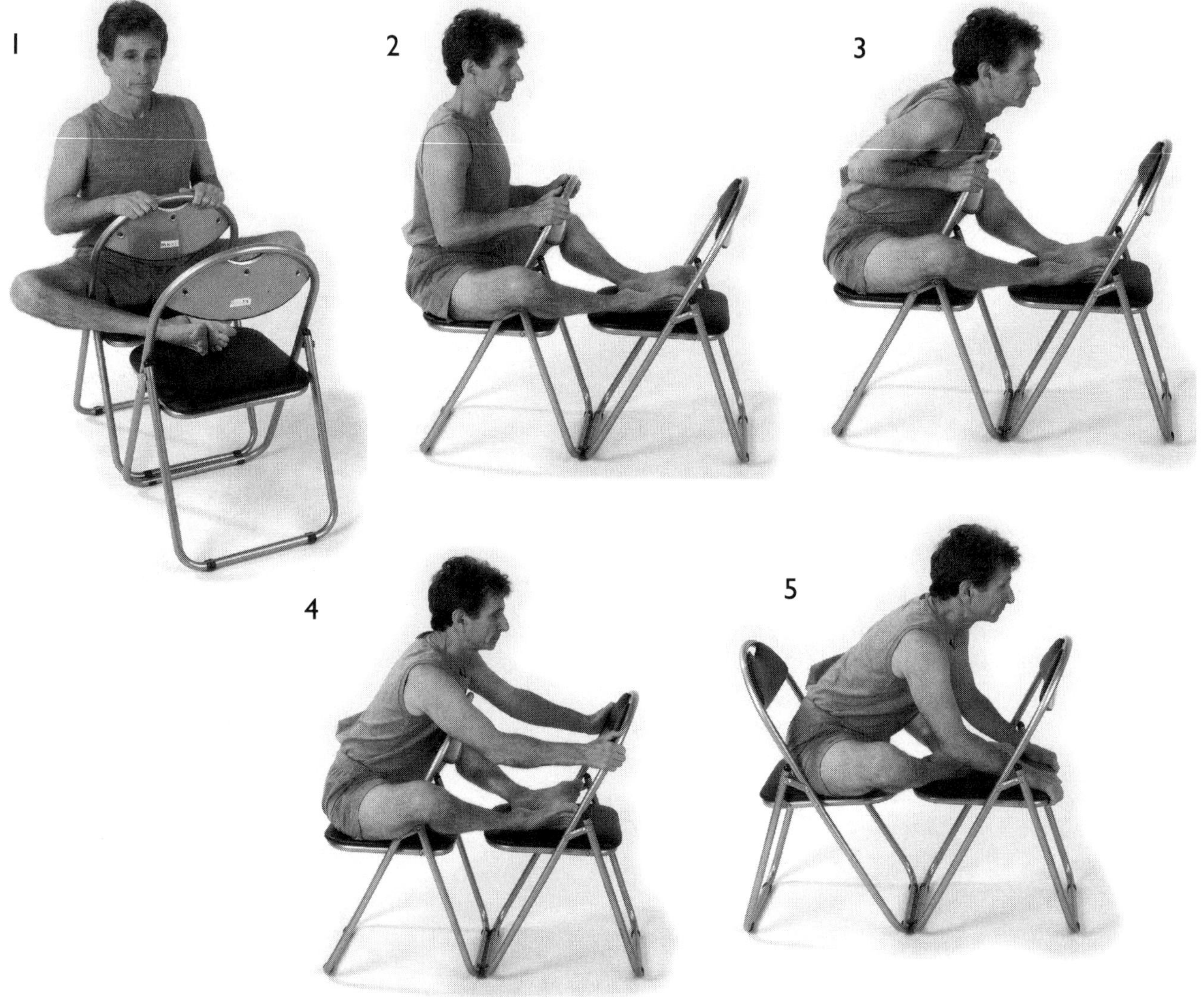

Entry-Level Bhujapidasana

1. Line up two card chairs front to back.

2. Straddling the foremost chair, move close to the chair directly behind it. [1]

3. Bring the right heel onto the seat of the hindmost chair, then the left heel. Rest the sides of the feet, in contact with each other, on the chair seat. [2]

4. Smoothly inhale and grasp the seat back of the foremost chair.

5. With exhalation pull the chest toward the chair back, arms horizontal. [3]

6. When this pose is no longer challenging, hold the back of the hindmost chair. [4]

7. To progress further yet, put both hands on the seat beside and behind the thighs, and lift the body upward.

8. Turn the chairs so that they face each other, pulling forward on the back of the opposite chair's seat to flex the torso. [5]

9. When this is no longer a challenge, go to the intermediate pose.

Intermediate-Level Bhujapidasana

1. Use two blocks approximately 4 inches high. **[1]**

2. Bring the knees out and the feet forward and toward each other.

3. Place the arms at the inside of the knees, fingers facing forward, elbows bent 30 degrees. **[2]**

4. If the blocks are too low, it will prompt falling forward. If they are too high, the next part will be impossible. Put more and more weight on the palms, lifting first one foot and then the other. **[3]**

5. If it is impossible to lift both feet, place only the fingertips on the blocks and try again. If this does not accomplish the objective, then raise feet one at a time, breathing calmly for 10 seconds with each foot. **[4]**

6. Otherwise do this once with both feet aloft for 10-20 seconds, interlocking ankles. **[5]**

1

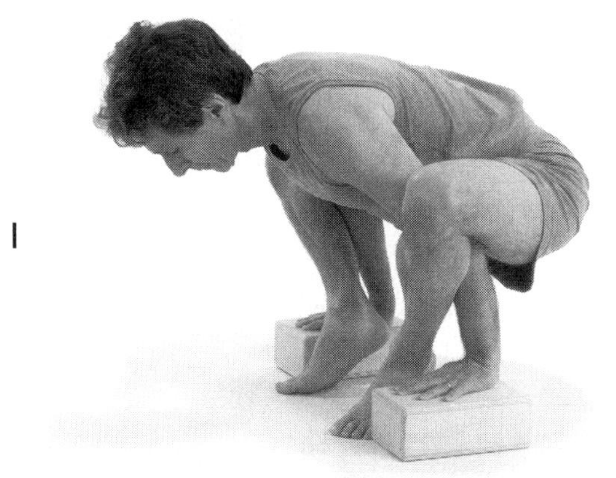

2

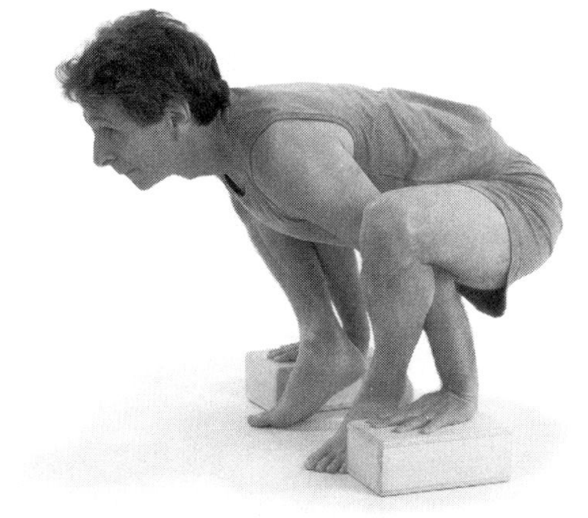

3

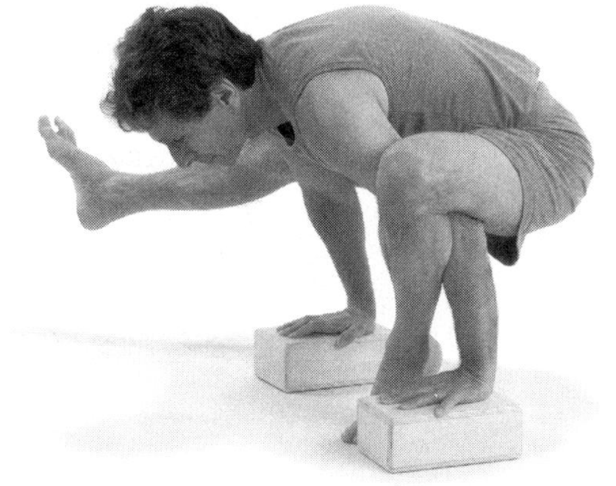

4

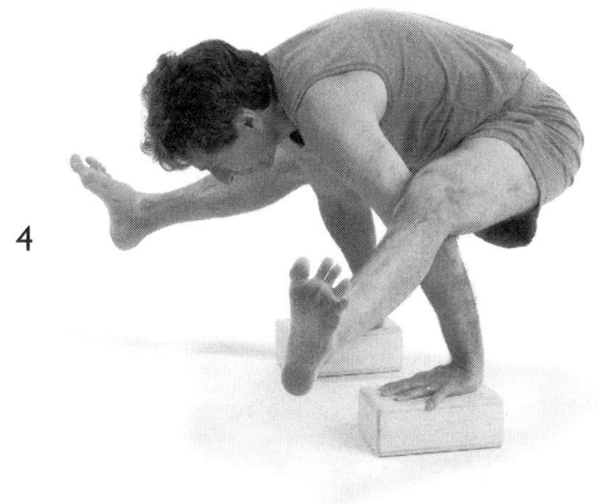

5

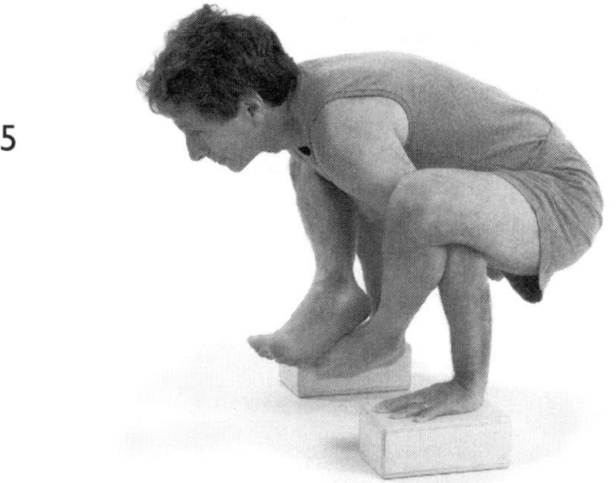

SARVANGASANA/ HALASANA

Shoulder Stand/The Plow

1. Use blankets as pictured.

2. After 1 minute slowly breathing in Savasana, place the palms at the kidneys and bend both knees as far as possible toward the chest.

3. Pressing forward with both hands, raise the torso and both legs to vertical, bending the elbows and supporting the trunk with the hands on the kidney region of the back.

4. Only the head, the neck and the apex of the shoulders should be in contact with the floor. Fix the eyes on the toes and breath quietly for 30 seconds to 1 minute.

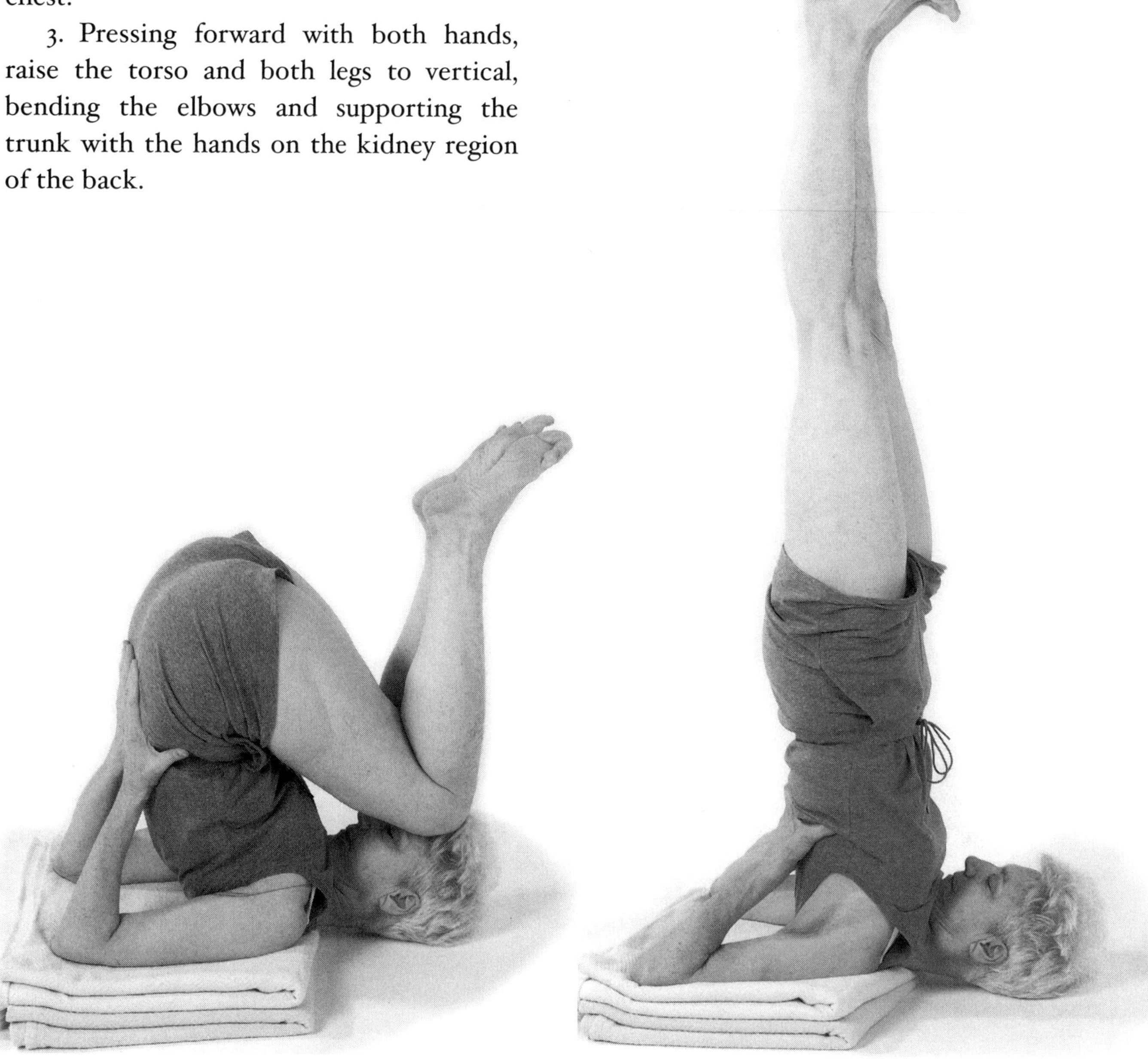

Halasana

Begin with Sarvangasana, through direction 3 on the previous page.

4. Extend your arms behind you, fingers interdigitated. Exhale and bring the straight legs forward over your head and down to the floor, making an acute angle with the torso.

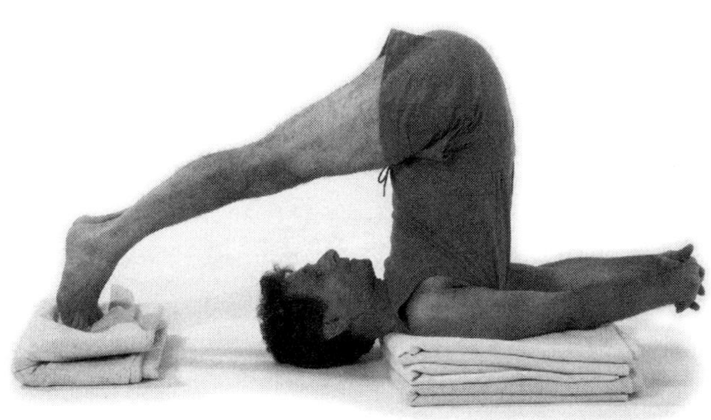

5. Raise up the ischial bones, arching the lumbar and thoracic spine slightly.

6. Open the chest and breathe calmly for 10-20 seconds.

Entry-Level Sarvangasana

1. Lie on your back beneath a card chair.

2. Breathe softly for 30 seconds.

3. Bend both knees. One by one lift the calves onto the card chair.

4. You have the option to raise the arms up with inhalation and lay them down in parallel above the head, palms up.

6. Exhale and breathe quietly for 1-2 minutes.

For individuals significantly challenged by this posture, Vitari Karani is a suitable lead-in. See the inclined pose in Chapter 7.

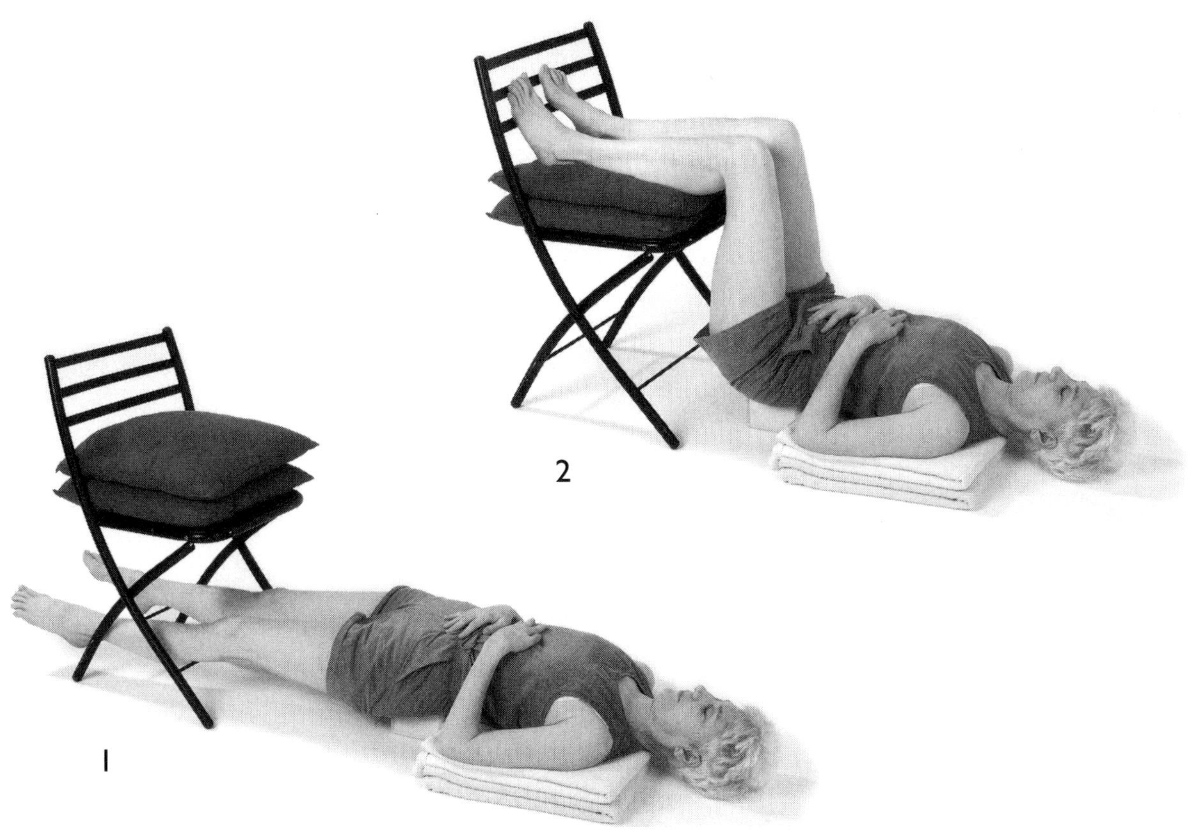

Intermediate Sarvangasana

1. Assume Savasana diagonally beside a card chair.

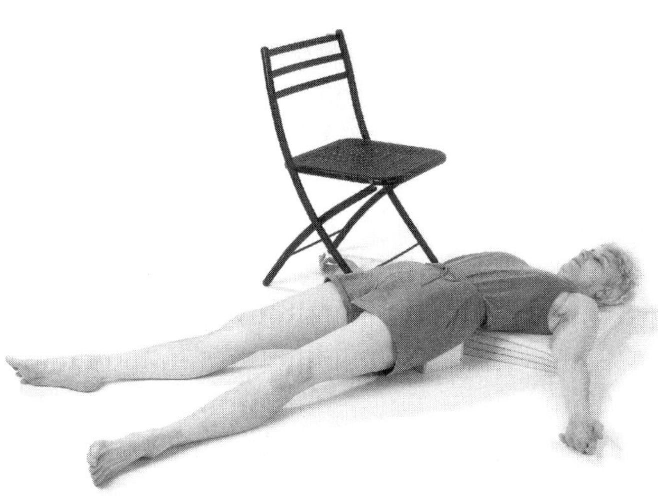

2. Press palms down, swing the torso and "climb up" the seat of the chair with both legs while gripping the back legs of the chair from underneath.

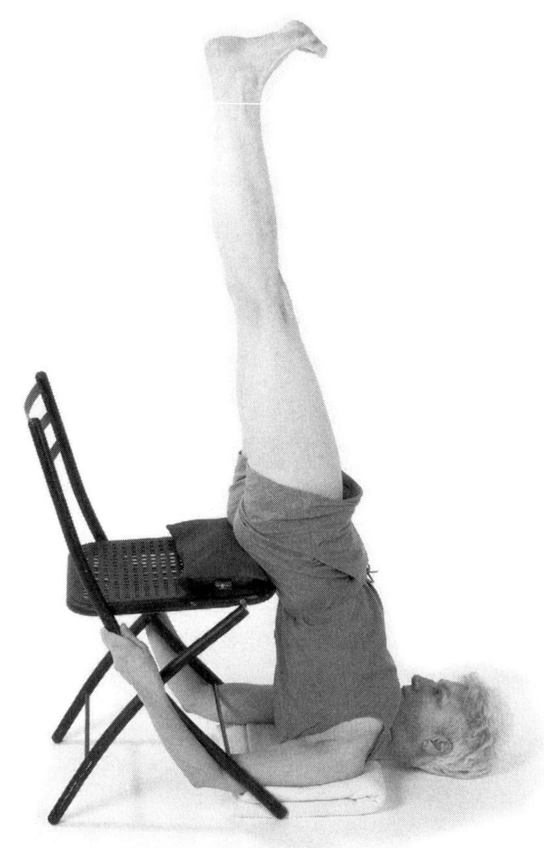

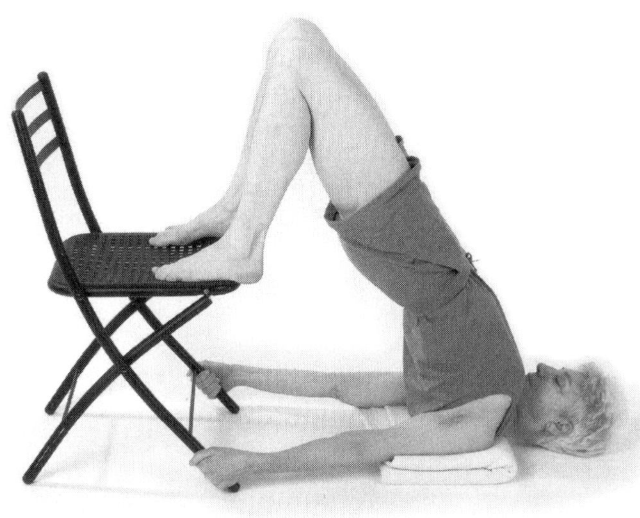

3. Straighten the legs and torso vertically. Pull the chair toward you and use the edge of the seat of the card chair to hold the sacrum in its forward position.

4. Transfer your weight carefully onto the head and neck and apex of the shoulders.

5. Lift the heels and pelvis upward, rest the eyes on the toes, the only part of the feet that should be visible, and breathe quietly for 10-20 seconds.

Entry-Level Halasana

Another surprisingly simple way to perform the pose uses a strap.See the series of photographs on the facing page, which include doing this pose with a partner.

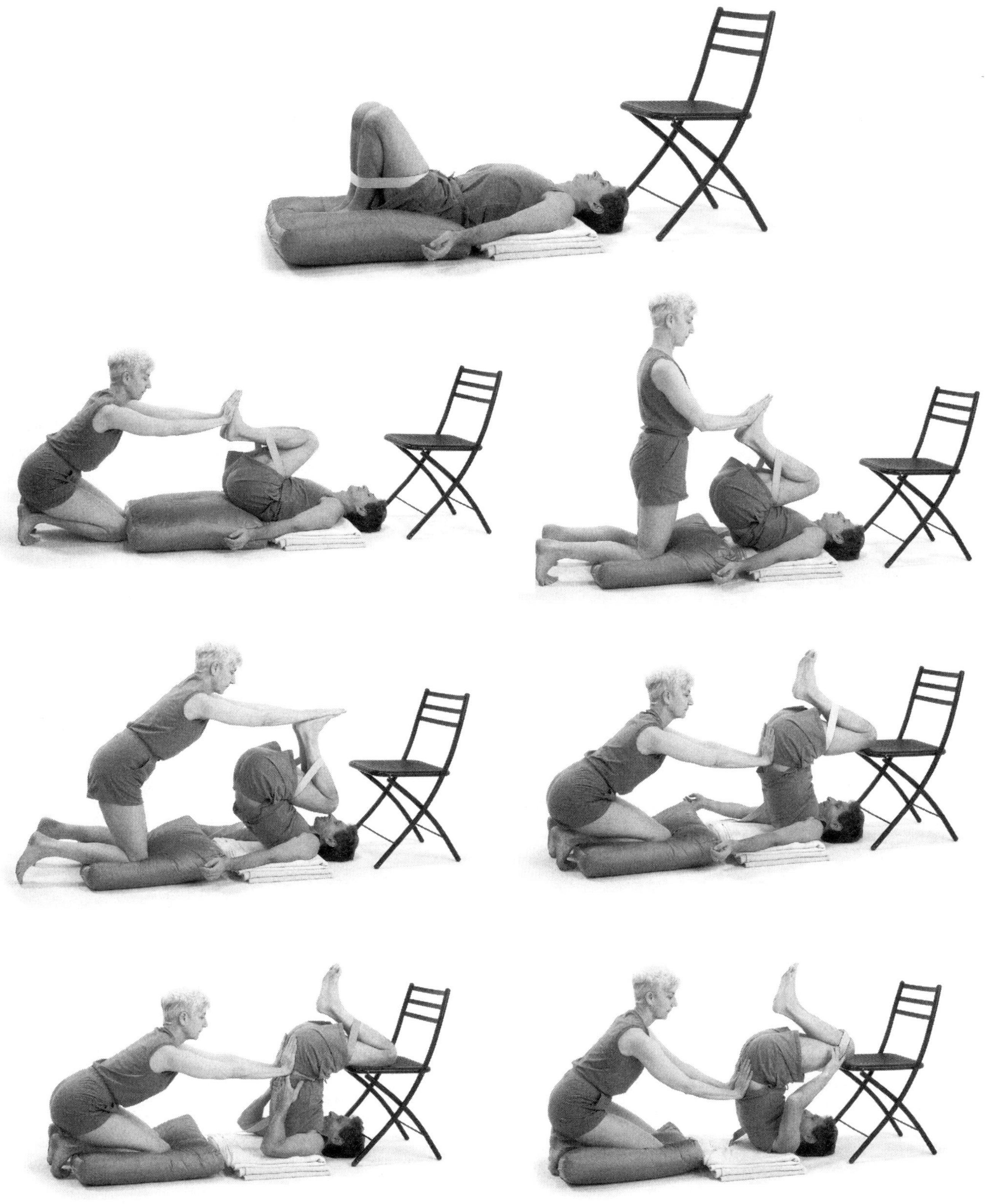

Intermediate-Level Halasana

1. Lie down in savasana, head toward a card chair.
2. Breathe quietly for 30 seconds.
3. Turn the palms down.
4. Bending the knees and simultaneously pressing downward on the floor with your forearms, bring the thighs over your head as the lumbar spine comes off the floor. You may need a helper.

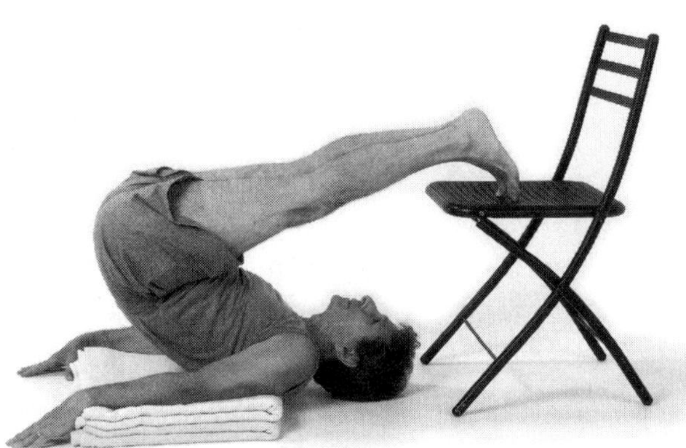

5. Rest the feet or shins on the seat of the chair. A helper, blankets and/or cushions may be needed to sustain the pose.
6. Straighten the knees to tolerance.
7. Breathe evenly for 1-2 minutes, attempting to make the legs straighter and to bring the torso up further in a mild but sustained and coordinated effort.

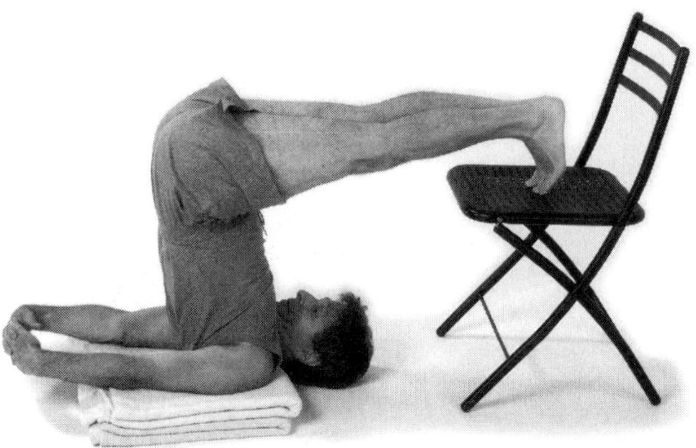

SVANASANA

Dog Poses

URDHVA MUKHA SVANASANA

Upward-Facing Dog

1. Lie in prone position with toes pointed and feet one foot apart. **[1]**
2. Elbows bent, palms on the floor at shoulder-level, with fingers pointing toward the head, inhale, raising up first the head, the throat, **[2]** then the chest, abdomen, pelvis and legs, bringing the head and chest as far back as possible.
3. Only the palms and dorsal feet are on the floor, toes still pointed back. **[3]** The legs are as straight as possible; the entire body including the buttocks and the lumbar, thoracic and cervical spine arch backward as far as possible. **[4]**
4. Breathe deeply and slowly for 10-20 seconds.

5. Now return to prone position, hands feet and head as they were at the start of Urdhva Mukha Svanasana in step 1.
6. Take two breaths.
7. Pressing forward on the floor with both hands and straightening the elbows and wrists and forward raise the hips and chest ever farther from the floor.

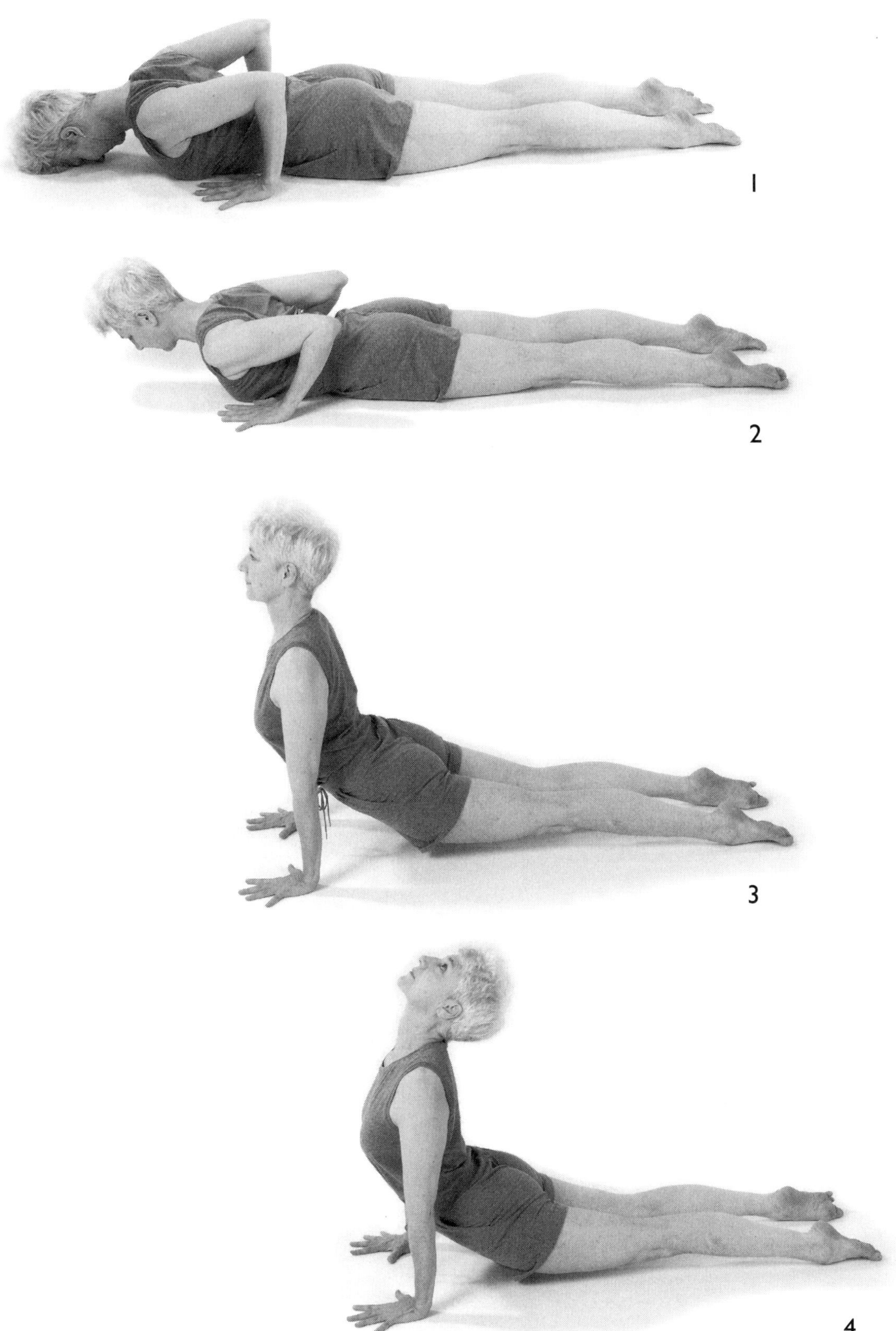

1

2

3

4

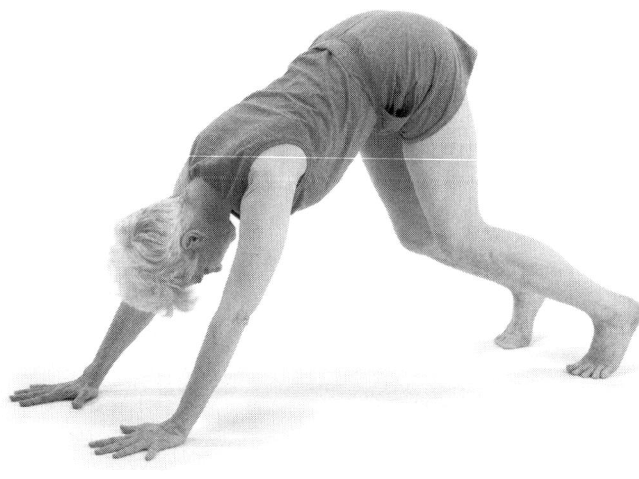

8. Straighten the backs of the legs, toes still parallel, but now pointed in the same direction as the fingers, heels on the floor, knees and thoracic spine maximally extended, shoulders retracted, the top of the head toward or near the floor.

9. Breathe deeply, calmly, and slowly for 1 minute.

10. First lift the head, then carefully lower your head and chest and abdomen to return to the prone position on the floor.

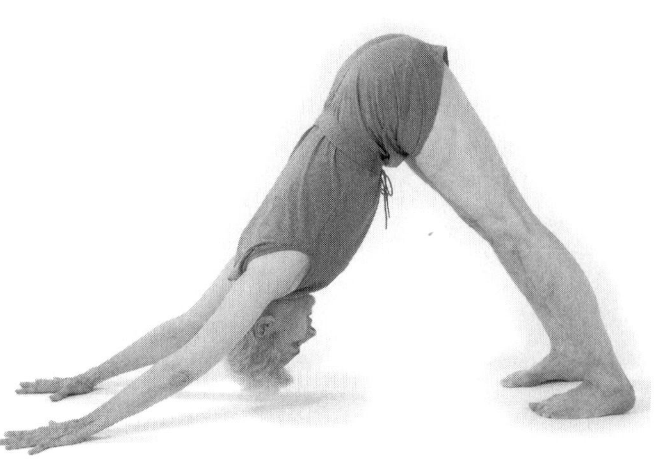

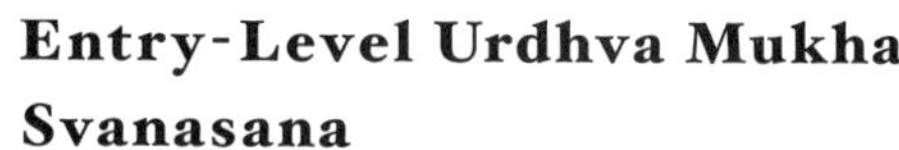

Entry-Level Urdhva Mukha Svanasana

1. Lie in prone position with toes pointed and feet one foot apart.

2. Flex the left arm, palm down, and press the floor, rolling longitudinally into the supine position.

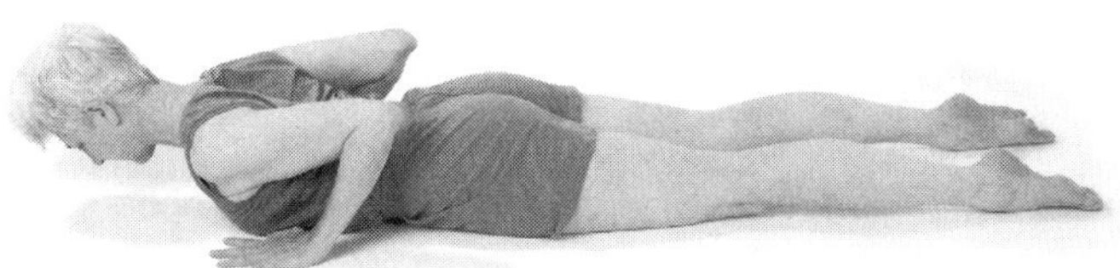

3. Press downward with the palms, pulling the shoulder blades back, together and toward the pelvis.

4. Relax the abdominal muscles, but straighten the knees and tighten the buttocks as much as possible.

5. Breathe quietly, being careful to balance the pressure on the two hands and the dorsal parts of both feet.

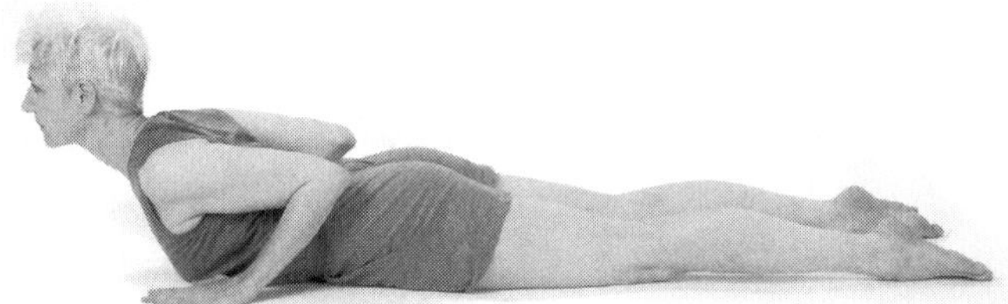

Reverse Downward-Facing Dog

1. Carefully return to the relaxed prone position.

2. Flex the left arm, palm down, and press the floor, rolling longitudinally into the supine position.

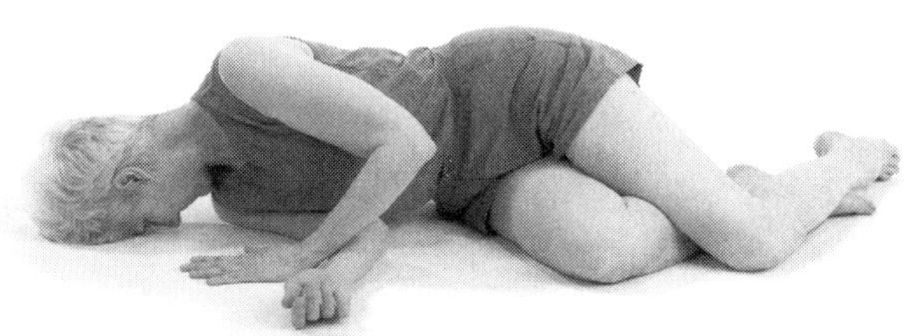

3. Now raise the arms overhead, so that both are parallel, palms upward, and stretch maximally from the waist to the fingertips.

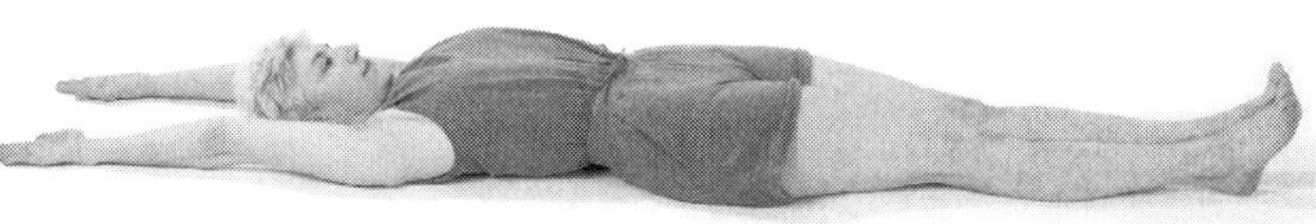

4. Breathe in a controlled, even manner for 1 minute.

5. Now flex both knees, feet still on the floor, and lift one and then the other, or both of them, as possible, straightening the leg(s) and bringing the toes down (stretching the Achilles tendons) in parallel at maximal elevation of the heels.

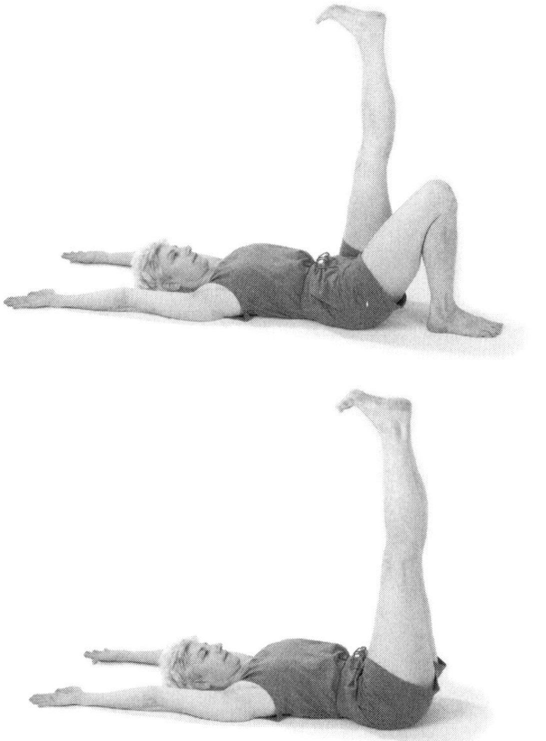

6. Breathe quietly for 10-20 seconds.

7. Then flex the knees, return the feet, then the backs of the legs to the floor, relax the shoulders and remain supine for another minute resting.

8. Finally bend the left knee, pressing the foot on the floor to roll longitudinally to the right, back to prone position.

Intermediate-Level Urdhva Mukha and Adho Mukha Svanasana

1. Lie in prone position with toes pointed and feet one foot apart.

2. Elbows bent, palms on the floor at waist-level, with fingers pointing toward the head, inhale slowly and evenly, raising up first the head, then the neck, then the throat, then the chest.

3. Retain the navel's contact with the floor at first as you arch the neck and chest back as far as possible.

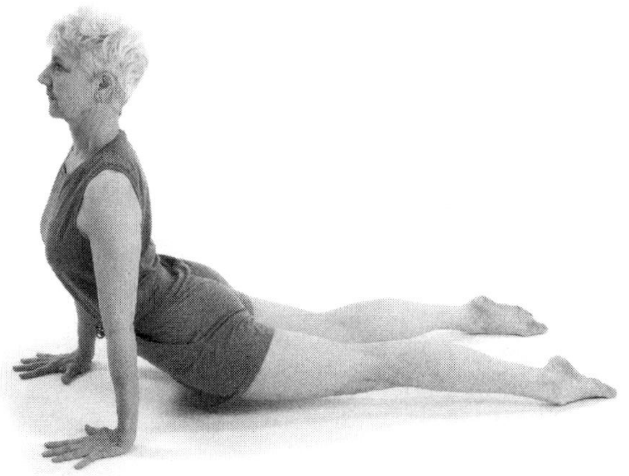

4. Press the palms downward. Pull the shoulder blades back and raise your torso.

5. Relax the abdominal muscles, but straighten the knees and tighten the buttocks as much as possible.

6. Breathe quietly, carefully balance the pressure of the breath on the abdomen, and weight on the two hands and the dorsal parts of both feet.

7. Return to prone position by gently lowering the chest, throat, neck and head. Relax the buttocks and leg muscles.

THE WALL DOG

A Standing Intermediate for Both Dog Poses

1. Take one quiet breath, then rise. Stand two feet from a wall or door, facing it. Feet should be parallel and 8-18 inches apart.

2. Place your palms on the wall above your head, fingers pointing upward, making a 45 degree angle between the wall and the wrists. **[1]**

3. Balance your weight evenly on the two feet, and maintain that balance while you draw the hips and buttocks backwards, and lean forward, approaching the wall with your armpits, lessening the angle between the wrists and the wall to a minimum. **[2]**

4. Equalize pressure on the two hands. Bring the shoulder blades back, together, and down, stretching the entire front of the chest and abdomen from the throat to the pubic bone. Emphasize arching the thoracic spine, not the lumbar spine, though both are concave in this position.

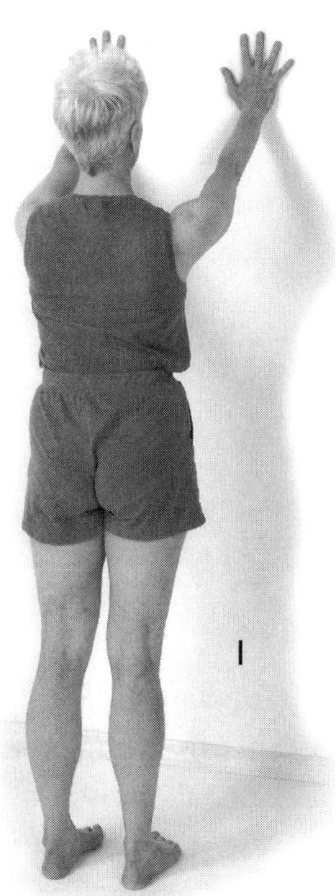
1

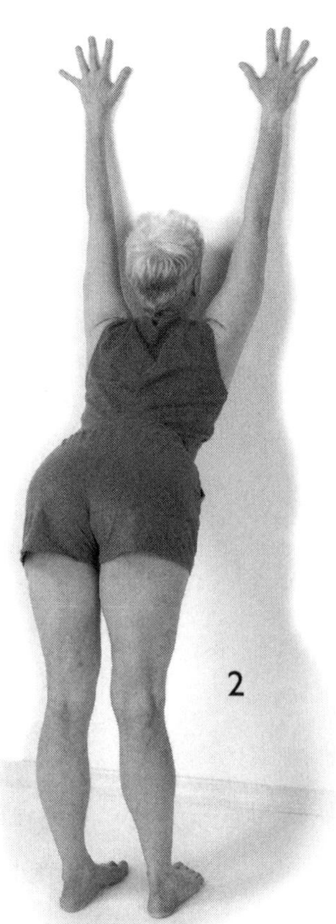
2

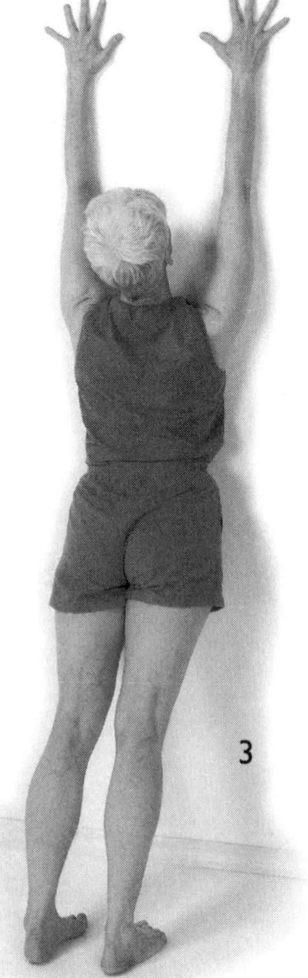
3

5. Breathe calmly and symmetrically for up to 1 minute.

6. Then smoothly reduce the pressure on your hands and return the shoulder blades to their resting position. Bring the head and chest back to vertical and pull the hips and buttocks toward the Tadasana position. **[3]**

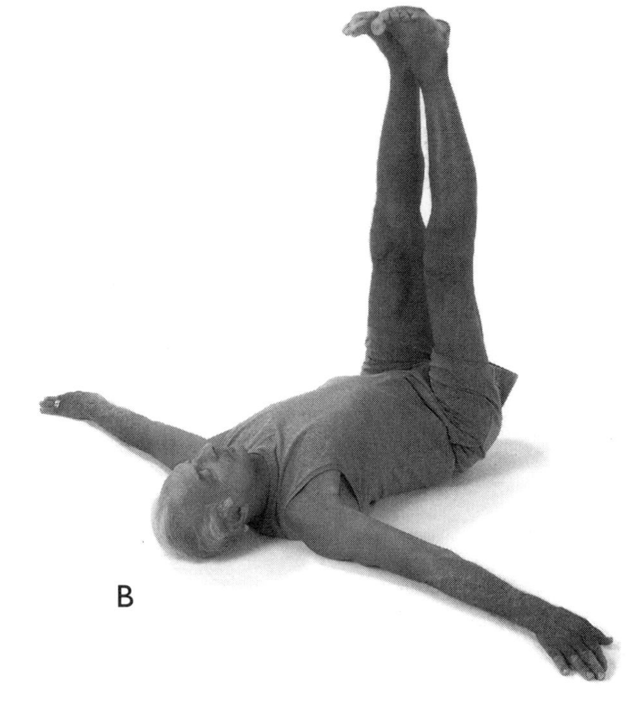

B

JATHARA PARIVARTANASANA

Abdominal Turning Pose

1. Lying in Savasana, abduct the arms 90 degrees, palms upward. **[A]**

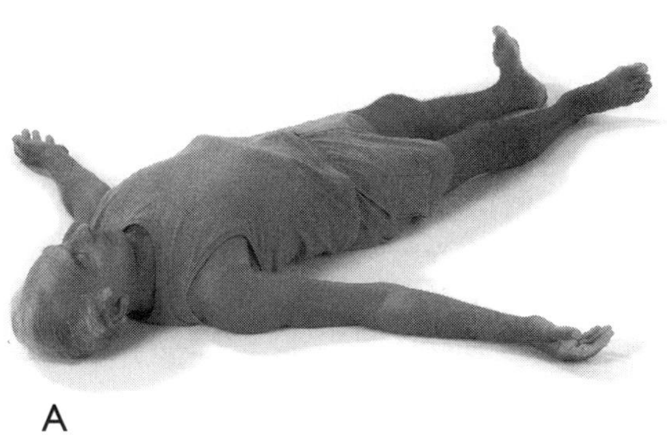

A

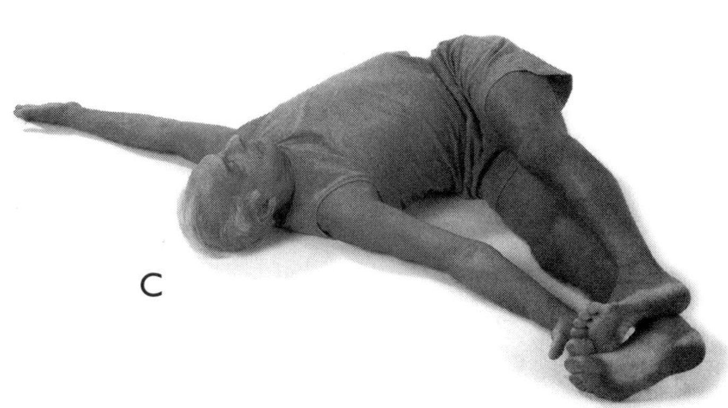

C

2. With toes pointed, knees straight and ankles in contact, raise both legs together to vertical. In lower back pain, both knees can be bent in raising, then the knees straightened when the thighs are vertical.

3. Make your soles horizontal. **[B]**

4. Take a calm breath and turn palms upward.

5. First move your hips slightly to the left as you inhale.

6. With exhalation lower both legs to the right, so that they are in contact both with each other and the floor, parallel to the right arm. Press downward with the right hand to retain contact of the left shoulder with the floor also. Keep as much of the thoracic and upper lumbar spine as possible in contact with the floor. **[C]**

7. Breathe calmly for up to 1 minute.

8. Then, pressing with the right hand and forearm, raise the legs back to vertical.

9. Take a breath.

10. With exhalation, perform the same lowering on the left, keeping floor contact for the right shoulder and thoracic spine with left hand pressure.

11. After the legs are on the floor and parallel to the left hand, breathe calmly and symmetrically for 1 minute.

12. Then raise the legs to vertical again.

13. Bend your knees and lower your legs to the floor.

14. Return your arms to your sides, return to Savasana.

Entry-Level Jathara Parivartanasana

1. Lying in Savasana, abduct the arms 90 degrees, palms upward.

2. With toes pointed, knees bent and ankles in contact, raise both legs together to vertical. Take a calm breath.

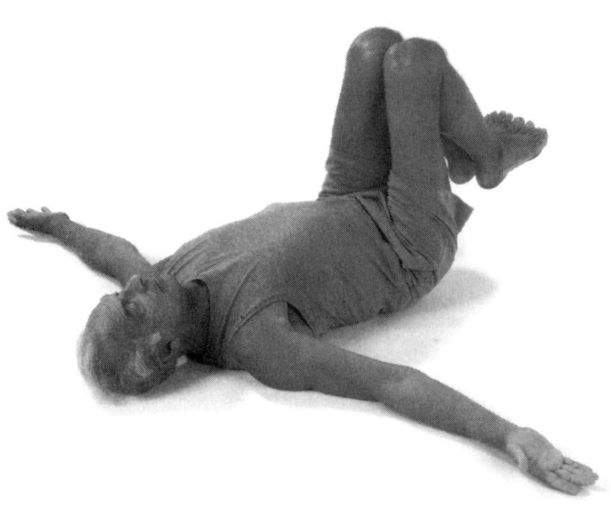

3. Tilt your pelvis somewhat to the left.

4. Lower both legs to the right as you exhale. The legs should be in contact both with each other and the floor, with cushions that have been properly placed, in a position as close to parallel to the right arm as possible.

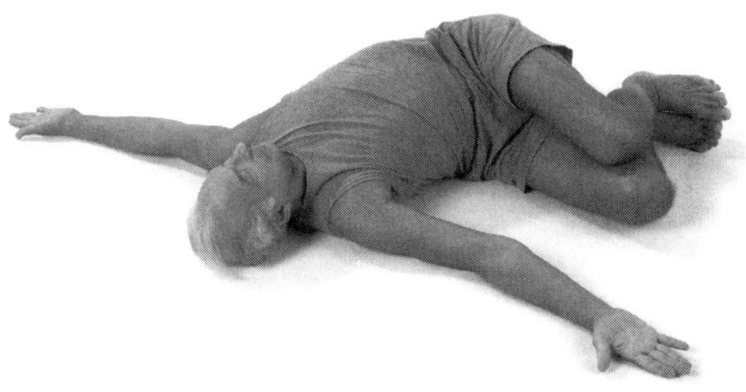

5. Press downward with the right hand to press the left shoulder down in contact with the floor, or as close to it as possible. Keep as much of the thoracic and lumbar spine as possible in contact with the floor.

6. Breathe calmly for 10-20 seconds.

7. Then, pressing with the right hand and forearm, raise the bent legs back to vertical.

8. Take a breath.

9. After tilting the hips somewhat to the right, exhale as you lower the legs to the left, keeping floor contact for the right shoulder and thoracic and lumbar spine with left hand pressure.

10. After the legs are on the floor (or cushions) and parallel to the left hand, breathe calmly and symmetrically for 10-20 seconds.

11. Then raise the bent legs to vertical again, and slowly lower them. When the soles are resting on the floor, slide the legs back until your knees are straight.

12. Return the arms to the sides.

13. Breathe calmly in Savasana for 20-30 seconds.

Intermediate Jathara Parivartanasana

1. Lying in Savasana, abduct the arms 90 degrees, palms upward.

2. With toes pointed, knees bent and ankles in contact, raise both legs together to vertical.

3. Take a calm breath.

4. Then tilt the hips somewhat to the left.

5. With exhalation lower both legs to the right, so that they are in contact both with each other and the floor, thighs parallel to the right arm. See picture on page 228.

6. Extend or flex the knees according to the strength and flexibility of the practitioner's abdominal musculature.

Note: As practice continues over weeks and months, gradually straighten the knees, beginning with the sideward lowering phase, then in raising them from the side, and, if there is no back pain, later extend the knees in raising and lowering the legs from Savasana at the beginning of the pose, and back to it at the end.

7. Press downward with the right hand to keep the left shoulder in contact with the floor also. Keep as much of the thoracic spine as possible in contact with the floor.

8. Breathe calmly for 1 minute.

9. Then, pressing with the right hand and forearm, raise the bent legs back to vertical. Take a breath.

10. After "cocking" the hips somewhat to the right, perform the same lowering on the left as you exhale, keeping floor contact for the right shoulder and thoracic spine with left hand pressure.

11. As with the right side, gradually extend the knees as practice continues and strength allows.

12. After the legs are on the floor and parallel to the left hand, breathe calmly and symmetrically for 1 minute.

13. Raise the bent legs to vertical again.

14. Slowly lower them to the supine position.

15. When the soles are resting on the floor, slide the feet back until the knees are straight, return the arms to the sides, and remain there.

16. Breathe calmly in Savasana for 20-30 seconds.

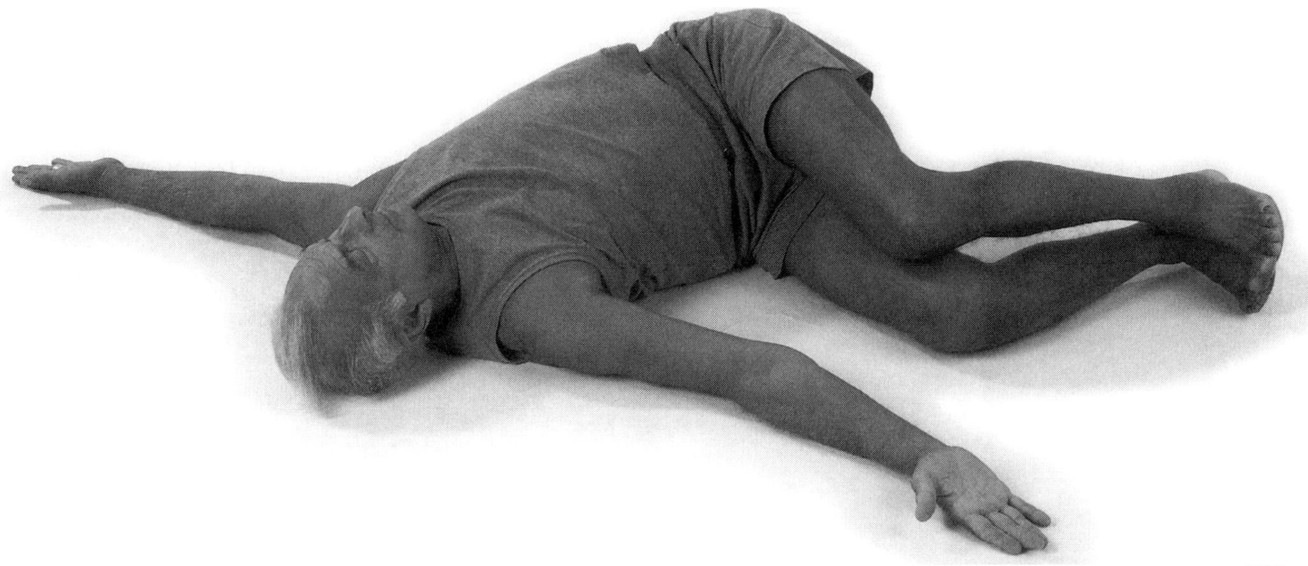

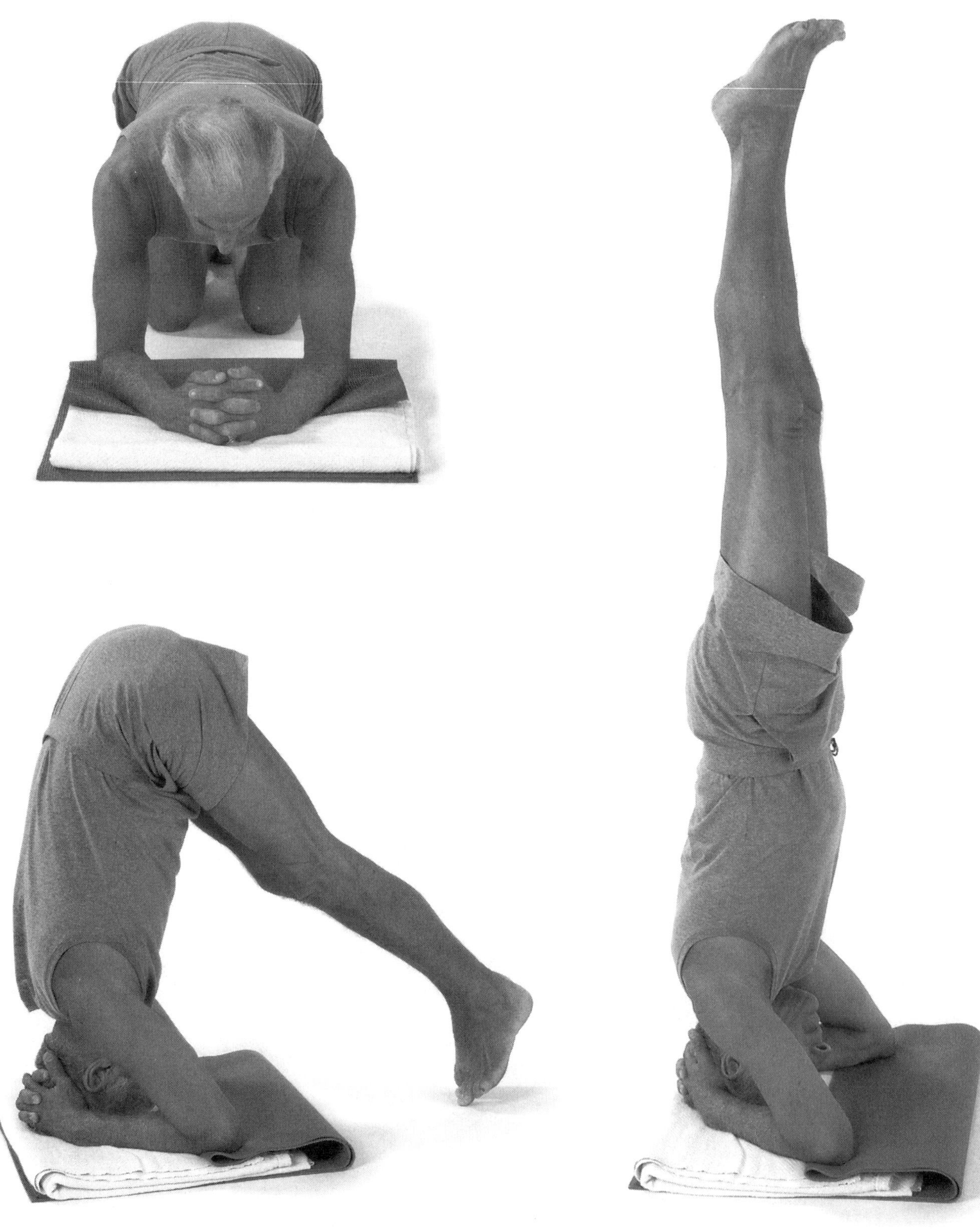

Sirsasana Headstand

1. Kneel near a folded blanket.

2. Clasp the hands, interlocking the fingers, making an equilateral triangle with the clasped hands and two elbows as vertices. Keep the heels of the hands close together and wrists vertical throughout the pose.

3. Place the very top of the head in the center of the triangle formed by the forearms, straighten the knees, and walk in until your weight is predominantly on the head and forearms.

4. Breathe calmly for 20 seconds, and on inhalation, raise the straight legs together to vertical. Retract and raise the shoulders, but otherwise, all the weight should be supported by the top of the skull. Point the toes, narrow the body, pulling in the stomach, to avoid arching the back. Open the chest and extend the hips.

5. Resist the fear of falling backward. The fear promotes a tendency to keep the hips flexed and bear too much weight at the elbows. If in fact one does fall backward, simply loosen the hand grip and curl your back to roll innocuously into a supine position. Assistance of another person is advised at first.

6. When beginning, remain in the pose for 10-20 seconds and increase gradually to 5-6 minutes over the next year. Periodic checks with a teacher are strongly advised: A person may go seriously awry without them.

7. Exit the pose by lowering the still-extended legs from the hips until the toes reach the floor. Then bend the knees to the floor. Undo the hands and place the palms on the floor beside the ears, as far apart as the shoulders. Raise your head.

8. Remain for 10-20 seconds before arising.

Entry-Level Sirsasana

1. Kneel on a low, stable plinth, chair or sofa, knees at the edge with a firm but soft and nonslipping surface on the floor below. **[1]**

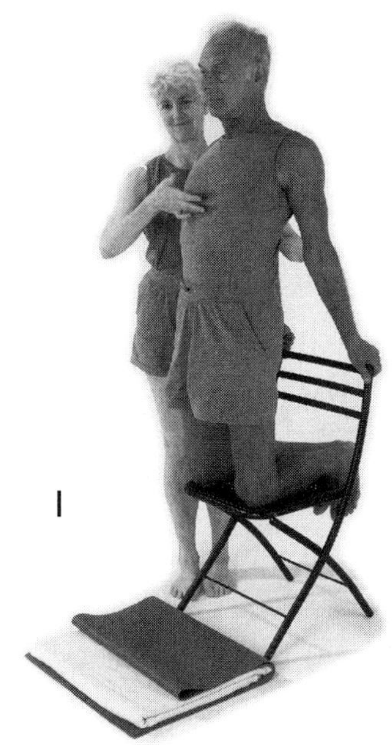

1

2. With the help of another person, place palms on the surface one by one. **[2]**

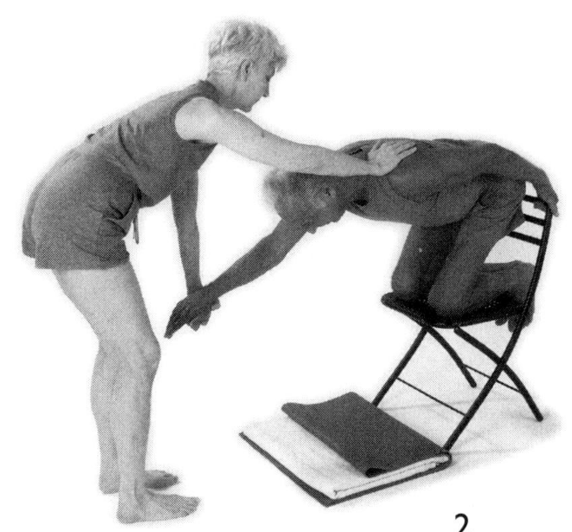

2

3. Breathe calmly for 20-30 seconds.

4. Gradually lower your head until the very top of it rests midway between the palms, slightly further from the furniture than the hands. Distribute the weight evenly between the hands, and also between the knees, shins and feet. **[3,4]**

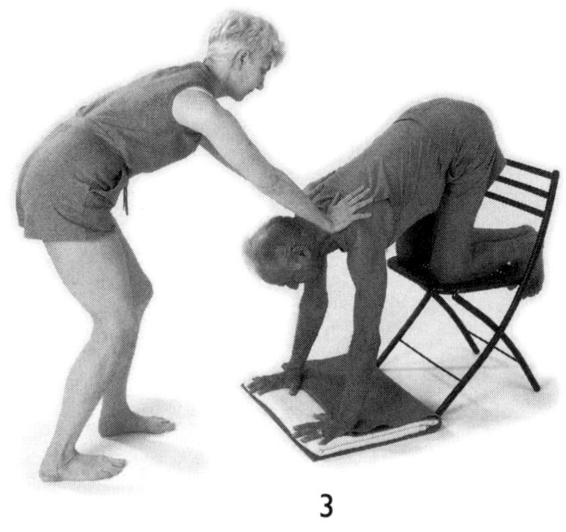

3

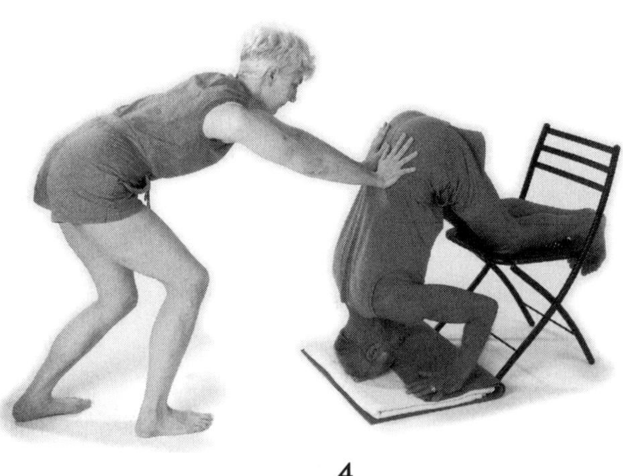

4

5. Interlock hands, making an equilateral triangle with your head at the center. Straighten the legs as much as possible, the helper standing behind and restraining the thoracic spine to prevent rolling forward onto the floor. **[5,6]**

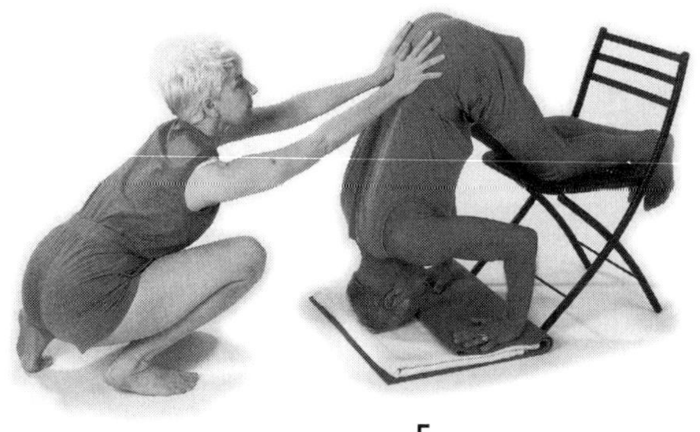

5

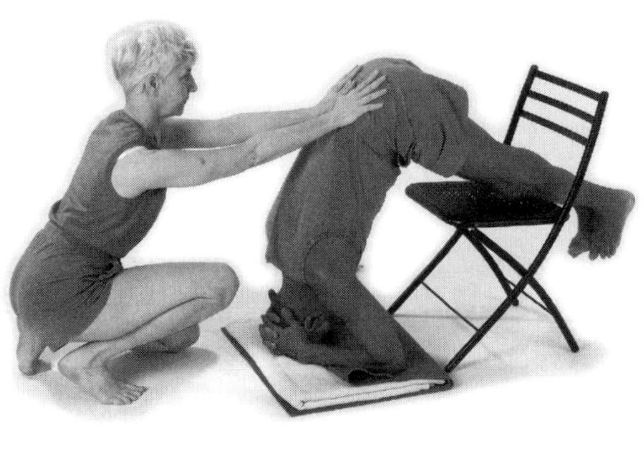

6

6. Point the toes. Raise the right leg as far toward vertical and as straight-kneed as possible. **[7]**

7. Breathe calmly for 10-20 seconds at first, gradually increasing beyond 3 minutes. Return the right leg to the plinth or furniture.

8. Repeat the procedure with the left leg, complete with breathing.

9. Then flex the knees and hips further, using assistance as necessary to return to kneeling on the plinth or couch. Follow this by placing the knees one by one on the floor, slowly moving your hands away from the furniture as you do so. **[8,9]**

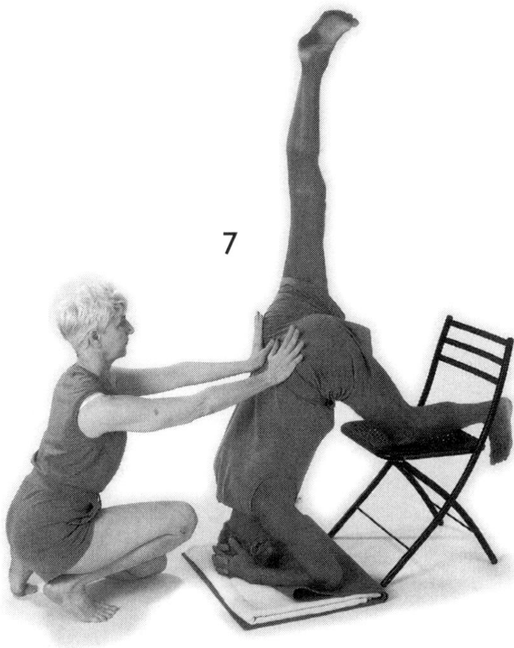
7

Intermediate-Level Sirsasana

1. Place a blanket in the corner of a room or against a wall.

2. Kneel near the blanket, shoulders four or five inches from the walls.

3. Clasp the hands, interlocking the fingers, making an equilateral triangle with the clasped hands and two elbows as vertices. The wrists should be 2-3 inches from the walls. [1]

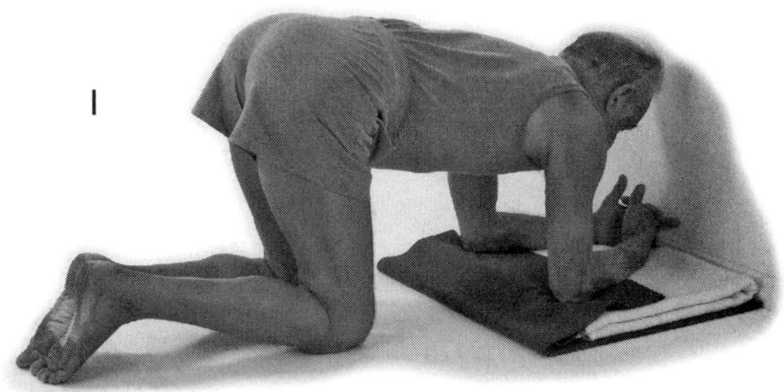
1

4. Keep the fingers tightly interlocked and the heels of your hands close together throughout the pose. [2] Place the very top of the head in the center of the triangle formed by the forearms.

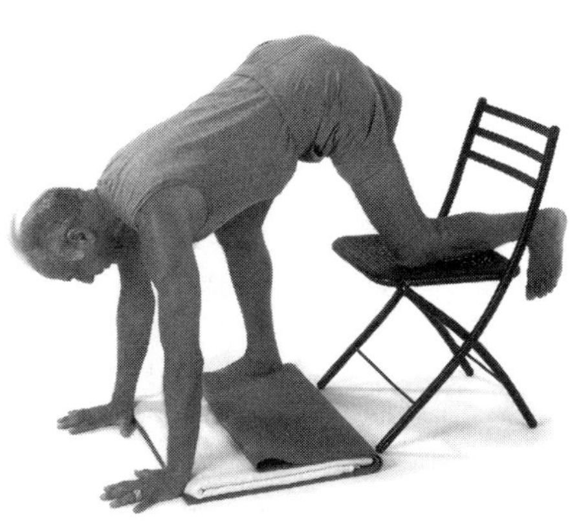
8

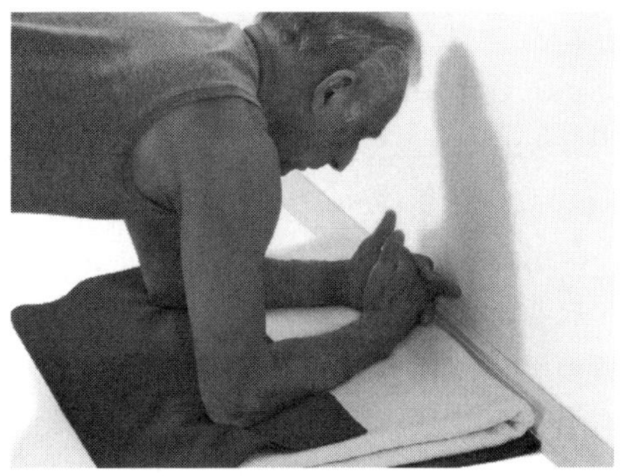
2

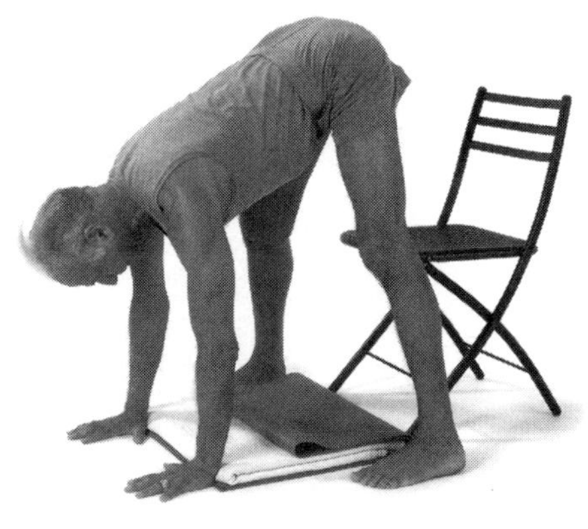
9

5. Straighten the knees and walk in until the weight is predominantly on the head and forearms. [3]

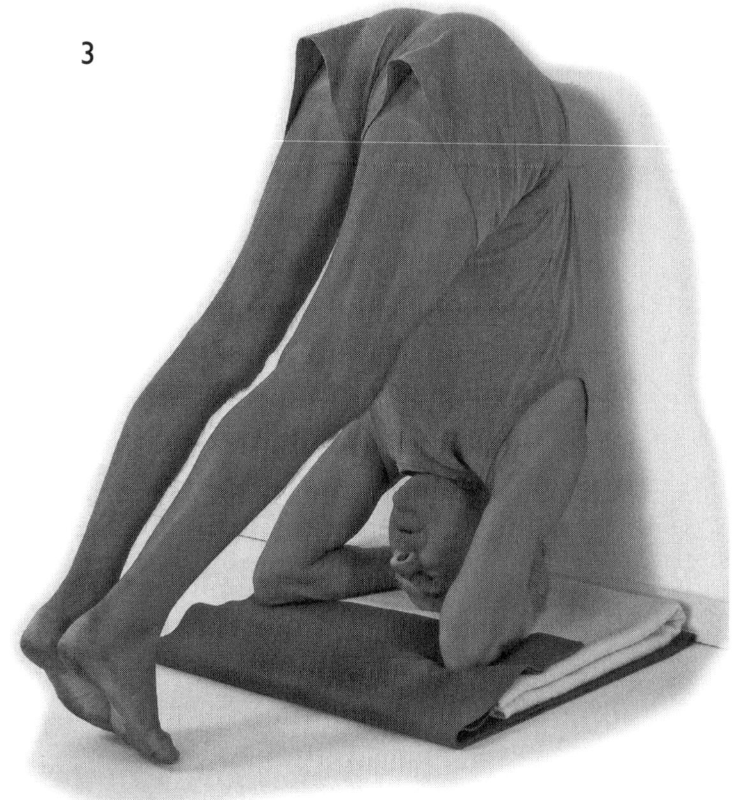
3

6. Breathe calmly for 20 seconds, and with the assistance of another person raise your legs on inhalation, knees bent to tolerance, to vertical. It is best to raise them together, but it is easier to do so one at a time. **[4]**

7. Balance yourself with the outside of the heels against the walls.

8. Retract and raise the shoulders. Most of your weight should be supported by the top of the skull.

9. Point the toes, bring the buttocks back close to the walls and pull in the stomach to avoid arching the back. Open the chest and extend the hips. **[5]**

10. Most importantly, keep on the top of your head. Balancing nearer the back of the head is dangerous for the neck; balancing too much toward the forehead is tiring and poor posture. You cannot fall backward here, so make use of your heels' contact with the walls to develop a straight line from shoulder and lumbar spine through the hips and legs.

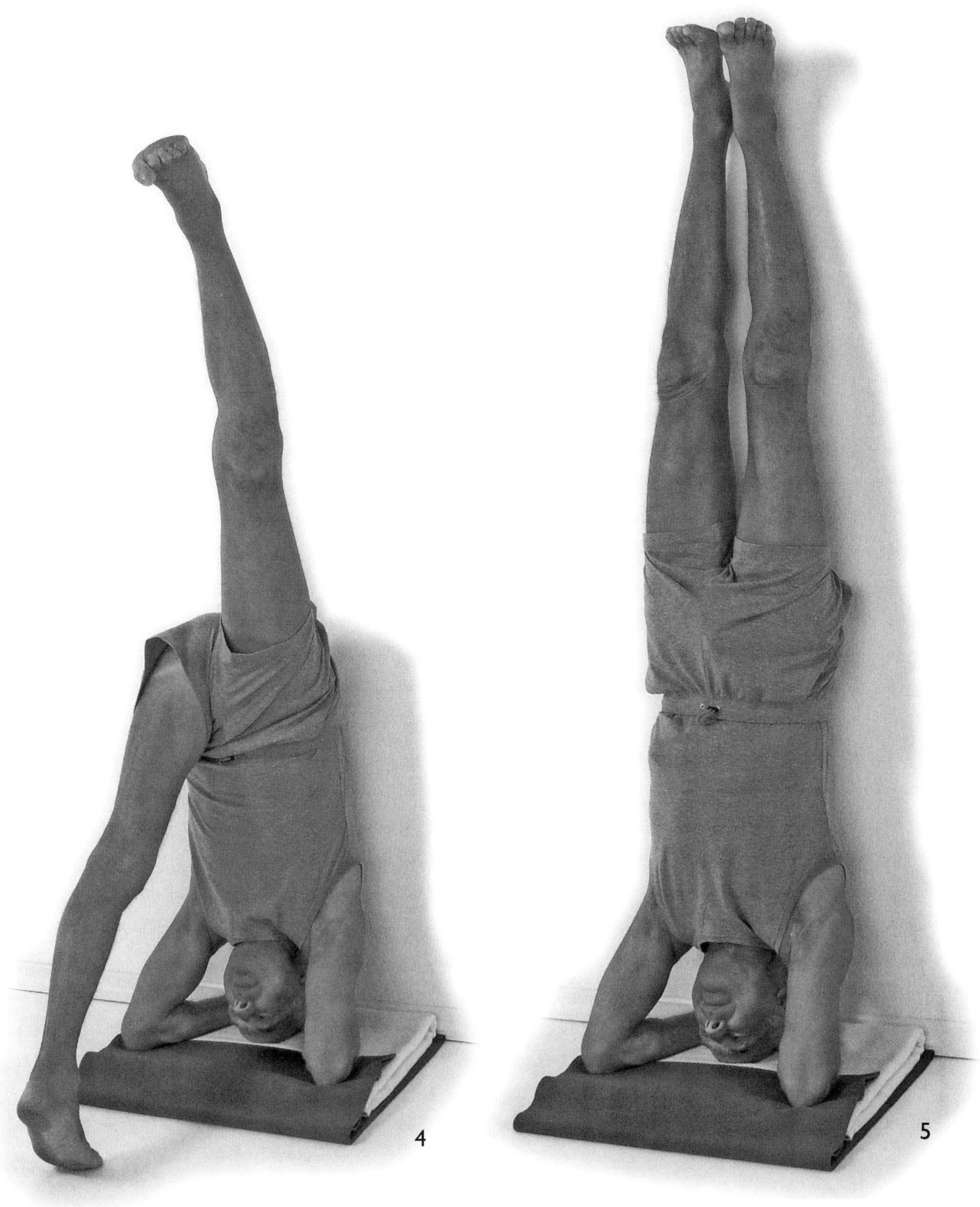

12 Confidence and Calm

Yoga poses serve to improve patients' confidence, because they are effective in reaching the goals set out in this book, and can be, to one degree or another, self-administered. And where confidence grows, can calm be far behind?

One difficulty commonly encountered by people with MS is the emotional upset and free-floating anxiety that comes from a feeling of relative helplessness: This is as intense in patients with relapsing and remitting MS as those with the so-called "progressive" type. In each case there is suspense, a salient element of not-knowing when or whether something new will appear on waking the next morning. It is as though the illness, itself an inanimate thing, had a mind of its own, and a mysterious inscrutable method to its unkindness.

The significance of having some control over one's own body and therefore greater control in one's own life hardly can be exaggerated. The doubting fears and initial trepidation of people facing possible embarrassment or "public pain" have been described so well in Dickens' fiction that it needs no further focus here. A more analytical view is found, for example, in Donald L Nathanson's *Shame and Pride*. (30) But the type of inner security that comes from Yoga may be echoed in Herman Hesse's Siddhartha's "I can wait, I can fast, I can think." The yogi with MS can rejoice and add "I can stretch, I can balance, I am calm."

Work among patients with Alzheimer's disease has amply demonstrated how anxiety worsens that cognitive handicap. People's memories fade, and their acuity is made blurry by tenseness and a sense of alarm. Once experienced, the unfortunate victim is doubly victimized: Franklin Delano Roosevelt once said: "We have nothing to fear but fear itself." The anxious Alzheimer sufferer recalls with sharp dread the memory deficit, raising the anxiety before which surviving memories flee still further out of reach. This begins a vicious cycle of heightened anxiety about forgetting, which makes remembering harder still.

The practice and application of Yoga may be compared to an entire pharmacopia, or a refined set of tools. There are poses and processes for many different purposes, with specific means to aid alertness or hasten sleep, improve calm and still increase agility, counter spasticity yet promote strength. Any level of accomplishment and independent practice raises self-control and self-mastery, increasing confidence and lowering anxiety, contributing to the stable inner environment consonant with that sweet reasonableness we associate with the higher workings of human beings.

An illustrative example might help here. One major problem encountered by people with multiple sclerosis is scissor-gait. Walking involves swinging one leg forward while the other supports you. Contraction of the swinging leg's adductors, sartorius and gracilis bring it in so closely that it catches the back of the stance-phase ankle and calf as it swings by.

Now what actually happens when you walk? Since both legs are (roughly) the same length, some tilting of the pelvis, flexing of the swinging leg's knee, and dorsiflexion of its foot are necessary for it to get past the standing leg. **[1]** So the abducting muscles of the standing leg tilt the pelvis to let the swinging leg move past it. This stretches the adductors enough to trigger the hyperactive reflex that makes them involuntarily contract. And this brings the front of the swinging ankle to hook around the back of the standing leg, causing gross imbalance and dangerous falls.**[2, 3]**

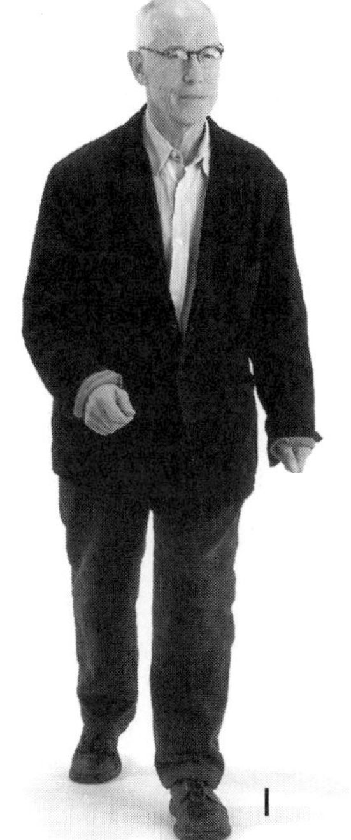

1

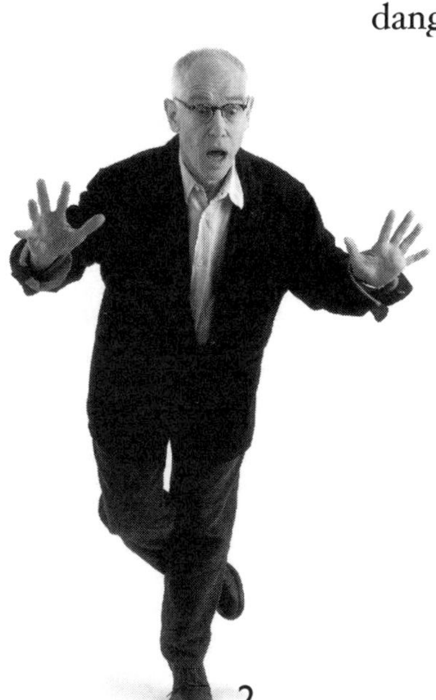

2

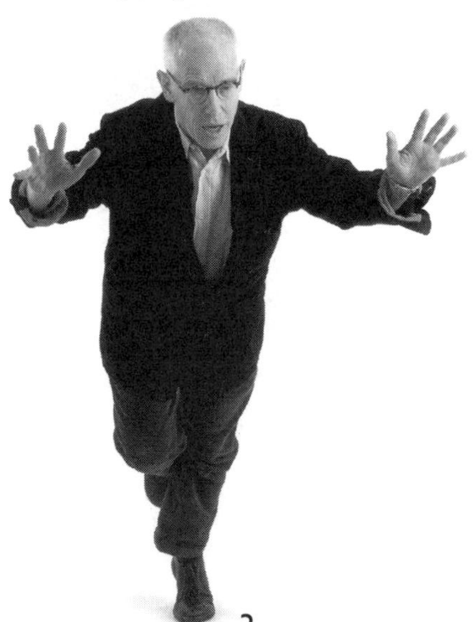

3

Reduced ankle range of motion means the leg actually has to swing out further to clear the floor. This exaggerated abduction triggers the adductors' reflex on the swinging leg as well.

The same hyperactive mechanism may react to reverse the natural forward rotation of the pelvis itself on the swing-leg side.

The way yoga activates the golgi and intrafusal systems to modulate spasticity does not work in reciprocal motion such as walking. The velocity-dependent intrafusal system has dominance in reciprocal activities, since no contraction persists long enough for the golgi tendon organs to damp it down, and the myotatic reflex is overcome by synergic patterns of spasticity.

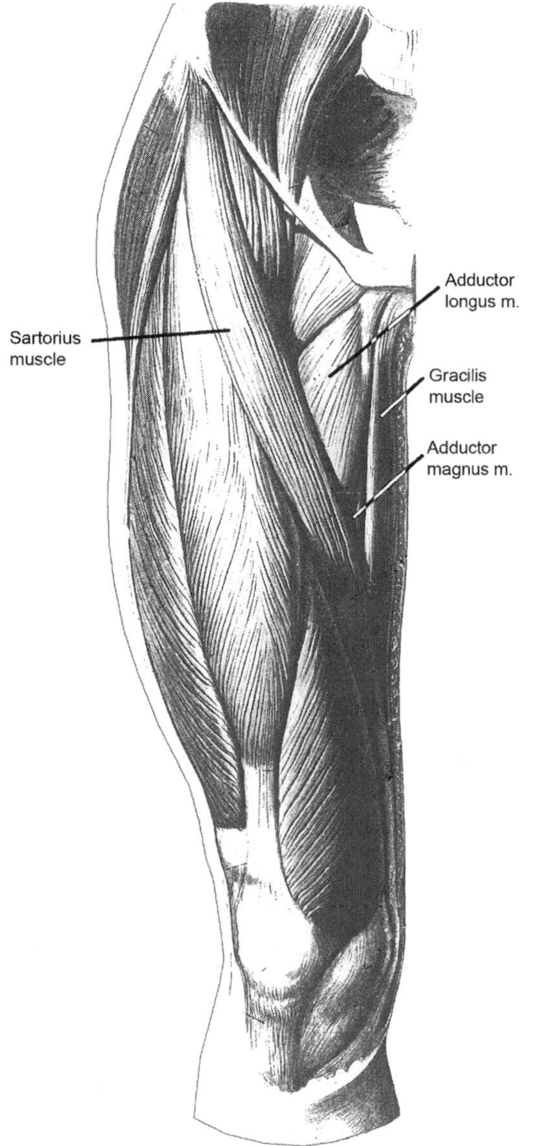

In this situation yoga helps in more basic ways, stretching the gastrocnemius muscle to increase dorsiflexion and facilitate the swinging foot's clearing the floor, stretching the adductors so that their natural resting length is greater. Poses such as the "dog pose" and the standing poses accomplish the first; the angle poses such as Konasana and Baddha Konasana bring about the second. This will enable walking to take place with the legs less sharply abducted, and with muscles less prone to trigger the hyperactive reflex.

The overall strategy here is to (1) Improve the range of motion of all joints involved so there is no muscle group obliged to overstretch in compensation; (2) Gently stretch and thereby lengthen every muscle in the chain; and (3) Arm the patient with suitable exercises and attitude to maximize the calm and thereby minimize the hair-trigger these exagggerated contraction-responses are otherwise more apt to have.

In the reciprocal and weight-bearing movements of walking, the adductors "gang up" on the ambulatory person, both stance- and swing-phase groups producing reflex adduction just before the middle of swing-phase. The yogic response is like the Romans of old: divide (the problems) and conquer.

13 Advanced Balance

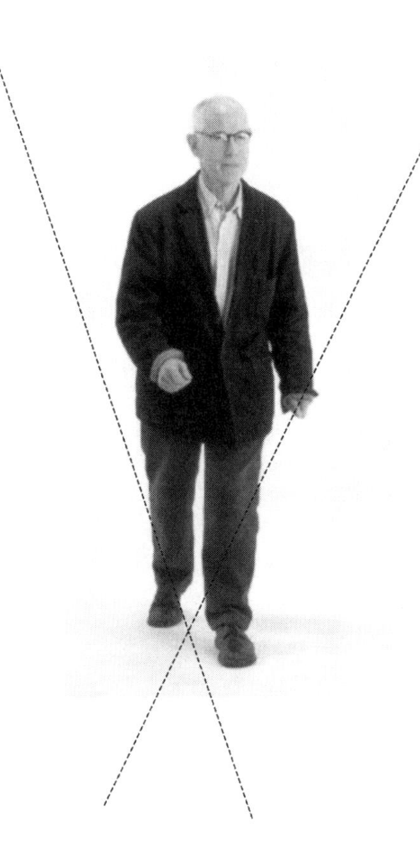

All other things being equal, there are three systems that people use to maintain balance: The inner ear gives a sense of acceleration in any dimension, cutaneous and proprioceptive information relating to floor forces come from the feet and ankles, and visual data reveals our position and any change in it relative to our environment.

Safety in ambulation is often measured by how far a person can deviate from a perfectly perpendicular position and maintain their equilibrium.

This "cone of balance" depends not only on the three determinants of balance itself, but on the personal resources available: how quickly and how well does the individual respond to signs of disequilibrium? How much weight can he or she sustain with knees bent 20 degrees, how far does the right ankle flex or extend?

Compromised equilibrium in MS and related conditions can result from reduced range of motion, weakness, dyscoordination, spasticity, and sensory dysfunction either of the cutaneous, proprioceptive or visual systems, or the inner ear.

A person's balance is reduced when any of these factors is compromised, but compensation through focused analysis of other inputs, or sharpening of the perceptions themselves may be very effective. Just as a person with hearing loss will "read lips" to augment his or her data-set about what's being said, a person with compromised feedback about the terrain from his or her feet and ankles will "overuse" eyesight. That is why it is easier for all of us to stumble in the dark.

Unfortunately, in neurological conditions such as MS, stroke and peripheral neuropathies, multiple systems can be affected. Still, in the majority of individuals, adaptation and compensation for impaired feedback is a solid strategy to improve equilibrium and balance. This is the purpose of the asanas that are presented here.

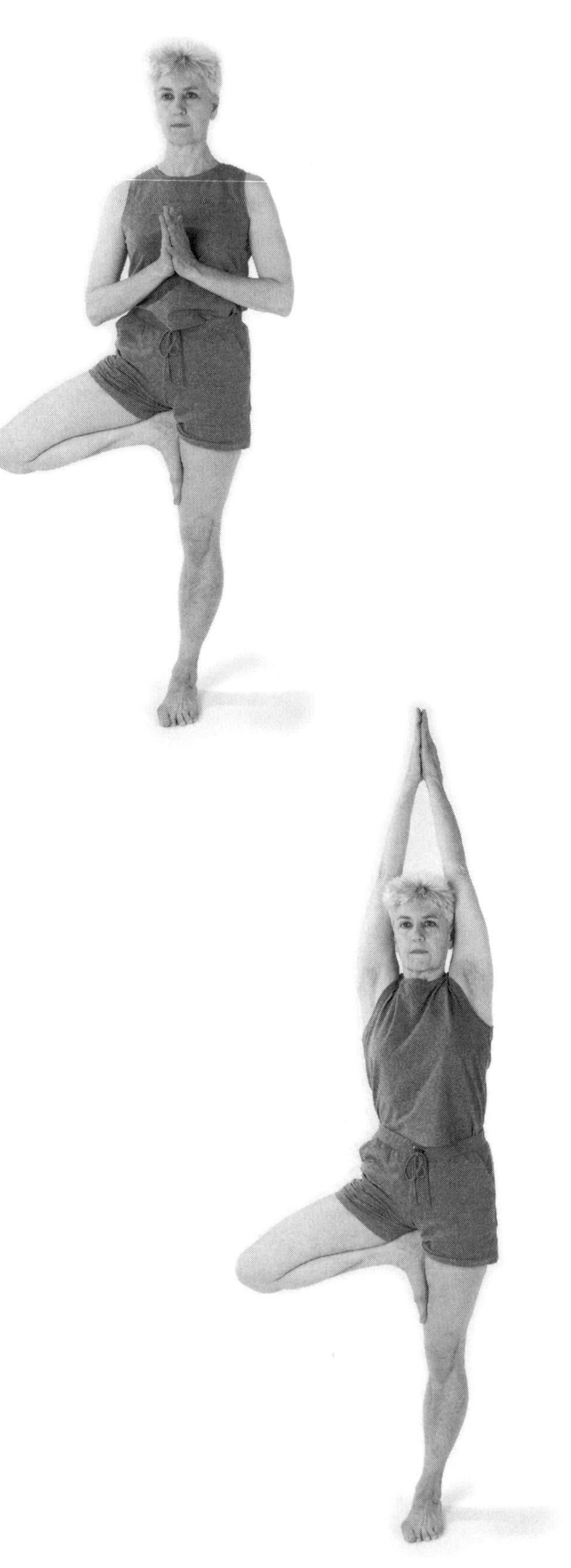

VRKSASANA

The Tree

1. Stand in Tadasana.
2. Abduct the right leg and flex the knee, bringing the heel to rest as high as possible on the inner left thigh. The toes should point down toward the left ankle.

3. Breathe evenly and quietly for 10-20 seconds, seeking the same solid and even balance that was present in Tadasana.

4. Raise the arms from your sides slowly, revolving the palms inward until they meet directly overhead. Fix your vision on a point in front of you.

5. Stretch upward from the heel to the fingertips, especially the backs of the legs and spine, and the thumb side of the hands.

6. Inhale, and remain in the pose for another 10-20 seconds.

7. Retain the balance while returning your arms to their resting position.

8. Place the right foot back on the floor and remain in Tadasana breathing calmly and balanced for 1 minute.

9. Then repeat this process with the feet reversed.

Entry-Level Vrksasana

1. Sitting squarely in wheel- or armchair, straighten the spine from coccyx to cranium.

2. Raise one or both arms overhead with inhalation, slowly revolving the palms so that the right palm faces left and vice versa.

3. Extend the maximally elevated arm(s) upward as much as possible, breathing calmly for 10-20 seconds.

4. Exhale as the arm(s) return to the arms of the chair.

One may use only one arm, or raise them to different heights as circumstances dictate. The straight back, the elevation of the arms with inhalation, and the focus on balance are the essential elements.

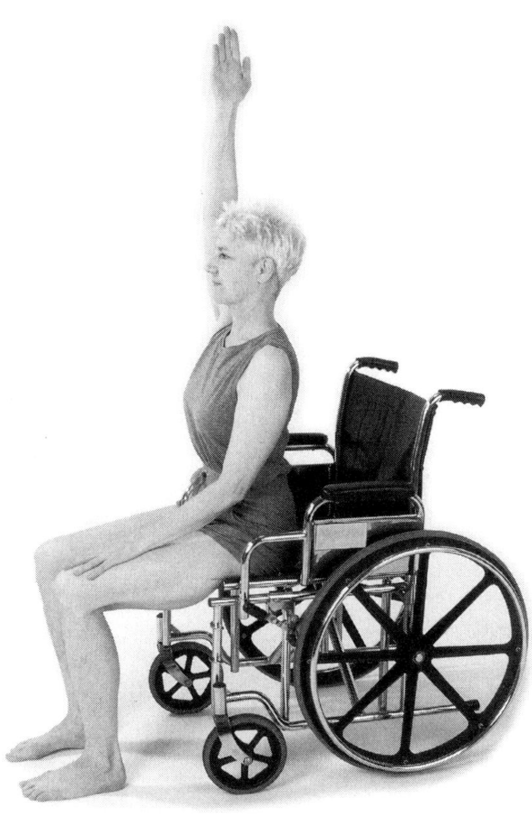

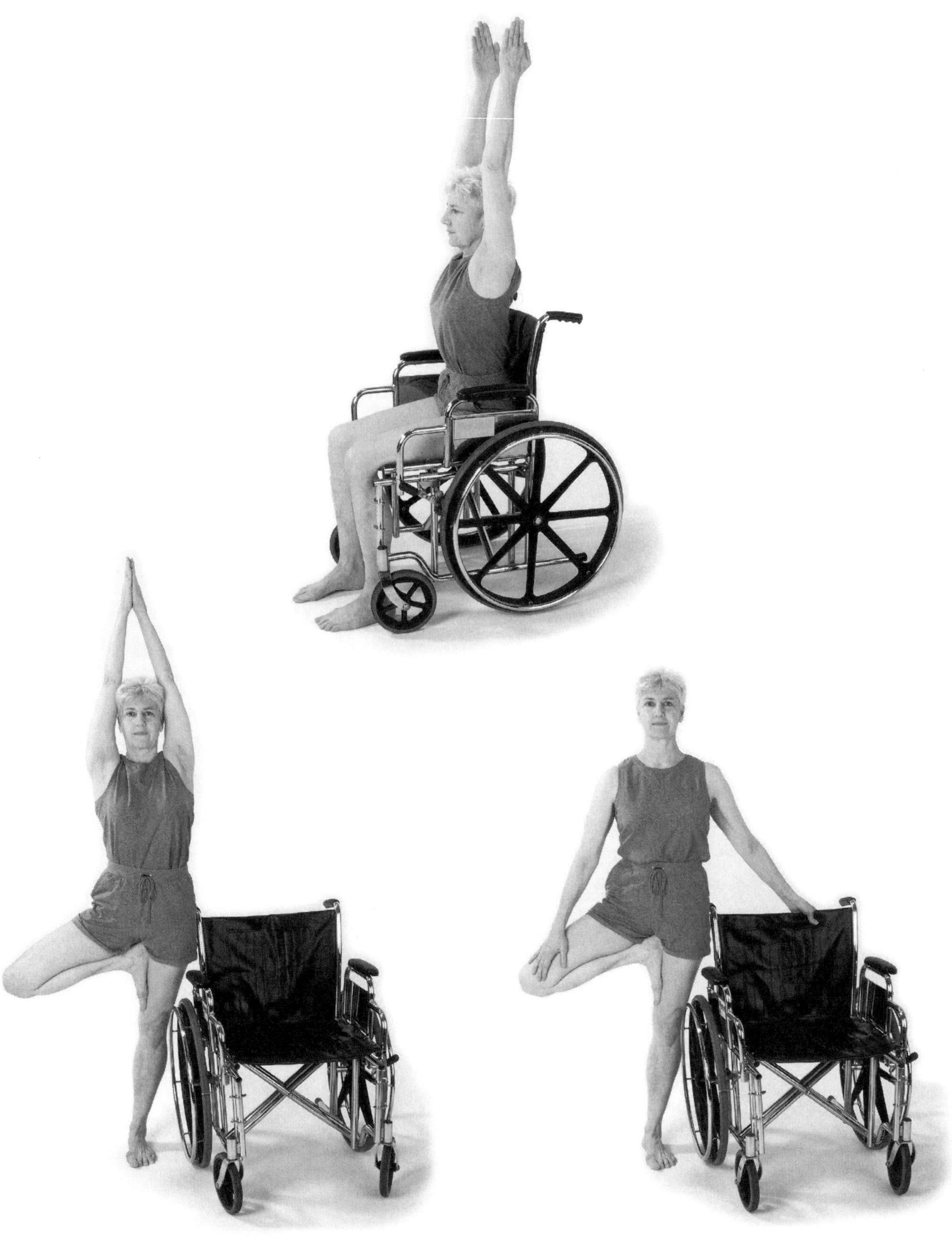

Intermediate Vrksasana

1. Stand next to a table, counter or chair in Tadasana.

2. Abduct the right leg and flex the knee, bringing the heel to rest as high as possible on the inner left thigh. The toes should point down toward the left ankle.

3. Breathe evenly and quietly for 10 -20 seconds, using the table or other object to maintain steady balance, but no more than necessary. Maintain the same solidity and calm balance that was present in Tadasana.

4. Raise the arms from the sides slowly, revolving the palms inward until they meet directly overhead.

5. Stretch from the heels to the fingertips, inhale, and remain in the pose for 10-20 seconds.

6. Retain the balance while returning your arms to their resting position, place the right foot back on the floor, and remain in Tadasana.

7. Breathe calmly, and balanced for 10-20 seconds.

8. Then repeat this process with the left foot.

ARDHA CHANDRASANA

Half-Moon Pose

This pose follows from Trikonasana, the triangle pose, which begins in Tadasana.

1. Spend 10-20 seconds in Tadasana, the mountain pose.

2. Then, inhaling, spring the legs to 3 1/2 feet apart. Turn the right foot out 90 degrees, and the left foot inward 30 degrees, stretching

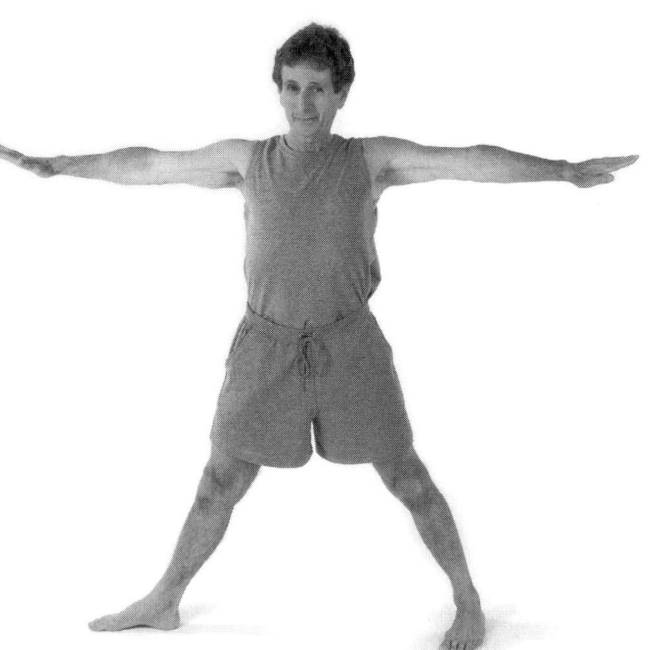

the arms horizontally as far apart as they will go. Puff out the chest, draw in the abdomen.

3. Descend toward the right calf. Exhale as you descend. Retain the alignment of the arms; keep the torso in the plane defined by the intersection of the two legs.

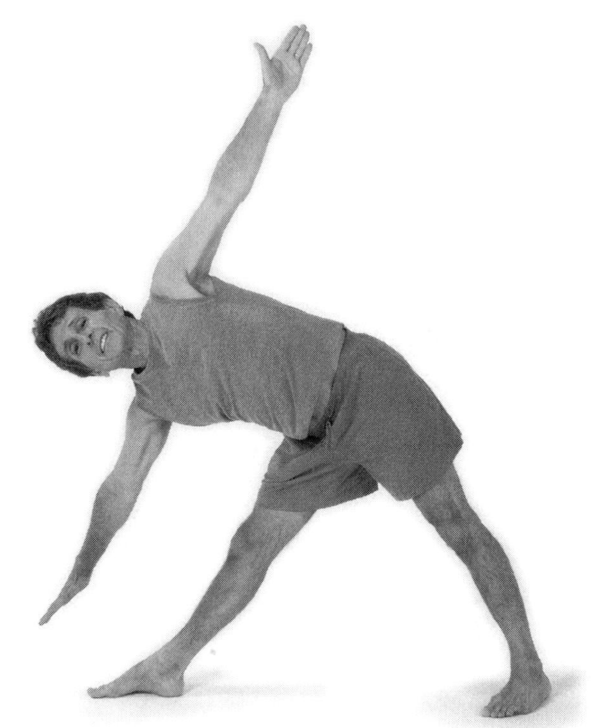

4. After the right hand reaches the floor, press backward on it to rotate the torso so that a line through the two arms would pass through the center of the earth.

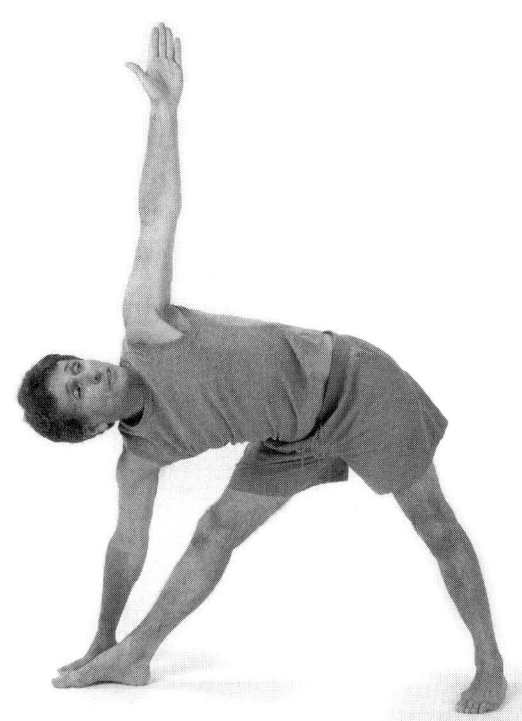

5. Keeping the left foot in place, rotate the left knee outward and curl the left buttock back, so that the lower torso is also brought in line with the same plane.

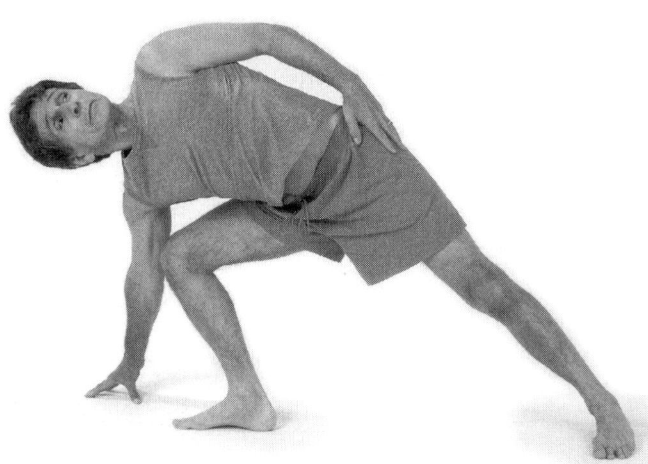

6. The action of the arms and the left leg will bring the right torso away from the root of the right thigh, and the left flank higher, widening the right groin and lengthening the left groin.

7. Breathe calmly and evenly, filling the right and left lungs equally, for 10-20 seconds.

8. With exhalation and bending the right knee, place the right palm or fingertips about one foot in front of the right foot, and slightly to the little toe side.

9. Let the left arm come down and rest the palm on the thigh.

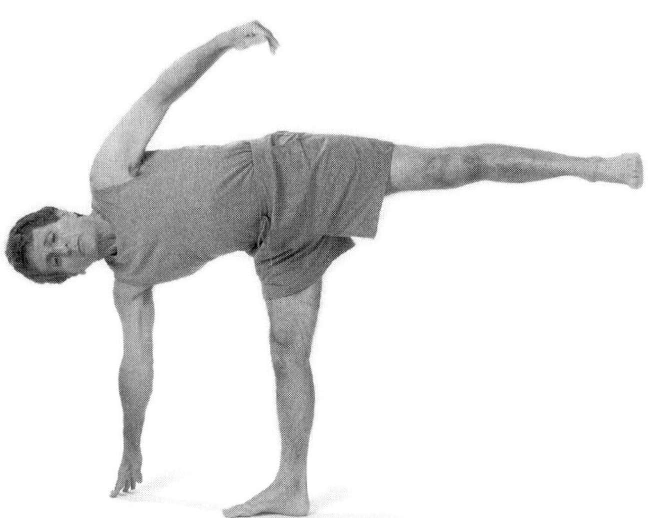

10. Breathe calmly for 10-20 seconds, then raise and revolve the left leg up to horizontal.

11. Straighten the knees and point the left toes forward.

12. Finally raise the left arm to vertical. The right eye should gaze at the left thumb, with all limbs and the torso in the same plane.

13. Breathe so quietly that no one, not even the breather can hear.

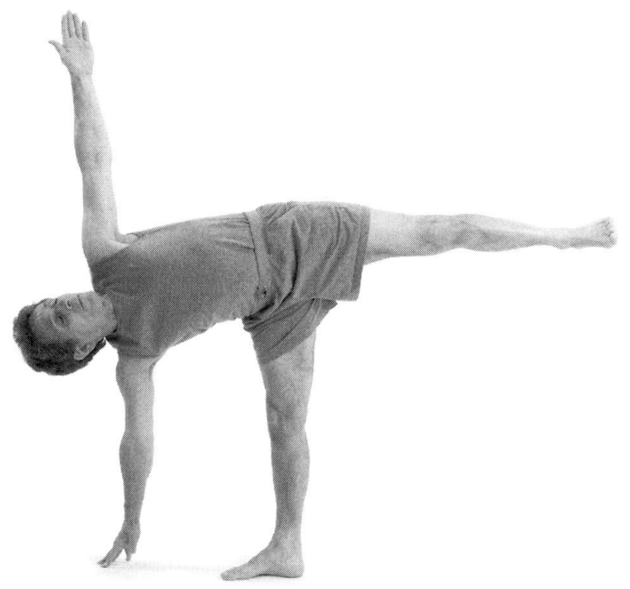

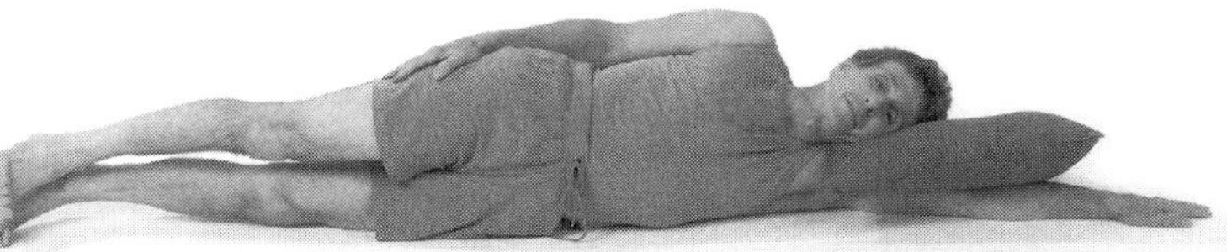

14. Now descend, reversing the steps that got you there, and repeat them on the other side.

Entry-Level Ardha Chandrasana

1. Using a reasonably firm flat surface, lie on the left side, shoulders perpendicular to the surface, right palm on right hip and left arm stretched directly beyond your head, palm down.
2. Take a few calm breaths.
3. Using the left arm for support, and possibly pillows, a bed board or a wall behind you, raise the right arm to vertical, palm facing forward.
4. Take a few more calm breaths, opening the chest and pulling in the abdomen.
5. If balance is adequate, raise the right leg in the same plane as the two arms and torso, revolving the toes to lie in that plane too. Use the left arm and leg for balance.
6. Extend the neck, still facing forward, and relax the soft and hard palate.
7. Breathe slowly and calmly for 10-20 seconds.
8. Then lower the leg, lower the arm, turn on the right side and repeat the process.

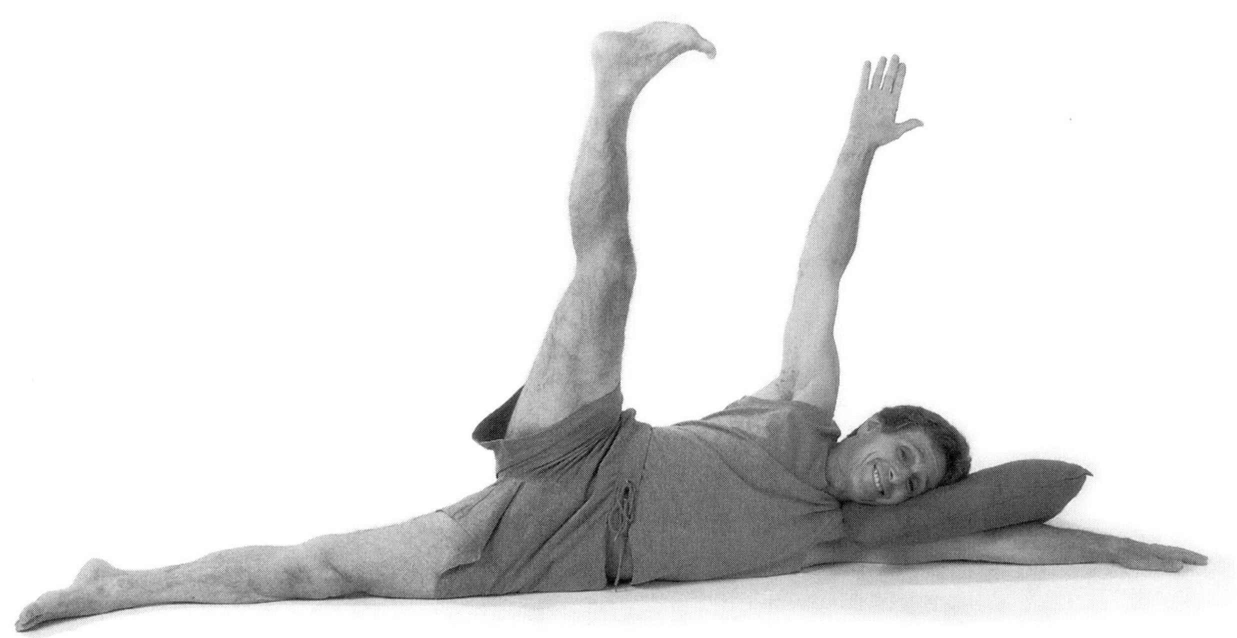

Intermediate-Level
Ardha Chandrasana I
(*Not pictured.*)

1. Alight on all fours, directly over an armless but strong child's chair that has been placed with its back against a wall. Balance weight evenly over the palms and knees and tops of the feet.

2. Breathe evenly for 10-20 seconds.

3. Raise the right arm up toward vertical, palm facing forward, and as the torso twists, raise and straighten the right leg to horizontal. Use the chair back for some support.

4. Breathe calmly for 10-20 seconds.

5. Then lower the leg and arm and alight in the opposite direction to perform the pose on the contralateral side.

Intermediate-Level
Ardha Chandrasana II

1. Stand with your back 2-3 inches from a wall. Spend 10-20 seconds in Tadasana, the mountain pose.

2. Then, inhaling, spring the legs to 3 ½ feet apart. Turn the right foot out parallel to the wall, and the left foot 30 degrees to the right, stretching the arms horizontally as far apart as they will go. The right buttock should be in contact with the wall, the left reasonably close to it.

3. Puff out the chest, draw in the abdomen and descend toward the right calf, retaining the alignment of the arms, and keeping the torso in the plane defined by the intersection of the two legs.

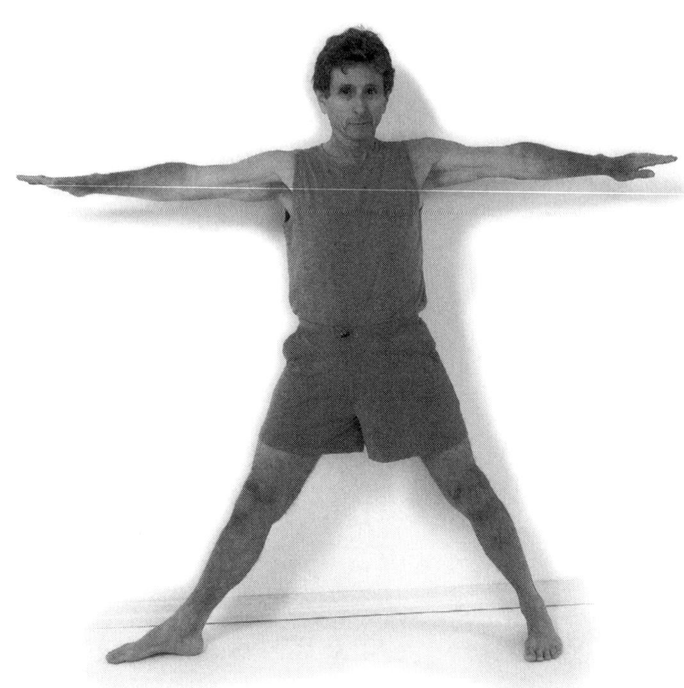

4. After the right hand reaches the floor, press backward on it to rotate the torso so that both shoulder blades are in contact with the wall.

5. Keeping the left foot in place, rotate the left knee outward and curl the left buttock back, so that the lower torso is also brought, in line with the same plane.

6. The action of the arms and legs will bring the torso away from the root of the right thigh, and higher, widening the right groin and lengthening the left groin, bringing the left buttock closer to the wall. Breathe calmly and evenly, filling the right and left lungs equally, for 1/2 minute.

7. With exhalation and bending the right knee, place the right palm about one foot in front of the right foot, with the little finger virtually against the wall. Let the left arm come down to rest the palm on the thigh.

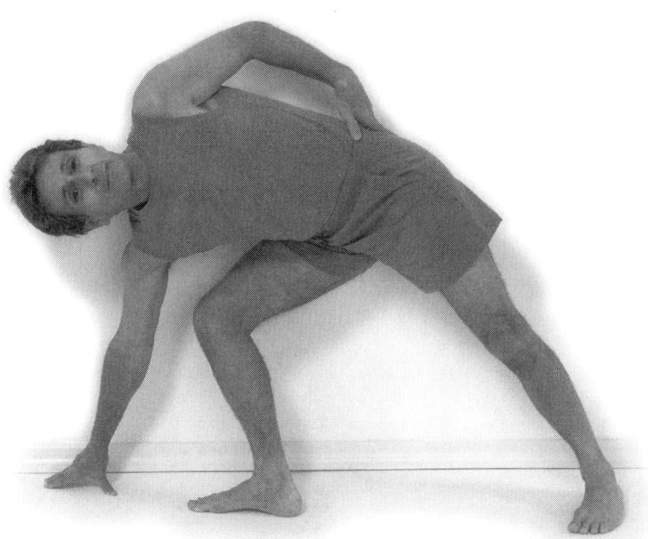

8. Breathe calmly for 10-20 seconds, then raise and revolve the left leg up to horizontal, keeping the knee straight and the toes pointing upward. Finally raise the left arm to vertical. The right eye should gaze at the left thumb, with all limbs and the torso in the same plane. Lightly press the wall with both buttocks and both shoulders. Remain in this position for 10-20 seconds. Breathe so quietly that no one, not even the breather, can hear. (See the picture on page 245.)

Eye-closed Tadasana

The Closed Eyes Mountain

Just as a runner may put weights around his ankle, putting himself at a disadvantage in order to strengthen his legs, a person with balance deficit may close his eyes in order to challenge that very faculty, sharpening his or her kinaesthetic sense and response to inner-ear stimuli. That is the point of this pose, which also bears close resemblance to the medical "Romberg test."

1. Stand with the feet close together and parallel, arms at the sides. Distribute the weight evenly: right to left feet, front to back, inside and outside of each foot. Splay out the toes and repeat the process. Draw in the abdomen, open the front of the chest,

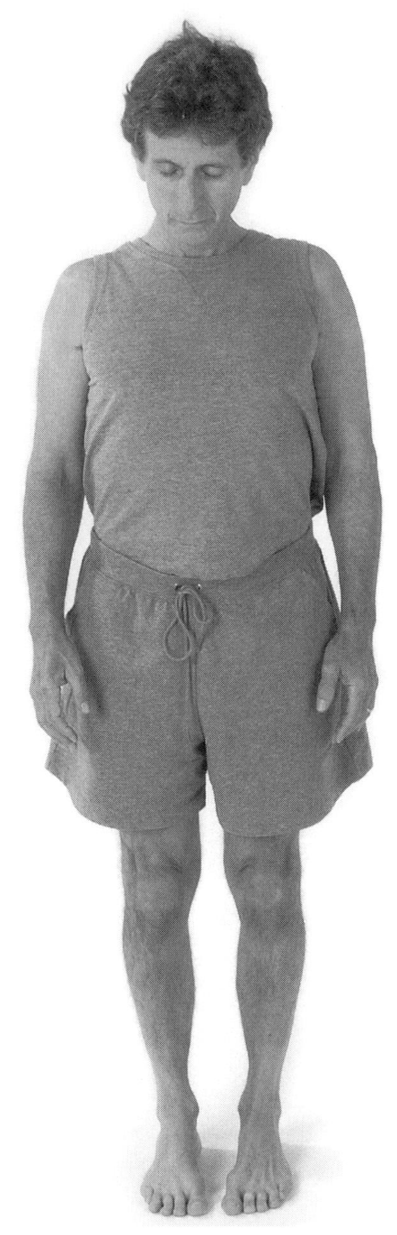

straighten the spine from the sacrum to the base of the skull, facing straight ahead. Totally still, concentrate thoroughly on motionlessness, except for calm breathing, for 1 minute.

2. Now draw and turn the arms upward until the palms meet firmly. With straight elbows, rest the biceps behind the ears. Raise the toes up so they no longer give any support.

3. Silently close both eyes and breathe evenly. Remain otherwise motionless, for 1 minute.

This is difficult at first. Leaning against a table or the back of a couch is a good way to start. Lean as little as possible, and soon one will not need to lean at all.

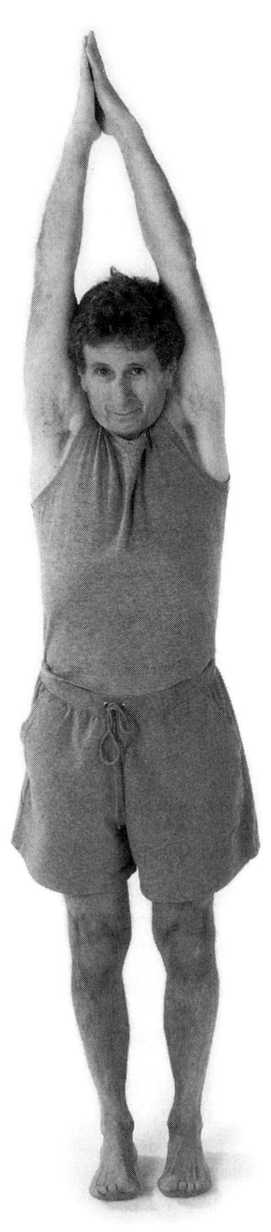

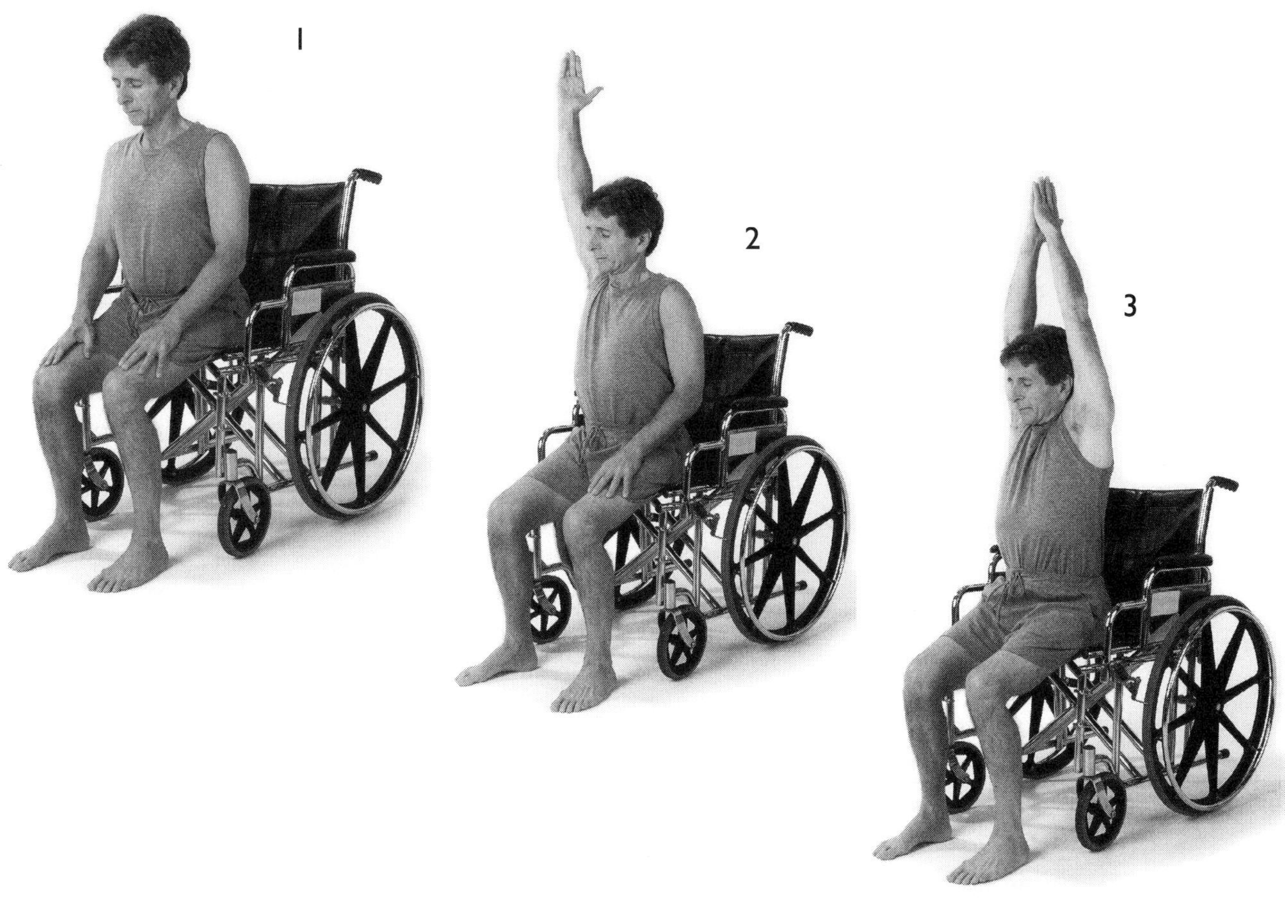

Entry-Level Eyes Closed Tadasana

1. In a wheelchair or armchair, sit erect and away from the chair back, with the hands on the thighs. Close your eyes.
2. Straighten the spine from the coccyx to the nape of the neck, drawing in the abdomen and opening the chest.
3. Align the shoulders and hip joints in one plane parallel to the chair back. [1]
4. Take a few calm breaths.
5. Raise the right arm directly overhead, elbow straight, palm facing to the left. [2]
6. Take stock of your balance and take a few calm breaths.
7. Retaining closed eyes, raise the left arm until the palms meet directly overhead. [3]
8. Take a few more calm breaths.
9. Now raise one or both thighs up off the chair, still with closed eyes, and breathe calmly.
10. Repeat the exercise beginning with the left arm and the opposite leg.

Intermediate-Level Eyes Closed Tadasana

1. Place a chair facing out from the corner of a room, with enough space to fit between the back of the chair and the corner.

2. Stand with shoulders near the walls, hands lightly on the chair back. Straighten the spine, retract the abdomen and breathe deeply several times, filling and opening the cheyst. **[1]**

3. After each of the following steps, close the eyes and draw a few calm breaths:

A. Balance the weight evenly from right to left foot, front to back, inside and outside of each foot.

B. Raise the right arm forward and upward to vertical, turning the palm to the left.

C. Elevate all the toes of both feet. **[2]**

D. Lower the toes and elevate the left arm so that the palm presses the palm of the right.

E. Raise the toes again. **[3]**

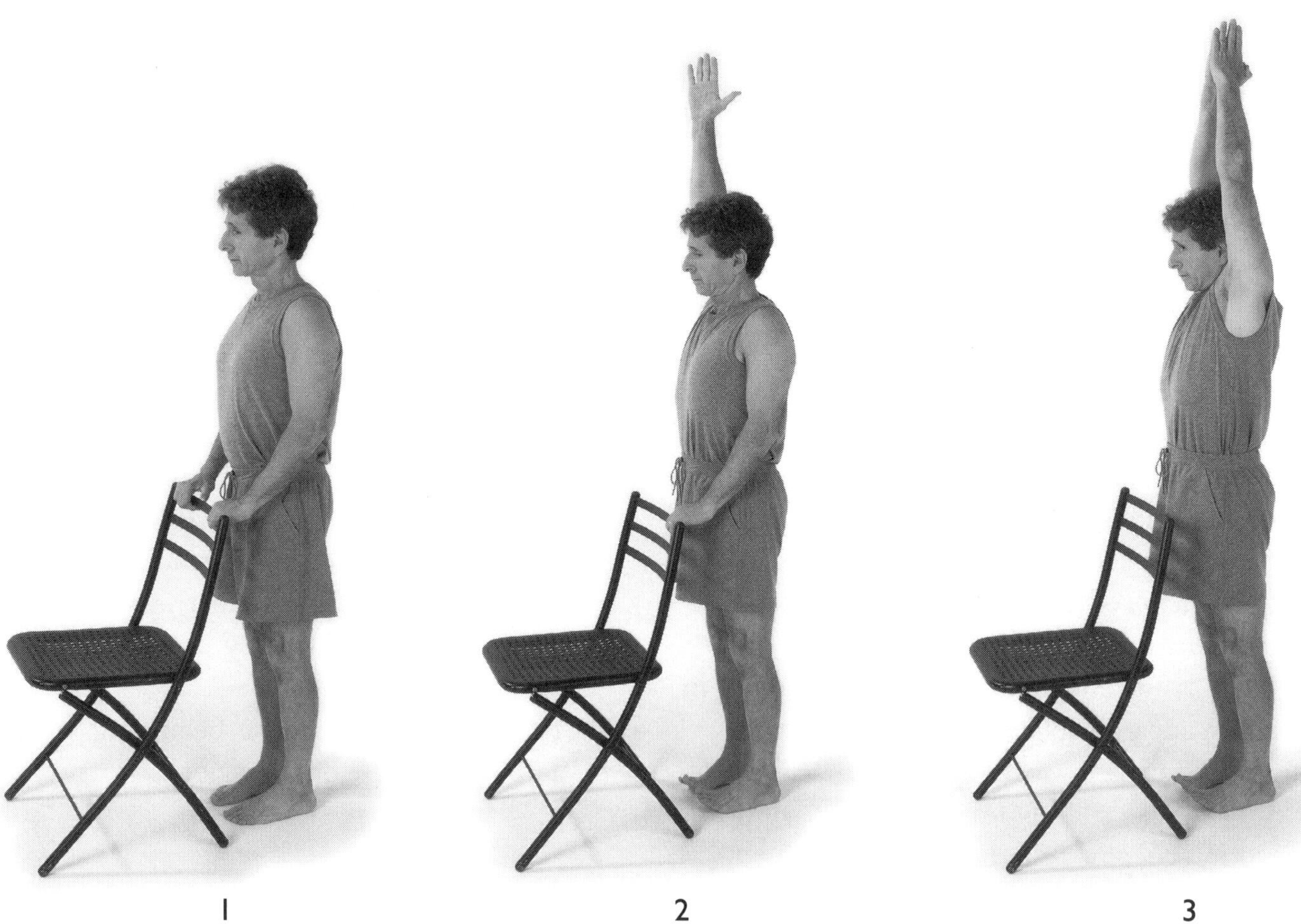

1 2 3

Pasasana

The Basket

1. Squat with soles of the feet entirely on the floor, inner knees and inner ankles in contact. **[1]**

2. Breathe quietly for 10-20 seconds, and balance.

3. Jut the left knee slightly forward, revolving the torso and inclining to the right so that the back of the left armpit is pressing the outside of the right knee. **[2]**

4. Now reach the left arm in front of the right and left knee, and then along the outside of the left thigh, while the right arm circles behind the left thigh and then both buttocks to join the left hand behind the left thigh. **[3]**

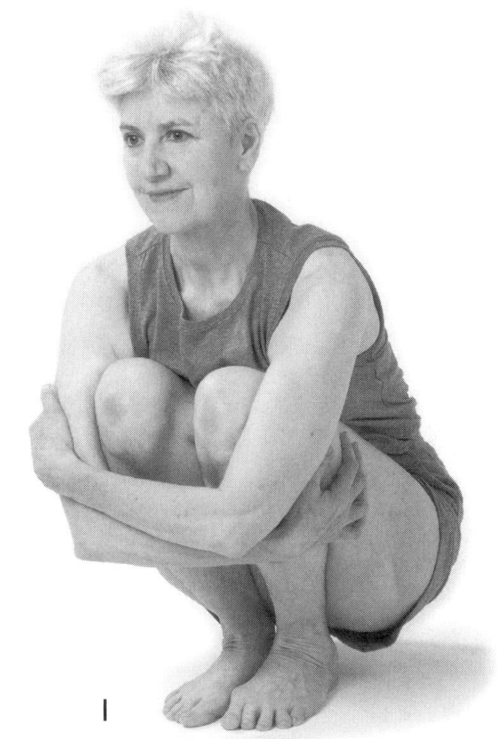
1

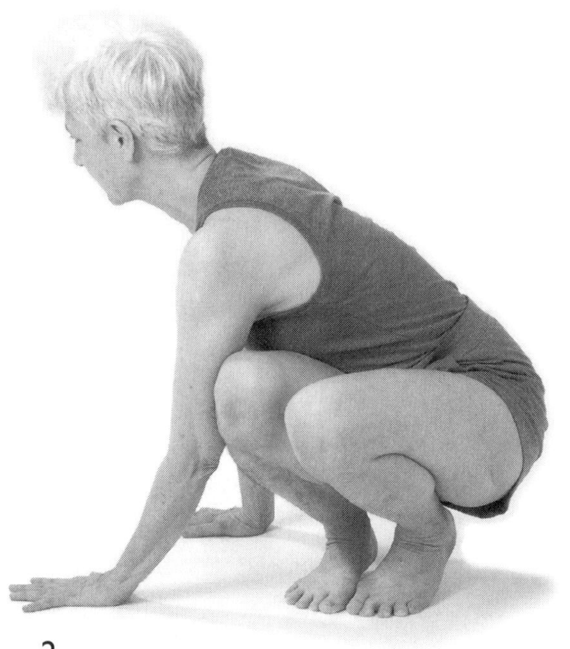
2

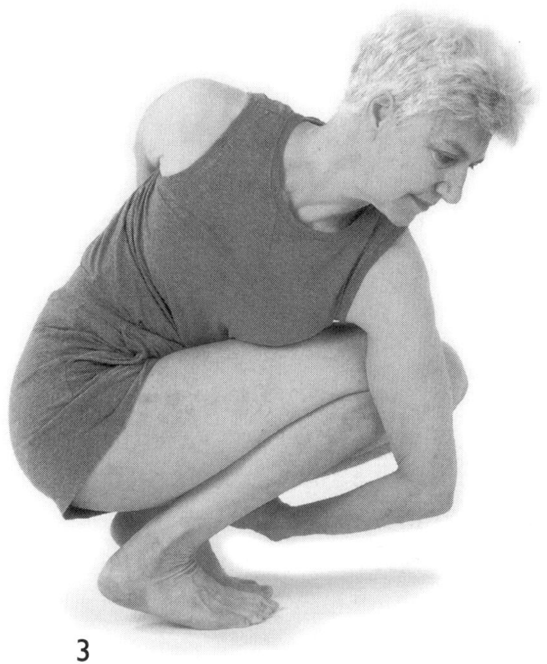
3

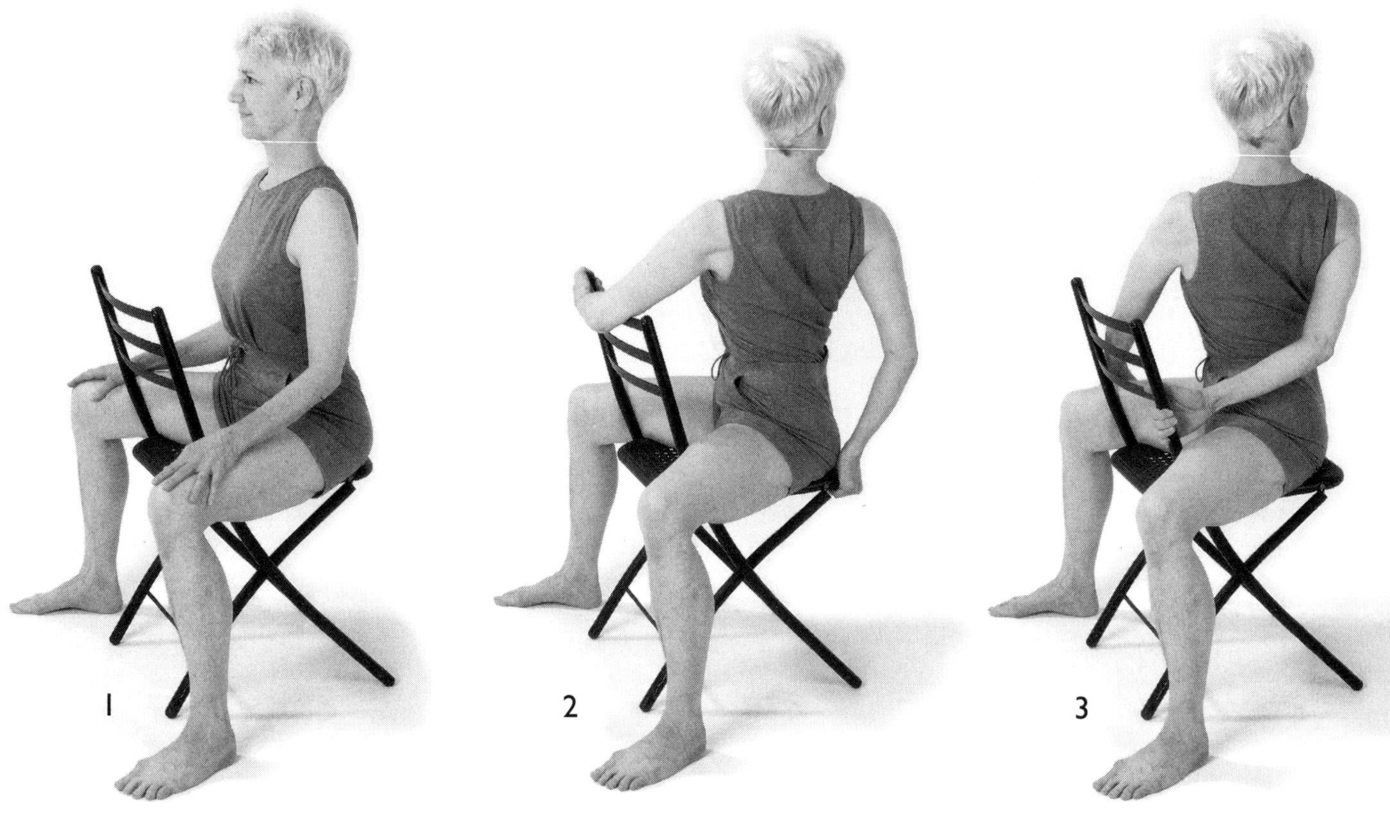

5. Use the back of the left arm and shoulder to twist further, and turn the head to gaze over the right or left shoulder.

Entry-Level Pasasana

1. Straddle the back of a chair or wheel chair. Be careful not to tip the chair. Settle both feet on the floor.

2. Straighten your back from the sacrum to the nape of the neck. Look straight ahead. **[1]**

3. Grasp the left arm of the chair with your left hand, circling the right arm behind and grasping the right arm of the chair. Retain the straightness of your back; keep your feet as squarely on the floor as possible. **[2,3]**

4. Lift the chest. Twist the torso and head reasonably far to the right, advancing the arms as possible.

5. Breathe as symmetrically as possible for 10-20 seconds.

6. Then reverse the arms.

Intermediate-Level Pasasana

1. Sit or squat as low as possible on a small armless chair or other support, with left arm and shoulder in contact with a wall, and torso perpendicular to it. Extend your arms horizontally before you **[A]**. Do not sit so low that the feet cannot rest squarely on the floor.

2. Inhale and exhale calmly.

3. Twist to bring the right armpit outside of the left thigh just above the knee. Support yourself with the right hand, pulling the right chest to the left, and bringing the right shoulder blade and ribs toward the wall. Use the left

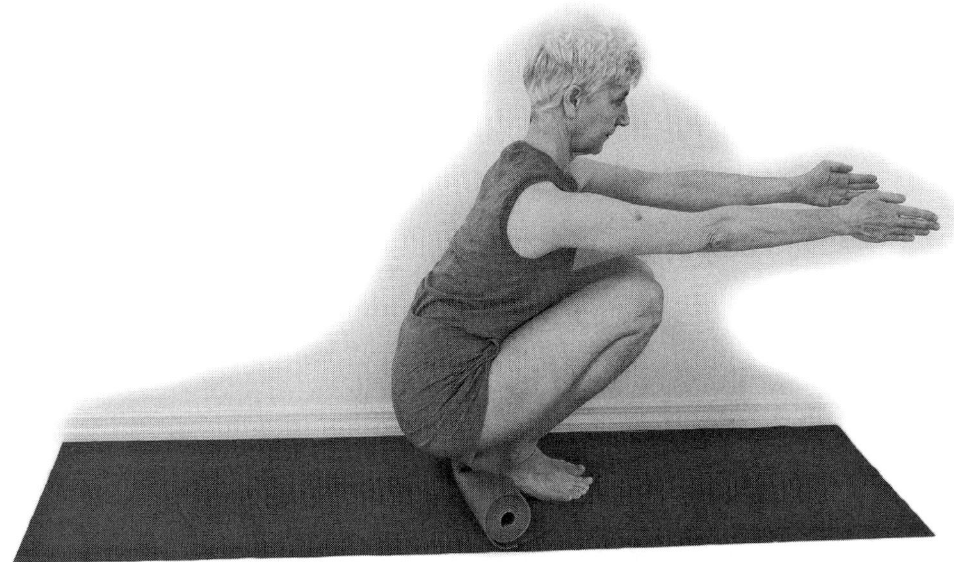

1

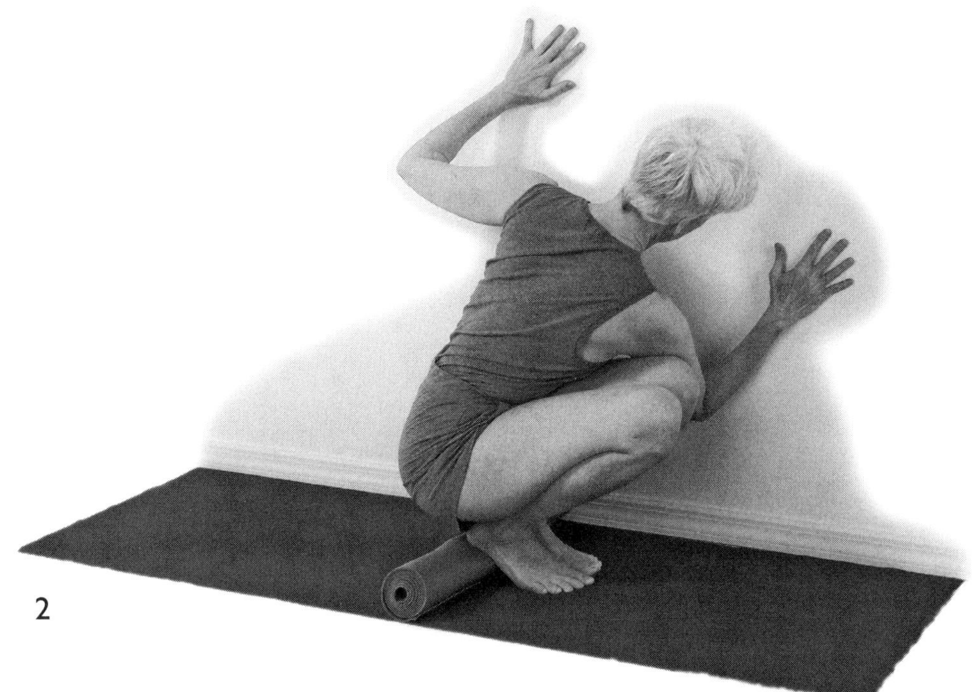

2

hand for further twist. Otherwise reach behind and beyond the buttocks to the left thigh, helping the right torso to approach the wall. [2]

4. Relax the adductors, breathe as slowly and symmetrically as possible for 10-20 seconds.

5. Release the pose by first releasing the left arm, using the right arm for support if needed, and by relinquishing the right hand's grasp on the wall beyond the left thigh or wall.

6. Then put the right shoulder and arm in contact with the wall, and repeat the pose.

Alternatively, this pose may be done with a roll perpendicular to the wall.

Vasisthasana

1. Begin with both hands and both feet on a flat surface, fingers pointing away from the feet.

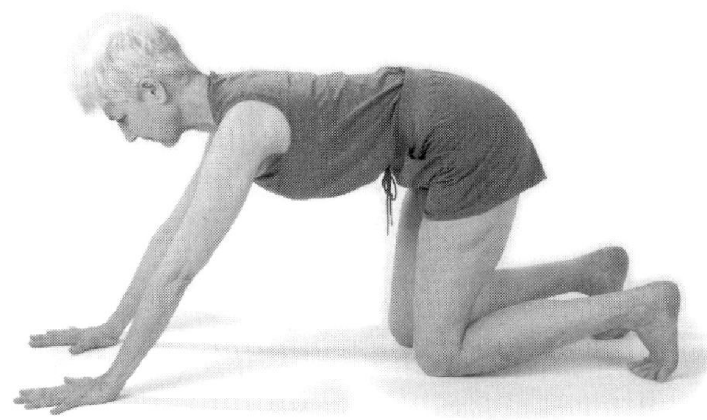

2. Rotate to the right side, bringing the left hand onto the left hip, and balancing weight on the hand of the straight right arm, and the little toe side of the right foot.

3. Straighten the entire body, from the right and left heel bones to the cranium, the left leg and arm close to the body. [1]

4. Breathe slowly and symmetrically for 10-20 seconds, then raise the left arm and leg until they are vertical and parallel.

5. After another slow breath, bend the left knee [2] and grasp its great toe with the first three fingers of the left hand.

6. Straighten the arm and leg again. [3]

7. Breathe calmly for 20 seconds.

8. Then release the grasp, lower the left leg and arm to contact the right leg and torso again, go back to all fours and swing the right side up, balancing on the extended left arm's hand and the left foot, to perform the mirror image of the same pose.

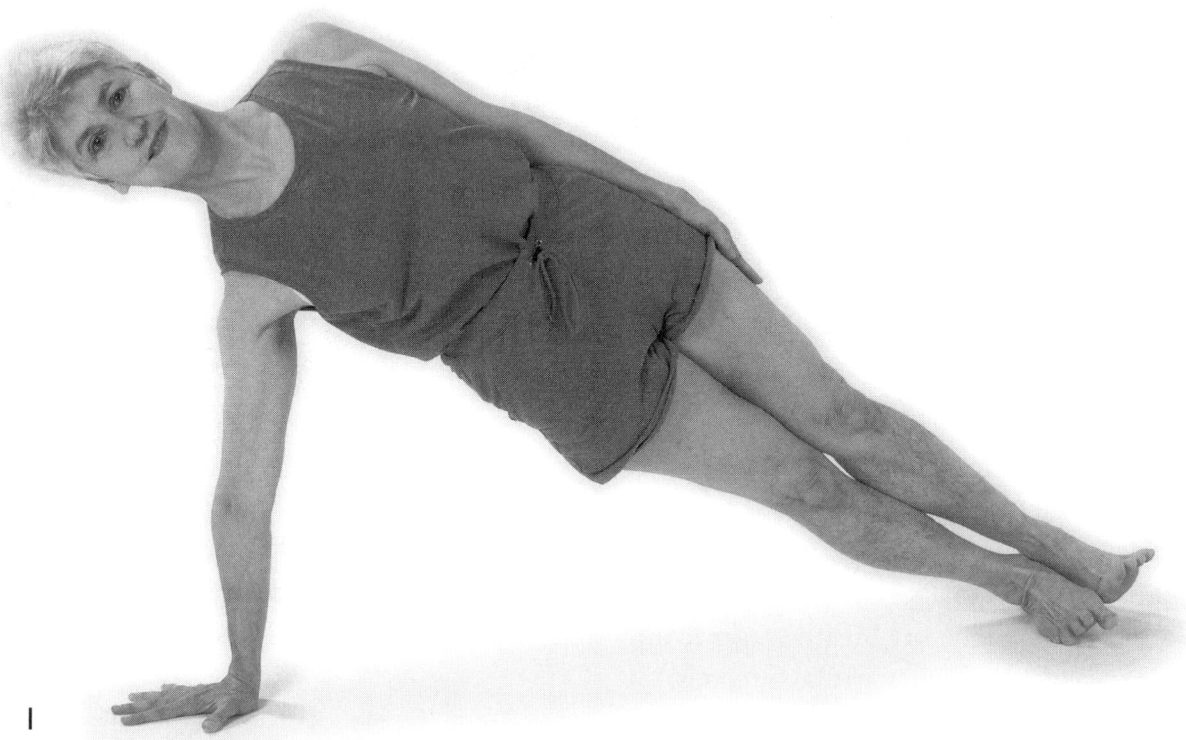

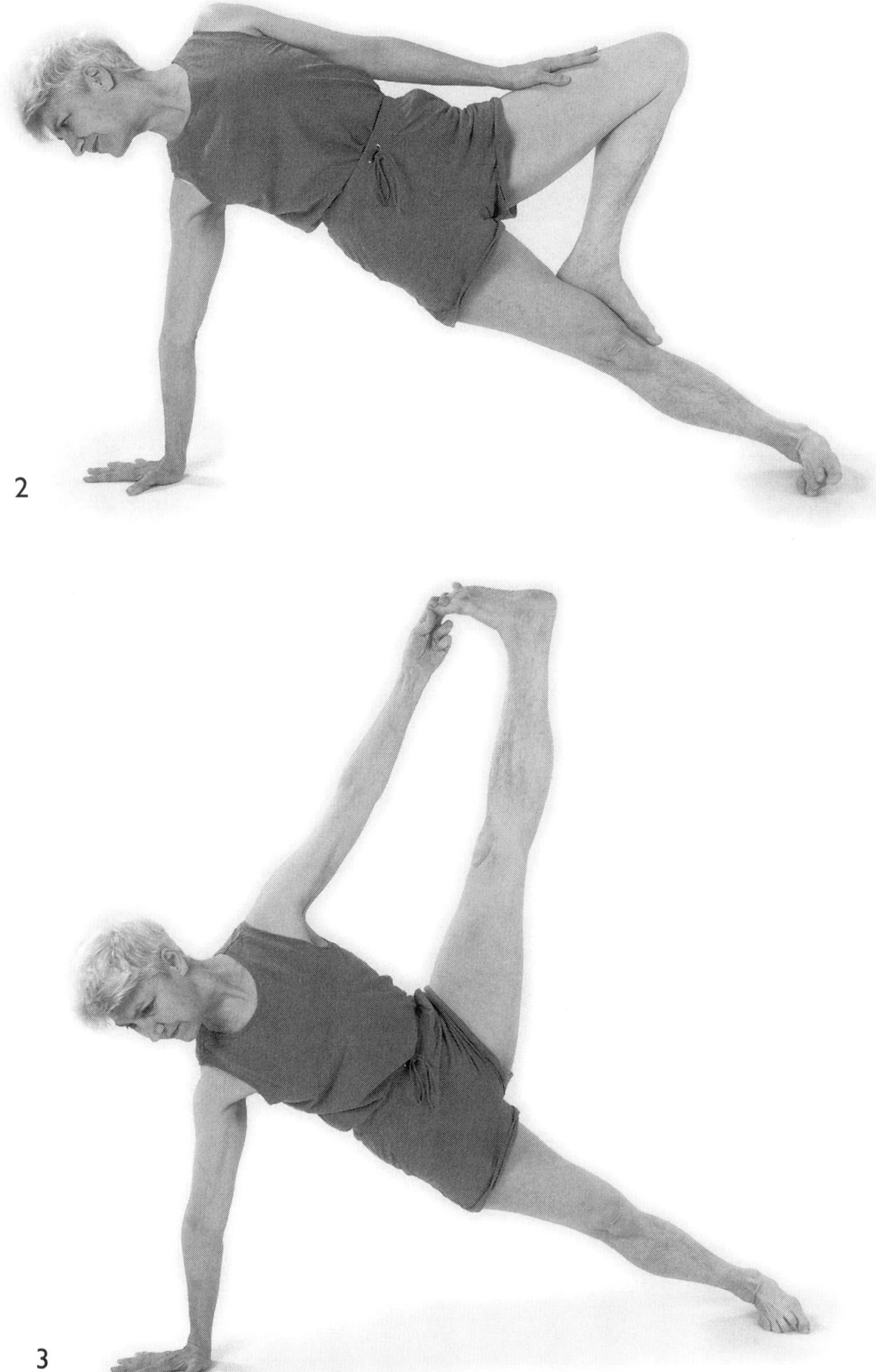

2

3

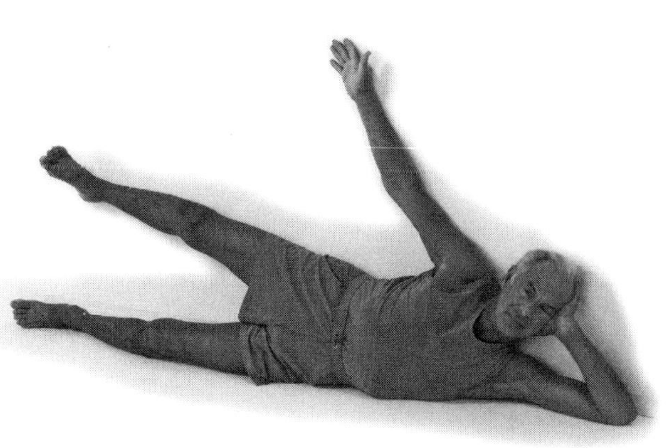

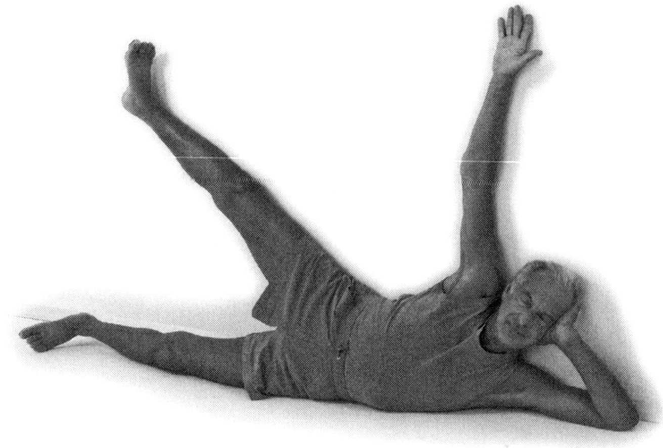

Entry-Level Vasisthasana

1. Securely prop the left ribs and thigh against a wall while lying on a flat surface. Use the left arm to support the head. Breathe quietly while raising the right arm and leg as high as possible, reaching upward with great effort.

2. Although working intensely, breathe in a relaxed manner for 10-20 seconds.

3. Repeat on the right side, but, in the presence of lumbar or thoracic scoliosis, perform only with convex side of curve as the upper side.

Intermediate-Level Vasisthasana

Perform the full original pose, Vasisthasana with the little finger of supporting hand, heel of supporting foot, and both shoulders, entire back and buttocks against a wall. (No picture.) In the presence of scoliosis, perform only with the convex side of the curve as the *lower* side.

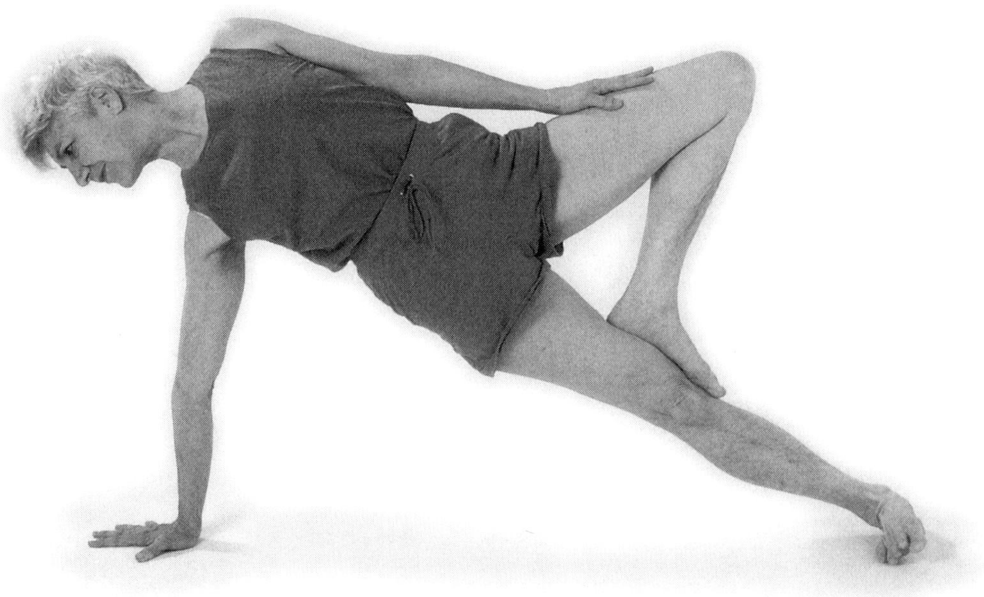

Breathing

While all of the problems we have dealt with are shared to one extent or another by each and every living being, breath control is somewhat unique in the degree to which the illness-free individual matches up with people with MS: few people have any degree of breath control.

This critical activity, in which the conscious individual meets up with the autonomic process that takes over whenever we are asleep, or when we are paying attention to something else, is the subject of an excellent book by B.K.S. Iyengar, titled *Pranayama*, to which all interested parties are referred.

Respiration and digestion are the two universal and necessary ingredients in metabolism, the process of being alive. Digestion goes on without our permission, whether we like it or not. Breathing will go on without our efforts, but we can easily alter it consciously, directly, and consistently. It is the estuary where conscious control meets the autonomic functions, and a portal through which we may enter our own unknown territories within.

It may be useful to begin breathing exercises with ten minutes of meditation. Dr. Herbert Benson and others, including the Maharishi Mahesh and their many predecessors have a developed a simple and effective methodology for taking up meditation.

1. Sit in a comfortable position.

2. Select a sound or phrase that is not emotionally charged (e.g., "Om," "One," "Inshallah," "Today.")

3. Close your eyes.

4. Say the sound or phrase to yourself every time you exhale.

5. Focus your attention on the phrase.

6. If your thoughts wander, passively return to concentrating on the phrase.

7. Continue for 10 minutes.

One way to continue into the breathing proper is Nadi Sodhana Pranayama. The best introduction to this type of alternate-nostril breathing, and many other techniques are the works of B.K.S. Iyengar.

For those interested in pursuing meditation, *Heart of Meditation* by Durgananda is highly recommended.

In this book we have introduced a number of asanas that are born of the uses that can be made of them by people with neurological deficits. All of us have profound and lasting deficits and deficiencies, which may be addressed and gradually remedied with proper attention and work.

The authors hope that the profound deficiencies of this attempt will be remediated by those interested parties that come after us.

Afterword

Eric's Story

I was raised in Avalon, on Santa Catalina Island, 26 miles off the coast of California. Los Angeles and environs were directly across the channel. It was paradise. It was like being at camp every day of the year. There were three boys and later a lovely sister. Everyone earned their livelihood from the tourists who came to the Island during the spring and summer and early fall. There were about 700 residents. Everyone knew everyone, and you learned to get along in such a tight social situation very quickly.

I was in college as a pre-law student, clerking for my uncle at his law offices, belonged to a fraternity, and dating. It was a very full schedule. I started to notice that it was getting difficult to read for any length of time. I was always tired and kept bumping into desks and corners. I came home for the summer and went right to work in the family business and also held down a part-time job in the afternoons at a local business on the front street. At night I was a relief waiter in one of the restaurants. This was a common practice as the locals needed to work double and sometimes triple shifts in order to make enough income to last the winter months when there was little or none of the tourist trade.

My uncle and aunt were the doctors in Avalon. There was a ten-bed clinic and surgery, which they operated with great devotion and dedication. It was my uncle who noticed I was staggering at times. He also noticed that I could not hold a focus, my eyes seemed to dance around sometimes. It was then that he sent me over to town (Los Angeles) for some tests.

In those days spinal taps were used to determine neurologic diagnosis. After several taps and observation of symptoms, it was determined that I had MS. There was no treatment, other than steroids and enforced rest. Today, with MRI and CT scans, the diagnosis is established quickly in the beginning stages and people can be helped with many new therapies and alternative techniques. I have made it a point to know where each and every plaque is located, what the possible effects might be, and how I am going to deal with it. I take full responsibility for my state of health. That includes diet, sleep, management of my day's activities, teaching, family activities, and being a full-time grandfather to four darlings.

With the choices offered at that time, it is no wonder that I started to look for solutions that were outside of the medical modality. Believe me, there were some humdingers. It would take another book to describe my journey. It became apparent that I was heading toward my discovery of Hatha Yoga. I was blessed to find Indra Devi, a teacher who was very compassionate. She sent me to Satchitananda, the teacher who had created Integral Yoga, who was located in Santa Barbara. I was developing a good solid base in Hatha Yoga, and doing a lot of investigating on my own.

In the mid 1960s I began to hear of B.K.S. Iyengar and his unique approach to Hatha yoga. I obtained his book *Light On Yoga*, and was fascinated with the application of his vast knowledge to various symptoms and diseases.

I wasn't able to meet him until the mid-1970s in Northern California. I became his student, followed his recommendations, and was thrilled to notice the improvement in the symptoms I was displaying at that time. It became possible for me to continue my studies with him in India. His great compassion and inspiration spurred me on to accomplish more than I ever thought was possible.

After ten years of study, I became certified to be one of his teachers. It was then that he suggested I begin to teach others like myself. I took up the challenge and my life unfolded to its true potential.

I am not cured. Iyengar yoga has become the tool with which I handle the day-to-day contingencies of living with MS. I am very proud to hold a Senior II teaching certificate from Mr. Iyengar personally, which has enabled me to travel far and wide teaching others the benefits of Iyengar Hatha Yoga.

The Flora L Thornton Foundation recently established the Eric L. Small Optimal Living with Ms Centers at UCLA, USC, Casa Colina, and Rancho Los Amigos which includes the Adaptive Iyengar Program specifically for clients diagnosed with MS and other neurological conditions..

Robert's Story

Robert came to my early morning class, referred by some mutual friends. He had been diagnosed three years before. His symptoms were fatigue, numbness in the legs, spastic hand-grip, diplopia, and the inability to concentrate for any length of time. There was a reluctance to share his problems with associates at work. He was afraid that he would lose his position and livelihood. He was becoming more and more isolated and depressed. His wife was a successful professional, and they had two young children. Their lives were moving on, and he felt inadequate and powerless. After a lengthy interview, he was convinced to give the adaptive yoga program a try provided his entering the program was kept confidential. We arrived at a series of asana and pranayama that he would be able to perform on a daily basis, coming to class once a week.

It should be pointed out that the series devised was for Robert. It is not possible at this point to recommend a series that was effective for an individual for the general population. This book is an offering from which students, teachers, and therapists may select what is appropriate, advancing as they, and especially therapists, see fit. The beauty of Iyengar Yoga is that it is very adaptable. When the instructor is certified at the proper level and has the experience to determine what will be effective, then both the student and the teacher/therapist are committed to the work. Both are responsible. The more responsibility the student takes in the management of his condition, the more the teacher and the student become partners.

There is a tendency in any diagnosis for the patient to hand over responsibility to the caregiver or health professional. The practice of yoga develops empowerment and confidence. Plus, there is no one who can measure the effects better than the students themselves. Sharing the work that has to be done is always more effective when students bring to the lessons feedback on what they've been doing and how they are doing it.

There are many levels in the practice of yoga. There is the physical accomplishment, the internal improvement of the organic body, and the physiological balance, all of which grow. All three levels are very subtle and take time to develop. Our society is motivated by quick results and the need to always move up the ladder of accomplishment faster and faster. We who have MS need to recognize that we place ourselves under unnecessary strain.

Part of any adaptive yoga program is to give the nervous system a rest. Several months into the program, Robert became aware that there were changes in his condition. First, on the advice of his doctor, he had reduced the medication for depression by half. He was taking a nap only once a day for less than 45 minutes, whereas before he was sleeping an hour in the morning, again in the afternoon, and retiring in the evening soon after dinner. The double vision only occurred if he became exhausted, or pushed beyond what would be considered reasonable. The numbness in the legs remained, but it was not the focus of his concern. His gait was steadier, with only a slight drag on the outer foot. He resumed his professional schedule with modification, and he had more energy and was able to spend more time with the family.

A while later, when a model was needed for a national publication, Robert volunteered without prompting and was comfortable with his commitment. He has been in the program for five years and has brought several newly diagnosed students to the studio. He tells them of his improvement and will often demonstrate his newfound abilities in his own practice. Change does not have to be dramatic. It only has to be a change.

John and Big John's Stories

No story about yoga and MS would be complete without including the stories of these two men. The Yoga and MS program found a home when the MS Achievement Center at UCLA began operations five years ago. There was a large, designated space with many windows overlooking a park-like view, equipment was provided by the Eric Small Trust, and a time was allocated just before lunch and right after the cognitive training class. It was a perfect opportunity to incorporate lessons learned from physical activity in the gym with the mental stimulation in the cognitive class

John was one of the first students in a wheelchair to enroll in the entire program. He recognized that what he was learning in the yoga class could be very valuable for managing the disease. Together, we developed a home practice for his particular range of motion, which he did every day without fail. With a great deal of hardship, he also attended every session.

John's increased physical ability was the first indication that he was on the right path. He developed more strength, more flexibility, and less spasm. John also reported that he was experiencing regular body and organ functions. The most improvement occurred in his attitude (which was good to begin with) and his zest for life beyond the wheelchair. He has been, and still is, an inspiration to all around him. I am very proud that he has become the spokesperson for our programs whenever we have visitors touring the facilities.

Big John entered our program several years ago. How he became involved in the yoga program is a story in itself. I would catch him wheeling around our area in his motorized chair out of the corner of my eye. He seemed to be listening and watching, coming closer each time, until I asked him if he was interested in joining us, and if not, please go somewhere else to do his wheeling around. Now, Big John always wore very bulky clothes, dark colors, and a grubby baseball cap pulled down over his eyes. Big John said that he would give our class a try, but he would not commit to becoming a member of the class.

Big John's range of motion was very limited, and he could not transfer from the electric wheelchair. He didn't realize at the time that he was perfect for our program. He had a background of acting and voiceovers, and showed that his mental facilities were mostly intact. We were able to demonstrate that there was a whole range of asanas that he could do from the electric wheelchair that would improve his general health and well-being. Many of them are described and illustrated in this book. Big John picked up the challenge and never missed a class if he could help it.

Within a few months the two men were the most enthusiastic members of the class. Not only that, they also participated in the MS Walk, raising funds and bringing sponsors into contact with the Achievement Center. Our goal was achievedusing Iyengar Adaptive Yoga to enhance the students' life in and out of the Center. Big John became a volunteer at the Center, teaching voice and diction. Not too long ago I met Big John in the lobby of the Center, and he informed me that he would not be able to attend the full yoga class because he had to prepare and rehearse for his class after lunch. How about that?

Footnote: I mentioned that Big John's appearance was rather lumpy and dark. Now he wears light-colored shirts, his hair is washed and cut on a regular basis, and he has a good relationship with the other members of the class and the general public. He manages all of this with only limited movement, and he has taught those who assist him at home how to carry on the yoga home-practice so that he can continue to improve his skills in managing life with MS.

Notes

1. Herndon, Robert M. (2006). *Handbook of Neurologic Rating Scales*, second edition. Demos Medical Publishing, New York.
2. Taimni, I.K. (1972). *The Science of Yoga*. Theosophical Publishing House. Wheaton, IL.
3. Iyengar, B.K.S. (1979). *Light on Yoga*, revised edition, Schocken, New York, page 31.
4. Ibid, page 30. Taken from *Hatha Yoga Pradipika,* Chapter I, verses 64-66.
5. Ibid, page 44-45. Taken from *Hatha Yoga Pradipika,* Chapter 4, verse 30.
6. Ibid, page 53. From *Sankaracharya Atma Satkam*.
7. McKenzie, Robin, and Craig Kubey. (2001) *7 Steps to a Pain-Free Life: How to Rapidly Relieve Back and Neck Pain*. Plume, New York.
8. Schatz, Mary Pullig. (1992) *Back Care Basics: A Doctor's Gentle Yoga Program for Back and Neck Pain Relief.* Rodmell Press, Berkeley.
9. Ekman, Paul, Joseph J. Campos, Richard J. Davidson, and Frans B.M. de Waal. (2003). *Emotions Inside Out*. Annals of the New York Academy of Medicine, New York, Volume 1000.
10. Ramirez, Martin, and Michael Cabanac. (2003). "Pleasure: the common currency of emotions," and Sullivan, Margaret W., David S. Bennett, and Michael Lewis, "Darwin's view: Self-evaluative emotions as context-specific emotions." In: Ekman, Paul, Joseph J. Campos, Richard J. Davidson, and Frans B.M. de Waal, *Emotions Inside Out.* Annals of the New York Academy of Medicine, New York, Volume 1000: 293-295 and 304-308, respectively.
11. Higgins, E.T. (1977). "Beyond pleasure and pain." *American Psychologist*, 52: 1280-1300.
12. Buonomano D.V., and M.M. Merzenich. (1995) "Temporal information transformed into a spatial code by a network with realistic properties." *Science* 267:1028-1030.
13. H. Cheng, Y. Cao, and L. Olson. (1996). "Spinal cord repair in adult paraplegic rats: Partial restoration of hind limb function." *Science* 273: 510-513; W. Young. (1996). "Spinal cord regeneration." *Science* 273: 451; and M.E. Schwab and D. Bartholdi. (1996). "Degeneration and regeneration of axons in the lesioned spinal cord." *Physiological Reviews* 76(2): 319-370.
14. Jones, Edward G. (ed.) (1991). *Cajal's Degeneration and Regeneration of the Nervous System*, Volume 5. Raoul M. May, translator. Oxford University Press, New York.

15. Roth, Jurgen, and Berger, E.G. (eds.). (1997). *The Golgi Apparatus.* Birkhauser, Cambridge; Sterr A., S. Freivogel, and A. Voss. "Exploring a repetitive training regime for upper limb hemiparesis in an in-patient setting: A report on three case studies," *Brain Injury*, 22:1093-1107; Sterr A, T. Elbert, I. Berthold, S. Kölbel, and E. Taub, "Longer versus shorter daily constraint induced movement therapy of chronic hemiparesis: An exploratory study," *Archives of Physical Medicine and Rehabilitation*, 83, 1374-1377; Sterr A., S. Freivogel, and D. Schmalohr, "Neurobehavioral aspects of recovery: Assessment of the learned non-use phenomenon in hemiparetic adolescents," *Archives of Physical Medicine and Rehabilitation*, 83, 1726-1733; and Sterr A., D. Schmalohr, S. Kölbel, and S. Freivogel, "Functional reorganization of motor areas following forced-use rehabilitation training in hemiparetic patients: A TMS study," *Biomedical Engineering*, 46: 102-108.
16. Kilgard M.P., and M.M. Merzenich. (1998). Cortical map reorganization enabled by nucleus basalis activity. *Science* 279:1714-1718.
17. Edelman, Gerald. (1987). *Neural Darwinism.* Basic Books, New York.
18. Oken, Barry. (2003). "Yoga reduces fatigue in multiple sclerosis." Presented at the American Academy of Neurology, Honolulu, Hawaii, April 3, 2003.
19. Christopher Reeves. (1998). "Reeve's special night raiseshope," *USA Today,* February 3, 1998; W. Young. (1996). "Spinal cord regeneration." *Science* 273: 451; Schwab, M.E., and D. Bartholdi. (1996). "Degeneration and regeneration of axons in the lesioned spinal cord." *Physiological Reviews* 76(2): 319-370.
20. Lazar S.W., C.E. Kerr, R.H. Wasserman, J.R. Gray, D.N. Greve, M.T. Treadway, M. McGarve, B.T. Quinn, J.A. Dusek, H. Benson, S.L. Rauch, C.I. Moore, and B. Fischl. (2005). "Meditation experience is associated with increased cortical thickness." *Neuroreport*, Nov 28; 16(17): 1893-1897.
21. Telles S, B.H. Hanumanthaiah, R. Nagarathna, H.R. Nagendra. (1994). "Plasticity of motor control systems demonstrated by yoga training." *Indian Journal of Physiology and Pharmacology,* April; 38(2): 143-144.
22. Stefano, G.B., T. Esch, P. Cadet, W. Zhu, K. Mantione, and H. Benson. (2003). "Endocannabinoids as autoregulatory signaling molecules: Coupling to nitric oxide and a possible association with the relaxation response." *Medical Science Monitor* April; 9(4) RA 63-75.
23. Cailliet, Renee (1997). *Foot and Ankle Pain.* F.A. Davis, Philadelphia.
24. Vedel, J.P., and J. Mouillac-Baudevin. (1969). Etude fonctionelle du controle de l'activite des fibres fusimotrices dynamiaques et statiques par les formations reticules mesencephalique, pontique et bulbaire chez le chat. *Experimental Brain Research* 9: 325-345.
25. Granit, R., and B. Holmgren. (1955). "Two pathways from brain stem to gamma ventral horn cells." *Acta Physiologica Scandinavica* 35: 9-108.
26. Granit, R. (1955). *Receptors and Sensory Perception.* Yale University Press, New Haven.
27. Ellaway, P.H., and J.R. Trott. (1978). "Autogenic reflex action onto gamma motoneurons by stretch to triceps surae in the decerebrated cat." *Journal of Physiology (London)* 276: 49-76.
28. Gurfunkel, V.S., M.I. Lipshits, S. Mori, E.V. Popov. (1976). "The state of stretch reflex during quiet standing in man." *Progress in Brain Research* 44: 473-486.
29. Wittgenstein, Ludwig. (2001). *Philosophical Investigations.* G.E.M. Anscombe, translator. 50th Anniversary Commemorative Edition. Basil Blackwell, Oxford.
30. Lanyon, L.E. (1989). "Strain-related bone modeling and remodeling." *Topics in Geriatric Rehabilitation* 4(3) 13-24.
31. Pead, M.J., R. Suswillo, T.L. Skerry, S. Vedi, and L.E. Lanyon. (1988). "Increased 3H uridine levels in osteocytes following a short period of dynamic bone loading in vivo." *Calcified Tissue International* 43: 92-97.
32. Nathanson, Donald L. (1992). *Shame and Pride.* W.W. Norton, New York.

Index

Note: Boldface numbers indicate illustrations